The Theory of Synergetic Spinal Mechanics and PPT Manipulation
Edition 2

The Theory of Synergetic Spinal Mechanics and PPT Manipulation
Edition 2
By J.R.Bayliss

Other publications by J.R.Bayliss:

DVD: Spinal Mechanics and Bony Locking *For Health Professionals*
by John Bayliss DO and Peter O'Toole
ISBN 978-0-9550936-0-0

First edition published 2007

Revised and updated edition 2 published 2008

ISBN 978-0-9550936-2-7

Published by: John Bayliss
3, Moor Lane
Chessington
Surrey KT9 1BJ
England UK
www.spinalmechanics.com

β

Data collected from thousands patient record findings over a 20 year period plus literally thousands of experiments and numerous mini research projects went into formulating the theories and practical application that are described and demonstrated in this book.

Acknowledgments

I would like to thank all the people who both encouraged me and took a role in helping me write this book:

Behind the camera:

    Lindsey Gleeson
    My sons, Daniel and James
    Peter O'Toole

The models:
In order of appearance

    Lisa Hood: *L3-right-right*
    Matthew Swan: *L3-left-right*
    Sam Lipop: *Walking backwards*
    Rafaela Arce Dantas: *PPT manipulations*
    Lindsey Gleeson: *Rib ergonomics/neck*
    Dan Hood: *Rib cage/Shoulder joints*

Sub-editing:

    John Day
    Lindsey Gleeson
    Terry Anderton

About the Author

J.R.Bayliss DO is a UK Osteopath who trained with the 'College of Osteopaths Educational Trust.' He has a background in psychology and engineering drawing and drew all of the illustrations.

Do you know the answers to these questions?

Test your knowledge on spinal mechanics

• 1) What is the reason people sway their hips from side to side when they walk?

• 2) Since ribs need to be parallel to function efficiently, how do the thoracic vertebrae side-bend without compromising them?

• 3) If the lumbar facets are concave and the thoracic facets convex, how do they mate and how does movement take place?

• 4) What single reason could explain why it has not been possible to correctly align the *sacroiliac joints with manipulation, using existing techniques?

• 5) In lumbar facet physiology, what mechanism causes the joints to side-bend one time and rotate another?

• 6) How do lumbar joints become locked against each other?

• 7) Why are left knee problems common?

• 8) Why is it not physiologically possible to backward bend the thoracic vertebrae and rotate? And what would happen if they could?

• 9) During walking, do the lumbar joints on the weight bearing side, side-bend and rotate to the opposite side or, rotate and side-bend to the same side?

• 10) How many forces acting on a spinal joint take place to lock the joint to the point of changing the chemistry of the local surrounding tissue? 0-1,1-2, 2-3, 3-4, 4-5, 5-6.

The answers to all these questions can be found in this book.

* M.C.McGrath *Musculo-skeletal Research Group university of Otago Dunedin, New Zealand from Clinical considerations of sacroiliac anatomy: review of function, motion and pain.* **"Manipulation of the sacroiliac joint has been shown to leave the position of the joint unchanged when compared with its pre-manipulated position"** *Page 22 Journal of Osteopathic Medicine volume 7 Number 1 April 2004*

Contents

True science begins from a starting point that is pure and uncontaminated from others misconceptions and prejudices. Bad science sets out from a mid-point and builds on the misconceptions and prejudices that have gone before, and that which has so far has failed to be demonstrated.

The science behind this book starts from the very beginning and provides a step by step set of new and practical theories on spinal mechanics and manipulation that can be demonstrated.

Recommendation:
To gain the most out of this book it is recommended that you hold the individual bones in your hands and play around with the joints as you read the chapters. Try out the walking and rotation theories on your own body. This way, the book will make a lot more sense to you and be easier to understand. Be very very careful if you try out the movements that cause subluxations, they can lock your back in an instant. (I found that out the hard way.) The responsibility is yours.

Chapter One
Rationale

In 2004 Peter O'Toole and I spoke about making a 10 minute film outlining the role side-shift plays in creating subluxations. From this meagre beginning and with Lindsey Gleeson's help, we ended up making a film on all aspects of spinal mechanics and subluxations, 1 hour 38 minutes long. We called the film 'Spinal Mechanics and Bony Locking *For Health Professionals*'.

In researching the subject of spinal mechanics for the film the best of the current and past theories were thoroughly scrutinized. But there was a real problem as none of the currently accepted theories could be shown to account for the 'real world' movements we take for granted. In fact I found that none of the theories could be shown to work either singularly, synchronously or synergetically, and none convincingly explained the mechanics of walking or rotation.

In other words when applying the currently accepted theories on spinal mechanics the engine was not driving the wheels. Therefore, it was hard to envisage how professions could base their manipulative therapies on theories that are questionable. In the end I decided to try and work out how the spine and sacroiliac joints articulate in 'real world' movements for myself. And what a task that turned out to be, because I did not foresee that I would have to formulate theories not only individually but conceptually.

This chapter explains the reasoning that led to my conclusions and why I felt the currently accepted theories were questionable and the approach I took towards making my own discoveries.

I have had people criticize my work, not because they disagree with my theories but simply because I have not referenced it to other peoples work or research. The reason for this is because I worked out the theories on spinal mechanics from the ground up, for myself, using engineering principles. The bottom line is that my theories can be readily demonstrated and provide a plausible explanation for how the whole spine works both at a segmental level and as a whole. When the technology becomes available to look at the segmental movement of the whole spine, further research can follow.

Based on my spinal theories, I worked out how joints subluxate. From this I was able to work out an entirely new method of effective manipulation that does not involve the use of excessive force or the sound of a click. It is a method that can be demonstrated to provide excellent results.

Considering Best Approach

I considered three different approaches:

•1 Do I take a sample of people and make notes of all the angles of their joints and then go back to the drawing board and try and work out how they got like that?

Comment
The sample people would need to be naturally 100% free of subluxations so as not to confuse the results, especially where X-ray and other imaging are part of the research.

It is extremely unlikely that such a sample of people exists; further, the imaging would need to take account of the whole spine in a weight bearing and mobile environment and not just a selected area of isolation. *This is where things went wrong before.*

Rationale
Whilst this is a frequently attempted and favoured method of research it would be very time consuming and would leave considerable room for error, because whilst I could palpate the joints and know their plane of movement, or see the X-ray/imaging results (if such equipment existed), it would still be conjecture as to how they got like that. In other words the theory structure leaves room for doubt and that would consign the theory to the dump.

•2 Do I go about thinking up an ideological theory and then set about proving it?

Rationale
This theory can be likened to a child who wants to build a red sports car. His first thoughts are on where to buy the red paint. Only when he has the paint, does he think he needs to design a car to match, and when that proves too difficult he thinks, perhaps he should try another colour. This again would be a non-starter and destine the theory to the dump.

•3 Do I start with an open mind, begin my experimentation by examining the articular surfaces of the bones and see what waits to be discovered? When I have come up with a working model, only then do I compare the results of my experimentation to the spines of real people, via movement tests, observation, palpation and imaging.

Rationale
This promised a scientific result that would be based upon solid engineering principles that could be readily replicated by others. This meant disregarding everything that went before and thinking dynamically; I chose this route. The palpation, X-rays etc and research would therefore come later.

The Spine and Sacroiliac joints work in Synergetic Synchronicity

It is impossible to look at a single joint or series of joints in a certain area such as the sacroiliac, lumbar, thoracic or cervical in isolation because the body does not work like that. The body works as a complete interacting mobile unit.

Where to start?

For me, there was only one place to start and that was by examining one of the most basic human movements; walking.

Leaving aside muscles, walking involves many different forces, the main ones being:

- Weight bearing and weight leaning
- Leg lifting and leg direction
- The changing angles of the ilia and hip joint
- The reciprocal action of the sacroiliac joints
- The lumbar vertebrae accommodation for this action and
- The action of side-shift

With so many forces to contend with, walking is a very complicated three dimensional movement that requires all the forces to work in harmony.

Later in this chapter I have explained why I think current theory models of the sacroiliac joints do not complement the walking action.

In the beginning

From observing the way people sway their hips when walking I realised that side-shift was an important factor, but what I did not realise until later was just how much of an important factor it was.

Once I understood the principles of side-shift, weight distribution and balance everything fell into place. I was able to experiment and begin to understand how joints work individually and how they synergetically interrelate with real world movements.

The joint that gave me the most problem understanding was L1. Every book I have read and all that I was taught at college described L1 as just another lumbar vertebra. It most certainly is not. It is one of the most complicated and multi-functional joints in the body.

It was only by understanding the importance of side-shift that I was able to work out how incorrect employment of this force causes subluxations to occur.

Where to start

I have read many books on spinal mechanics and there is not one of them where I have not had to re-read a certain paragraph repeatedly to make sense of what the author was saying. This was due to several factors, but the main one was that they were starting the explanation of their theories from a mid point. It was like coming into their version of a conversation that they had picked up on halfway through someone else's conversation. The conversation was so ambiguous that it was impossible to predict which direction it would take. This led to many varying theories from different factions. And no one theory could be said to be better than another. What the men of science wanted to know was what started the conversation in the first place, and that is what I set out to discover. For only then could we begin to predict what the final outcome of the conversation could be. Theories must start from a sound, demonstrable basis.

L3 as a possible starting Point

When describing the movement of the spine, the L4/L3 vertebral joint is probably the most recorded movement. In most pictures L3 is shown in lumbar extension (neutral and forward bending).

So here is one mid point in the conversation, so let us carry out some simple tests to see where this fits into the conversation.

The tests are designed in a way that can be easily replicated.

__Test A for rotation__

Ask a colleague to sit sideways on a plinth with their back straight and their feet firmly on the floor. Their weight must be equally balanced on both buttocks. Stand or squat behind the colleague and place your hands around their pelvis in such a way as to completely immobilize it. By doing this, lumbar rotation is isolated. If muscles are the singular cause of lumbar rotation the L3 joint will rotate.

Ask your colleague to rotate their lumbar slowly in either direction and be very careful not to force the movement. This will lever the pelvis, so take care to keep it immobile.

The result of this test is that the lumbar spine locks after only a few degrees of rotation.

__Test B for side-bending__

So we know the L3 joint cannot be rotated very far when the pelvis is immobilized. So let us test side-bending. If the test above is repeated but instead of rotation, side-bending is attempted, we find side-bending is also restricted to only a few degrees.

.

Tests to Show True Movements

Test C for combined side-bending and rotation

Next we need to check what happens in the lumbar when side-bending and rotation are combined with the pelvis immobilized. Again, be sure not to allow even small amounts of pelvic movement to influence your results. Ask the colleague to side-bend their lumbar as best they can and then attempt rotation to the opposite side. If Fryette's laws are correct this combination movement should account for real world lumbar flexion rotation. However, the amount of rotation possible is still minimal and the lumbar vertebrae quickly lock.

Test D for combined rotation and side-bending

The experiment can be repeated starting with lumbar rotation followed by side-bending to the same side, which according to Fryette is how the lumbar vertebrae rotate in extension. Also try the experiment leaning forwards but again you will discover that this does not improve rotation. The outcome of this test fares no better.

So what can be learned from these primitive experiments?

These simple tests indicate that isolated combinations of side-bending and rotation and vice versa in the lumbar spine most certainly do not account for the amount of lumbar rotation a normal person takes for granted in the real world.

Judging by the leverage placed on the pelvis during the tests, the pelvis could have a role to play in lumbar rotation. If so, we need to establish that role.

To find this out we need to experiment further.

Test E adding pelvic side-bending (Lumbar flexion)

With your colleague in the same position on the plinth as in test A, place a book approximately 25 mm (1 inch) thick under their right ischial tuberosity so as to side-bend the sacrum to the left. The weight of the body is thus taken on the left buttock. If the person sits up straight the lumbar becomes side-bent to the left.

Now ask your colleague to rotate to the right. Be sure to block all pelvic side-shift to the left.

The result is that your colleague will be able to rotate further to the right in the lumbar than when the sacrum was horizontal. The test proves that side-bending of the pelvis improves the degree of lumbar rotation.

However, observe that the circumference of rotation is still not what one expects in the real world of lumbar rotation. So another test is needed.

Criteria of the Pelvis

Test F adding side-shift left (Lumbar flexion)

With your colleague in the same position as in test E, with the book under their right ischial tuberosity and their weight on their left buttock, try this next test. This time do not attempt to immobilize the pelvis. Ask your colleague to side-shift their pelvis to the left, and observe that the lumbar rotates automatically to the right without any levered effort from the muscles in sufficient circumference to comply with real world movements.

Observe Thoracic spine

If you repeat test F with the person sitting up straight you will notice that the thoracic spine refuses to rotate right. Do not force it to rotate; the thoracic spine is designed to restrict rotation in thoracic extension(backward bending) because of the danger it poses. This blocking mechanism does not apply to rotation in thoracic flexion and neutral. We can demonstrate this:

While in the same position, side-shift the pelvis to the right. This causes the pelvis to automatically rotate right and become almost level. Observe that the thoracic spine now automatically rotates to the right together with the pelvis and lumbar. Along with this general collective rotation the thoracic vertebrae independently rotate right and side-bend to the left. Observe that this combination movement is of sufficient rotational circumference to comply with real world movement.

Conclusion:

What these basic tests tell us is that the previously mentioned conversation has a lot to do with the pelvis having the ability to provide the angle and side-shift required by the lumbar and thoracic vertebrae to provide movements we take for granted in the real world. The next stage then is to look at the workings of the pelvis.

The Pelvis

The pelvis is designed to accommodate the action of the hip joints, the sacrolumbar joint, the symphysis pubis joint and the sacroiliac joints. For a real world theory to apply to the pelvic articulations, the theory has to fulfil working criteria. These criteria are:

1 It has to account for the walking action of the legs.

2 It has to account for the way the vertebral spine moves to complement the walking mechanism.

3 It has to act as a precursor for the lumbar spine to side-bend and rotate in both forward and backward bending.

4 It has to act as a precursor for the thoracic spine to rotate in lumbar forward bending and neutral and block backward bending.

5 It should not dislocate when completing items 1, 2, 3 and 4.

Sacroiliac Theories

Nature leaves nothing to chance, all things have their place and function and interact perfectly in harmony with their surroundings. The world we live in is an unbelievable engineering feat and when you observe the human body you are taken aback by how perfectly it is designed. With such perfection, it is absurd that nature would design the sacroiliac joints with a built-in flaw that causes them to semi-dislocate every time a person puts their foot forward. Yet this, unbelievably is the basis of most of current sacroiliac theories.

When we walk behind someone and observe the action of walking, one of the most obvious movements is that the person sways their hips from side to side with each step. When the pelvis sways to the left the right leg goes forward and when the pelvis sways to the right the left leg goes forward. Yet this basic observation is not accounted for in any of the current sacroiliac theories. Let us look at one of the most popular theories:

The Nutation Theory.

To accept this theory you have to pretend that the surface of the iliac facets are completely flat as in **figure 'A'**, and assume that the iliac facets move in a bilateral forward and backward

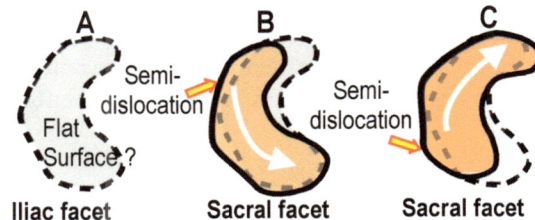

bending trajectory against the sacral facets. This movement is known as nutation, (nodding).

However there is a problem, because the path that the iliac facets follow causes the facets to semi-dislocate at the superior and inferior borders of the sacral facets, as shown in **figures 'B' and 'C'**. The idea of a rail running down the middle, would induce constant derailment.

If we indulge ourselves in this theory and imagine both innominates moving anteriorly against both sides of sacral facets at the same time, what would happen if such a movement was possible? Well, both legs would be weight bearing and parallel. How the person moves forward after this would be very interesting to witness. Presumably with the jump of a kangaroo.

If we entertain the idea that the nutation theory allows for each ilium to move independently on either side of the sacrum, the shape of the iliac and sacroiliac facets would guide one leg outwards and forward, whilst the other leg would be guided inwards and backwards?

Further, this theory makes no allowance for how the lumbar vertebrae rotate and side-bend to accommodate this action.

If one side of the ilium rotates in one direction and the ilium on the other side rotates in the opposite direction, the sacrum would have to remain level at all times. Trapped in the middle, the sacrum would be unable to side-bend and therefore would deprive the lumbar vertebrae of any means to accommodate the walking action or provide real world rotation.

Thoracic Articulation

Other popular current sacroiliac theories

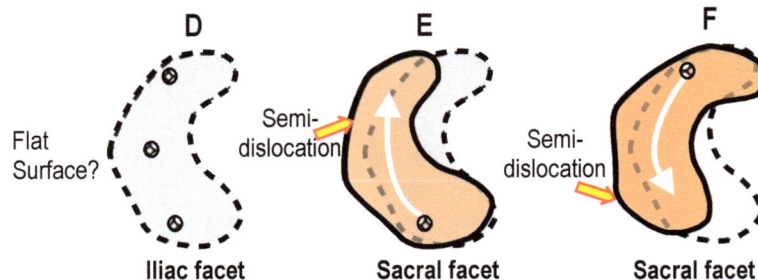

Figure 'D' roughly illustrates the axis points of the three pole theory. **Figures 'E' and 'F'** show what happens when the upper and lower points of axis are followed. Like the nutation theory they would cause the sacral facets to semi-dislocate over the anterior perimeter border of the iliac facets.

Sacroiliac joint conclusion

These theories do not fulfill the basics of a working criteria.

If you compare the angles of the facets in the 'nutation' or 'three pole' theories you will see a great similarity because both theories largely describe the same semi-dislocations. Both of these theories must have resulted from the research group subjects having subluxated sacroiliac joints and the researchers not taking this obvious point into account or looking at the how the joints integrate with walking and spinal movements.

As I said on page 4, to find a group of people 100% naturally free of sacroiliac subluxations is nigh on impossible. That is why I felt the only way to work out how the sacroiliac joints articulate is to work out the physiology with regard to the real world function of the joint.

Thoracic vertebral joints

According to Fryette's Laws the thoracic column side-bends and rotates to opposite sides in thoracic flexion and rotates and side-bends to the same side in thoracic extension.

Our simple test earlier in this chapter proved that the thoracic spine cannot rotate in thoracic extension (backward bending) and for a very good reason which is explained later in this book. The thoracic spine can rotate in thoracic flexion but the way it does this has little to do with Fryette's laws.

Conclusion

If the thoracic vertebrae really side-bent and rotated in thoracic flexion (forward bending) like the illustration in **figure G**, the attached ribs would be put under enormous torsion with every rotation.

Consider what would happen to the left rib if side-bending of this type was a valid movement? Supposing the angle of the left transverse process of a thoracic vertebra was 3 degrees, by the time the rib reached the apex of its conical curve, that 3 degrees would have increased by several degrees. This would put the inter-costal muscles under considerably stretch and if all the thoracic ribs were side-bent in a similar manner and held in this position for long periods, as happens in the real world, the inter-costal muscles on the left side would not be able to function optimally. Also like a see-saw, what goes up one side goes down the other, so the ribs on the right side would be compressed.

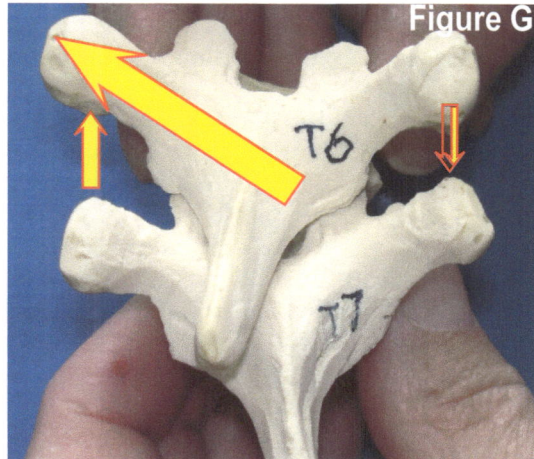

Figure G

Breathing is essential for life and therefore it is very unlikely that nature would evolve a design for the rib cage that hinders it. The musculo-skeletal frame is not designed with built in faults like this. So here is another example of a poorly conceived theory.

Overall Conclusion

As you can now see existing theories are seriously flawed, but numerous research papers have led to their general acceptance.

Personally I will not work with a theory I cannot trust, therefore I disregarded the books and research and investigated the bony movement of the spine for myself.

I started by looking at the whole picture, not an out of context focus joint with no regard to how that joint interrelated with the other joints of the spine and finished with two demonstrable models. I use the terms 'real world' and 'synergetic' with regard to the elements of the body and their relative and collective movements in order to differentiate between what actually happens in real life and what, largely as a result of conjecture and bad science, has been wrongly assumed to happen.

Research Background

The research group comprised of nine healthy people. Two of these were females aged between 28 and 45 years, and seven were men aged between 25 and 60 years.

One of the women and one of the men were considered to be L3-left-right and the others L3-right-right. Using Osteopathic techniques including PPT manipulation, as far as humanly possible all the sacroiliac and spinal subluxations were corrected before the research began.

The major bony landmarks* were used as reference points together with close observation. There was no difference in the findings, both men and women whether L3-left-right or L3-right-right performed equally well in the tests. Experiments were conducted to cover the tests in "rationale", the movements of rotation and walking and how to cause **subluxations. This ensured that each of the theories through practical application could be readily reproduced and demonstrated.

Using the structure of the theories described logically in the opening chapters, it was then possible to theorize how subluxations would take place if side-shift was misdirected. See pages 40 and 90.

Literally thousands of hours of experimentation using ***plastic bones went into calculating how the spine articulates and interrelates with the sacroiliac joint. I used my own body as a model and was only satisfied when the individual sacroiliac and spinal joints articulated in a way that reflected the real world movement I take for granted.

---

* P.S.I.S, A.S.I.S, Sacral Base, Femoral head, T.P's of L3 and L1/L2 and random thoracic T.P's
** The person was taken only to the point where the tightening of the subluxation began to bite.
*** I tried using real bones but they began to splinter and could not sustain the number of hours of experimentation I subjected them to.

Chapter Two
Side-Shift and the
Two Models

Overview

The workings of the spine can be likened in many ways to the workings of a grandfather clock. As the pendulum swings from side to side, so the cog wheels above turn clockwise and anti-clockwise. And from this long lever the precise time can be produced. However, if the pendulum or one cog wheel falters, it affects the function and efficiency of all the other mechanical parts. Ultimately the clock begins to malfunction and becomes unable to tell the correct time. The beauty of a pendulum action is that it takes very little energy to create a lot of power.

The synergetic principle theorizes that human motion is caused by a pelvic pendulum action. When working perfectly the sacroiliac and vertebral joints articulate synchronously, with precision and with minimal energy. However, like the grandfather clock, it only takes the pelvis or one joint to falter for the timing and function of the sacroiliac and vertebral spine to work imperfectly.

Terminology

The use later in this text of the word 'subluxation' is because part of the subject of this book is about bony locking and semi-dislocation. The 'Taber's Cyclopedic Medical Dictionary' definition of subluxation is 'a partial or incomplete dislocation' and this is the sense it is being used in.

An 'Osteopathic Lesion' or 'Chiropractic Subluxation' are broader terms that include both the subluxation and the resulting theoretical local pathology to the surrounding nerves, blood supplies, lymph, soft tissue and muscles etc.

Pendulum Vs. Balance

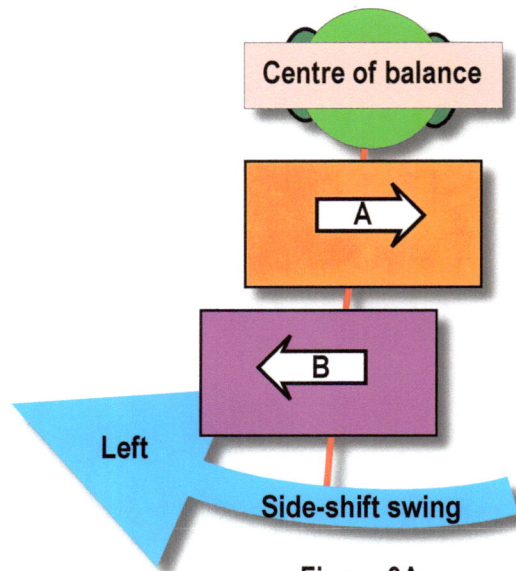

Figure 0A
posterior view

In order to survive, humans must be able to stand upright. To accomplish this they have been provided with a sense of balance and spatial awareness. The sense of balance and spatial awareness emanate from the middle ears and one of the prime functions of this mechanism is to keep the head level, and in the central axis.

At the origin of forward and backwards motion combined with rotation and side-bending movements, the pelvis has to sway side-ways, because, like a pendulum, it is the originating and governing force.

When the pelvis side-shifts left as shown in **figure 0A**, the inner ears create a powerful counter force in the opposite direction to maintain the upright position and balance of the body.

The magenta box labelled 'B' represents a typical vertebra closest to the pelvis. The pelvic side-shift drives it to the left.

Conversely, the orange box labelled 'A' represents a typical vertebra closest to the cranial counter-force of balance. As can be seen, the counter-force drives the vertebra to the right.

It is this meeting of the two directions that causes vertebral articulation. It is a very efficient method of creating movement whilst keeping muscle usage to a minimum.

Side-Shift

For survival the eyes must be kept level.

Figure 0B illustrates the main lines of gravity that are subjected to the vertebral column in neutral. The sacroiliac joints align closely to the lines of gravity under the inner ears. The mid point between the inner ears is situated at approximately the bridge of the nose and acts as the main point of balance. Point 'A' is the area where the lumbar vertebrae change to the thoracic.

Figure 0C illustrates the change in the lines of gravity when the pelvis side-shifts to the left, as in the action of walking. It can be seen that the lines of gravity from the inner ear and bridge of the nose overlap at point 'B' which, as will be illustrated later in this book, is an important requirement for balance. Smaller degrees of side-shift take place the closer they are to the bridge of the nose.

Therefore, it can be concluded that the lumbar facets have to move a greater distance than the thoracic facets during normal movements. For this reason the lumbar facets are larger than those found in the upper thoracic.

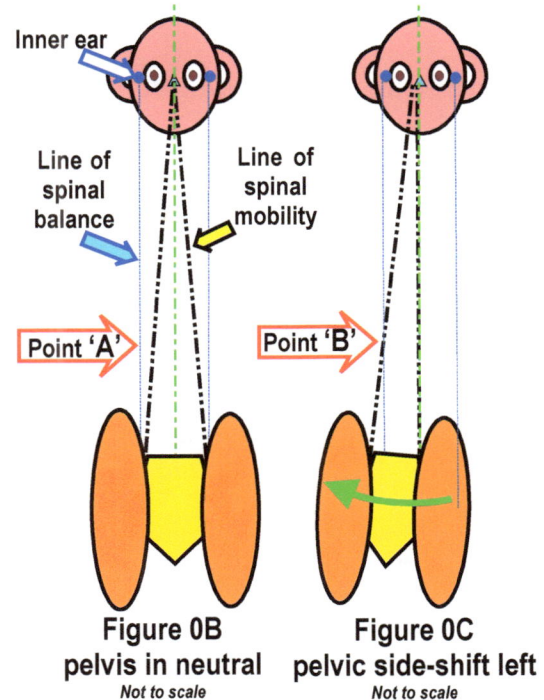

**Figure 0B
pelvis in neutral**
Not to scale

**Figure 0C
pelvic side-shift left**
Not to scale

The Two Models

In normal physiological rotation the third lumbar vertebra has limited options of movement. It can either side-bend to one side and rotate to the other, or it can rotate and side-bend to the same side.

Two options. For this reason L3 was chosen as the identifying description to associate the posture and mechanics during normal physiology and subluxation in the forward bending L3-right-right, (rotation right, side-bending right) pattern and backward bending L3-left-right (side-bending left, rotation right) pattern.

Most people in the western world conform to one of these two types, provided they do not have an anatomical leg length difference or spinal deformity, had surgical intervention, or have had their spine or pelvis subjected to direct trauma, etc.

People with L3-left-left and L3-right-left are rare, but they do exist.

L3-Right-Right

L3-right-right back view

Figure IA shows a picture of Lisa. Her back approximates the L3-right-right forward bending subluxation pattern.

At first sight her back looks fairly normal and typical of what you might see every day on a beach. However, when investigated more closely, it can be seen that there is a myriad of opposing forces. These will be pointed out and explained in more detail. Initially, observe some of the superficial markers:

Neck: Her neck muscles are pulling on the left and attempting to turn her head left.

Shoulders: Compare the uneven height and width of her shoulders and the unequal angles of her scapula bones. Her left shoulder joint is anterior and inferior in relation to the right shoulder.

Arms: Her right arm hangs at a different angle to her left and it can be seen from her flexed right elbow that her arm is posterior in relation to her left arm.

Hands: Notice that her right hand is internally rotated

Thoracic: Her thoracic region is generally leaning to the left. This gives the misleading impression that her pelvis has side-shifted to the right.

Lumbar: The left side of her lumbar is less tapered than the right.

Pelvis: Her left buttock is posterior in relation to her right and the fold of the left buttock is inferior.

Knees: Her left knee is flexed and turns inwards in comparison to her right knee.

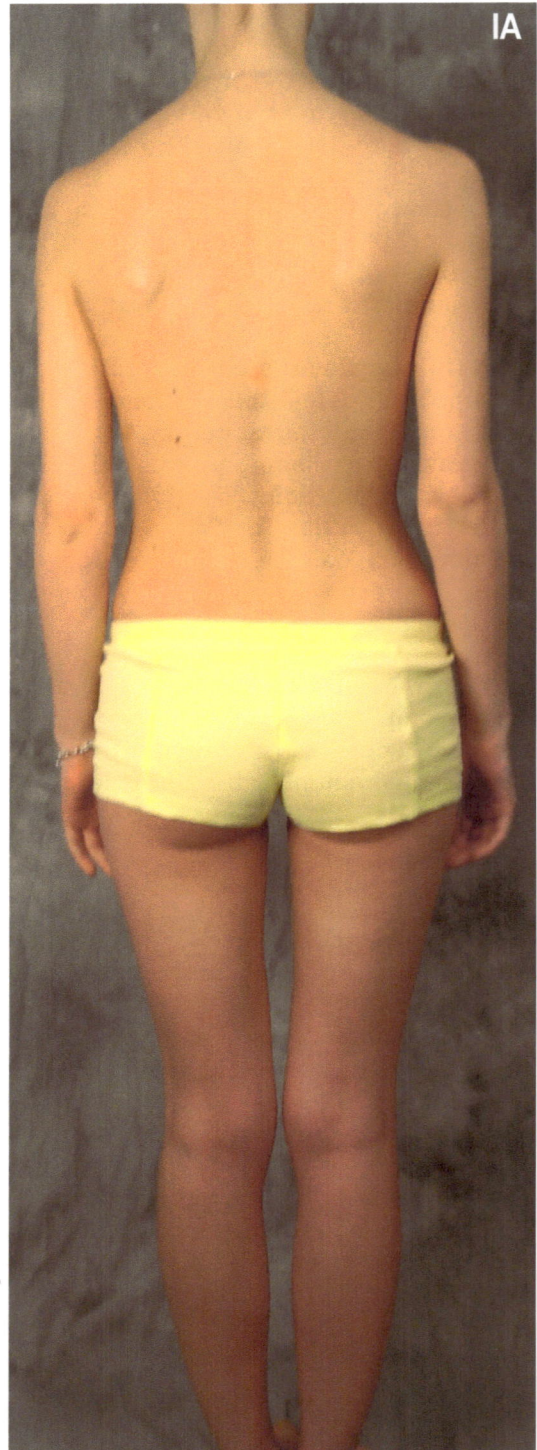

IA

L3-Right-Right: Side-Views

Figures **IB** and **IC** are two side-views of Lisa's torso.

The first observation to be aware of is that her whole posture is one of forward leaning.

Compare both pictures:

Her head. To look ahead her head has to backward bend which causes her jaw juts forward;

Her neck angles forwards;

Her cervico-dorsal junction is rounded;

Her torso is generally rotated left giving the incorrect impression that her left shoulder is the anterior shoulder;

Her arms. Notice that both arms of her hang at different angles and that her right elbow is posterior and mildly flexed.

Her shoulders are generally rounded. Her right shoulder is more anterior than the left;

Her upper thoracic area has a flattened shape and can be seen in **figure 1B**;

Her lower thoracic area also has a flattened appearance and can be seen in **figure 1C**;

Her lumbar area on both sides inclines forwards;

Her pelvis is posterior and leaning forwards.

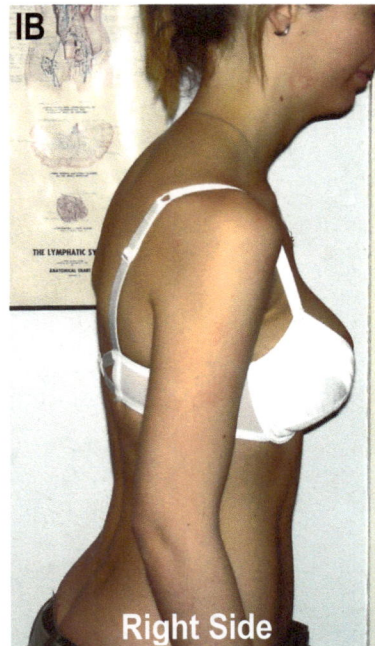

IB
Right Side

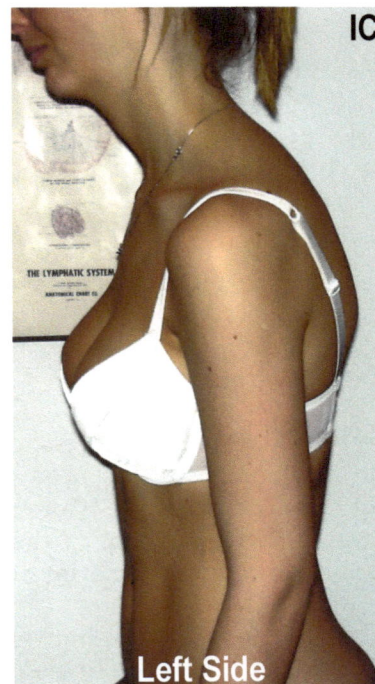

IC
Left Side

L3-Right-Right:
Calves and Feet

Figures ID and **IE** show that Lisa's forward bent posture creates a tightness in both of her calves.

Observe her heels in **figure ID.** It can be seen that her right achilles tendon inclines medially and that her left inclines laterally.

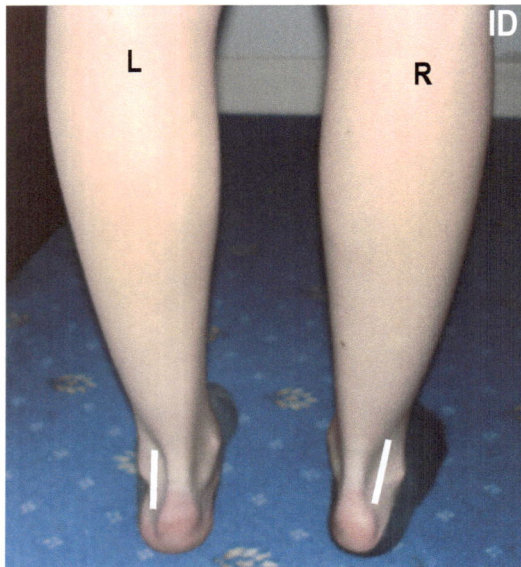

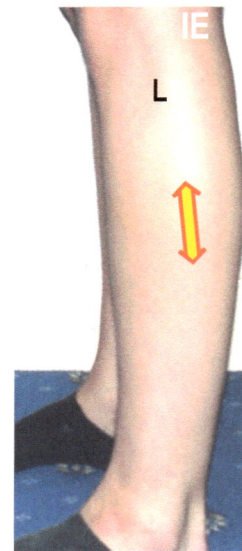

L3-right-right Feet

Figure IF shows an anterior view of Dan's feet. It can be seen that his left foot is splayed and has a dropped arch.

His right foot has a raised arch.

In this type of spinal subluxation pattern, weight is taken on his left foot in the area around his medial anterior metatarsals. Conversely the weight taken on his right foot is distributed in the area around his lateral posterior heel.

Note that his left foot rotates outwards and is generally posterior in relation to his right.

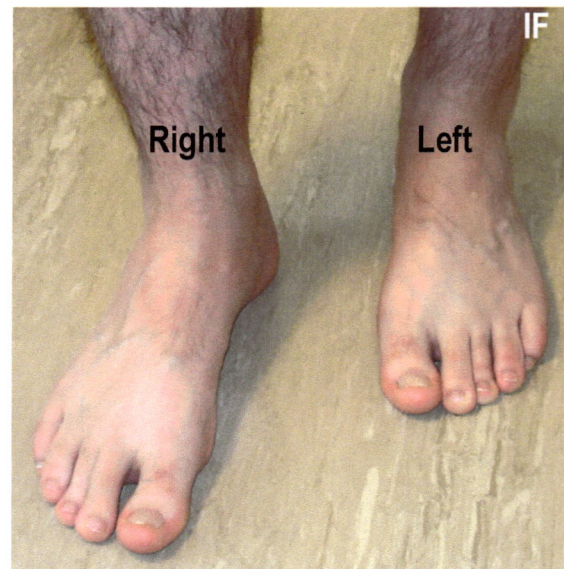

L3-Right-Right:
Knees, Neck and Head

L3-right-right knees

Observe the tracking of Lisa's knees, shown in **figure IG**. Her left patella is twisted medially and inferiorly.

Her right thigh at the distal end is angled medially and causing a shearing force on her right knee joint.

The opposing and twisting forces that distort her knee joints also puts considerable torsion and strain on both of her hip joints.

Her left knee is anterior in comparison to her right due to mild knee flexion.

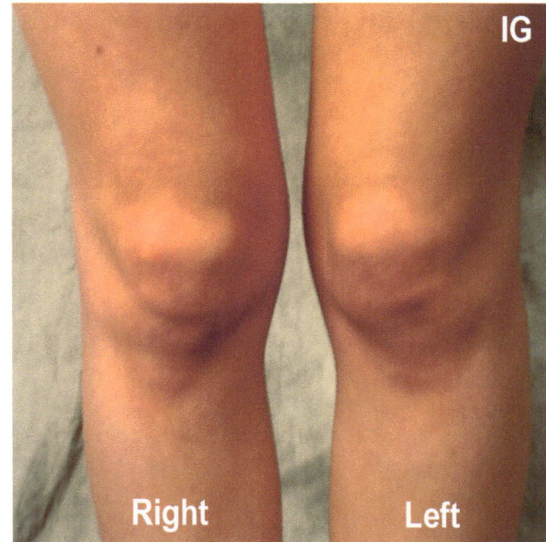

L3-right-right neck and head

Figure IH is another photograph of Lisa's back. In particular look at the angles of her shoulders and scapula again and observe the affect they have on her neck.

Notice that her left neck muscles are pulling, and that her head is rotated and side-bent to the left. This can be more easily appreciated by comparing the level and depth of her ears.

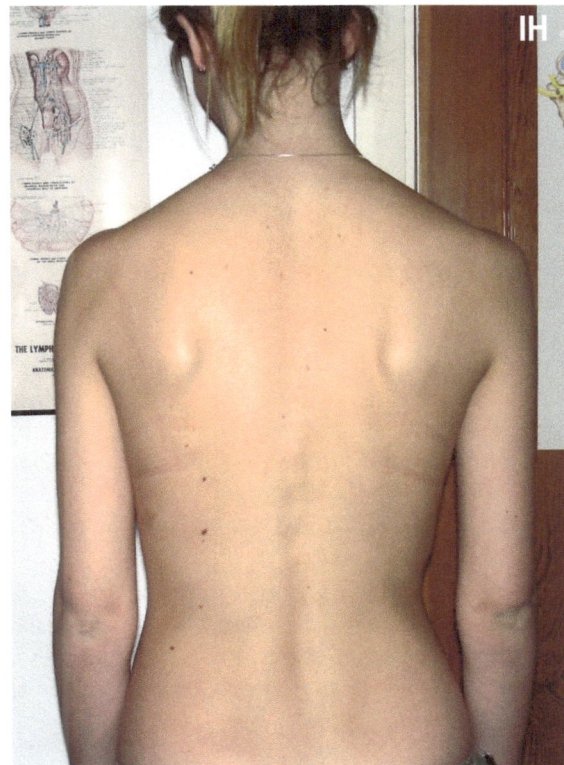

L3-Right-Right Assessment Clinical Assessment

L3-right-right plumb line from below

The purpose of a plumb line is to show the line of gravity. In a perfect spine the line of gravity would be down the centre of the body. When a plumb line is placed against Lisa's back as in **figure IJ**, the extent to which her upper torso leans to the left is highlighted. Observe her neck and see that the line of gravity passes to the right.

L3-right-right plumb line from above

If the plumb line is moved to the left to reflect the line of gravity passing through the middle of her neck, it can be seen from **figure IK** that it passes through her left sacroiliac joint, her medial left knee, calf and achilles tendon.

It is these areas that usually take the full forces of gravity.

L3-right-right clinical mobility neck

Figure IL and **IM** shows Lisa turning her head as far as she can to the left and then right, without rotating her torso. (Look at her pony-tail).

The limit to which she can rotate her neck to the left in relation to her torso is approximately 30 degrees and 25 degrees to the right. It is an illusion that there is more rotation to the right. This is due to the irregular symmetry of her shoulders. Maximum neck rotation for a young adult is approximately 70 degrees in both directions.

L3-right-right in forward bending.

Figure IN is of Lisa bending forward. In this forward bending test, observe the misalignment of her thoracic rib cage. Starting from L1, observe how her spine veers to the right and rotates to the left.

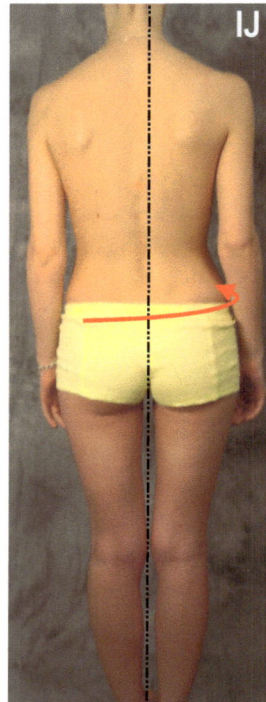

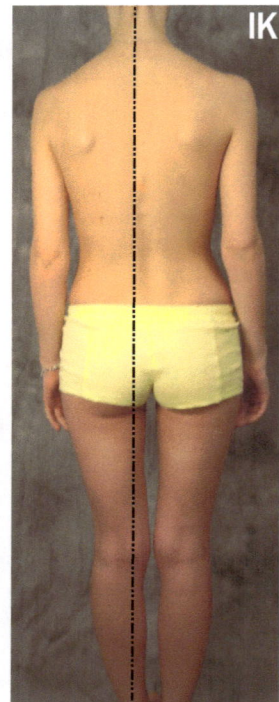

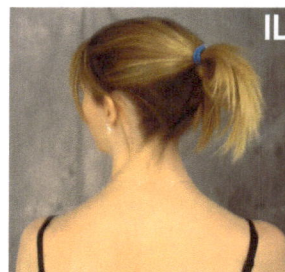

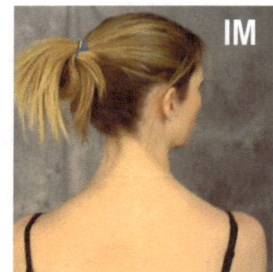

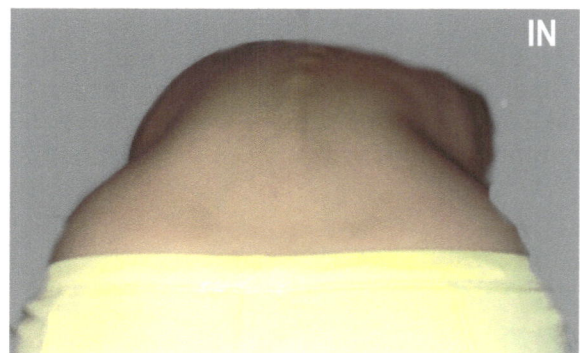

L3-Right-Right:
Clinical Observation

L3-right-right opposing forces

Lisa naturally rotated and side-bent her neck to the left because it was uncomfortable for her to straighten her head. **Figure IO** shows the main areas of torsion in her back. Observe that her left shoulder is more inclined inferiorly than the right. The medial angles of her scapulae have been highlighted to show their differences. The angles of the horizontal lines indicate some of the major opposing angles of her back.

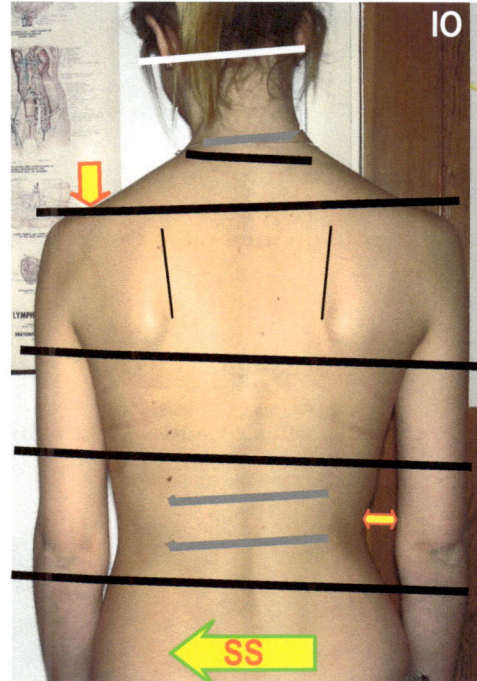

L3-right-right three blocks of torsion

Following on from the picture above, in **figure IP** her back has been divided into three blocks; the head, the rib cage and the pelvis.

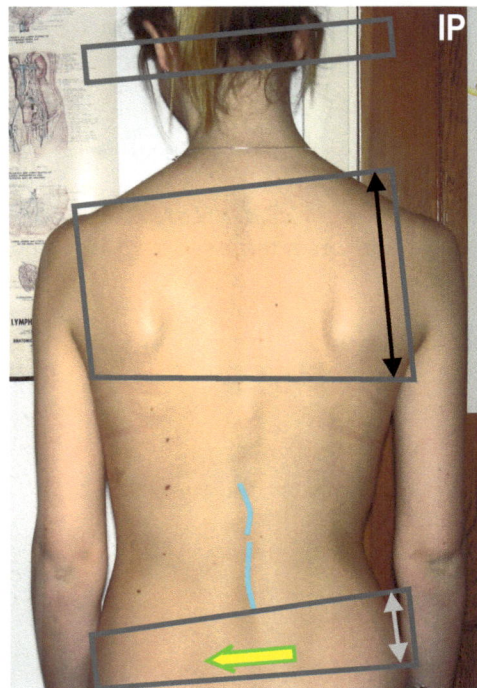

L3-right-right normal and reversed

Finally in **figures IR** and **IS**, Lisa's back has been shown normally and in reverse, to highlight the opposing shapes and bony forces at work. Our eyes are so used to seeing misaligned backs that it is only when we observe a back in reverse that the extent of the misaligned curves becomes obvious.

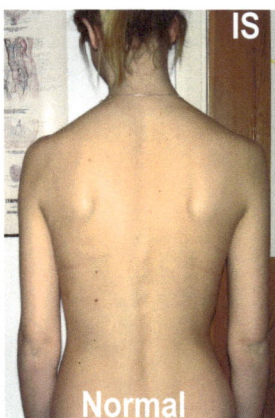

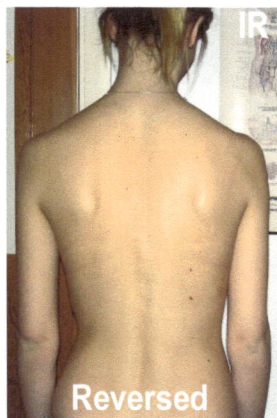

21

L3-Left-Right Model

L3-left-right posterior view

Figure IT is a photograph of Matthew's back. His type of back is representative of a fairly sizeable number of people in the western world.

The bony subluxation pattern within his back is predominantly backward bending and comes under the heading of L3-left-right.

In this type of pattern the shoulders are square.

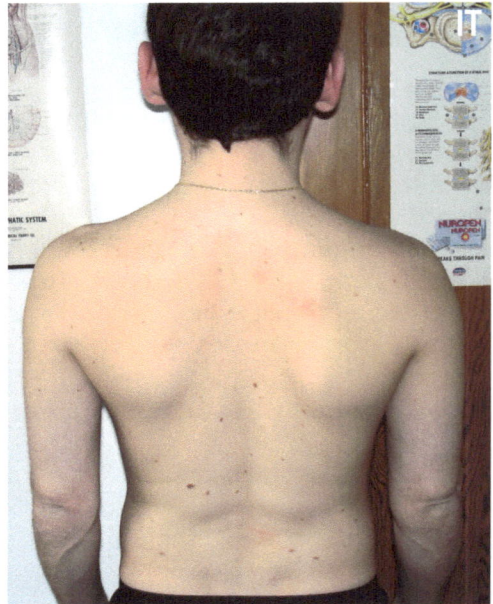

L3-left-right side view

Figure IU is a side-view of Matthew's torso. It provides a better appreciation of the backward bent curves of his posture.

Note, that unlike Lisa, his jaw is raised and his neck and head are generally posterior.

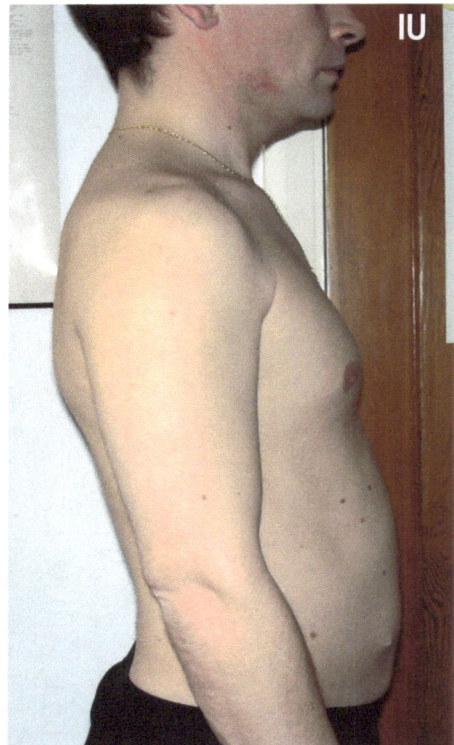

L3-Left-Right:
Clinical Observation

L3-left-right areas of opposing torsion

Figure IV of Matthew's back shows the areas of torsion drawn in.

It can be seen that his left shoulder, unlike Lisa's shoulder is higher than the right.

The medial borders of his scapulae have been highlighted. Notice that they are more vertical than Lisa's.

The direction of the transverse lines indicate the general opposing angles of his back at different points .

Note that the hang of his left arm is away from his body and is on the opposite side to that seen in Lisa's L3-right-right pattern.

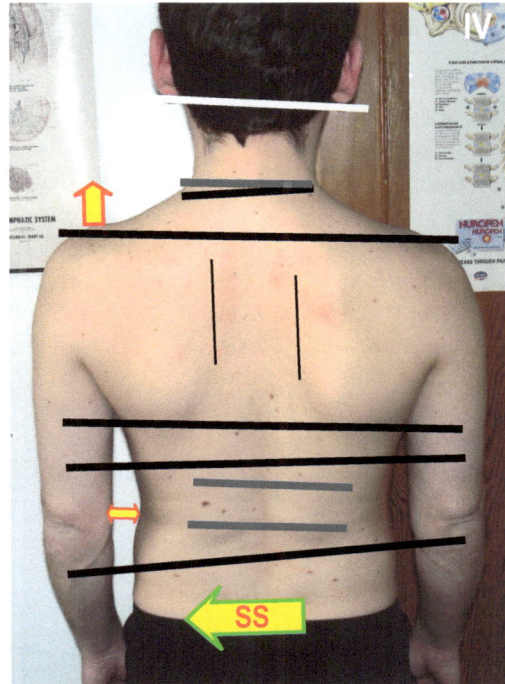

L3-left-right three blocks of torsion

Following on from the picture above, in **figure IW** Matthew's back has been divided into three parts, the head, the rib cage and the pelvis.

Each box represents a block of opposing angles.

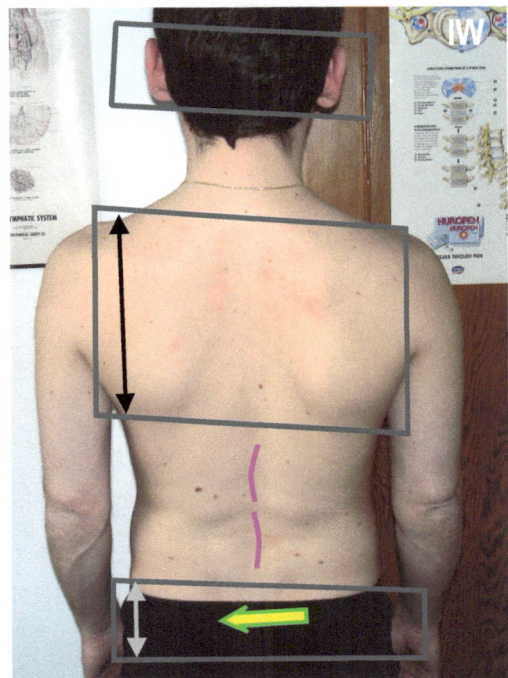

L3-Left-Right:
Feet and Reversed Torso

L3-left-right feet

Figure IX shows the placement of Matthew's feet. The angles of his feet typify the resulting torsion caused by the L3-left-right subluxation pattern.

These angles are less obvious than those created by the L3-right-right subluxation pattern. Observe that when Matthew's feet are together his left foot positions itself anteriorly, which is opposite to that seen in the L3-right-right pattern. His weight is taken medially on his left foot and laterally on his right. Notice the medial contour of his right achilles tendon compared to the straighter left.

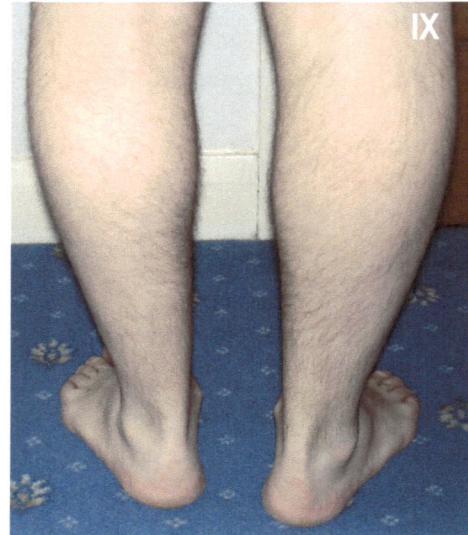

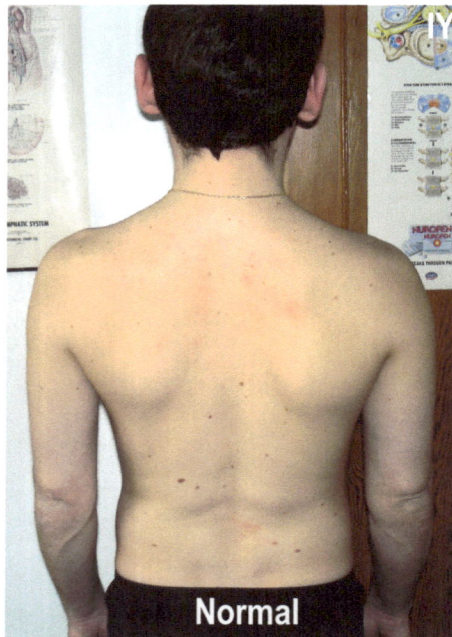

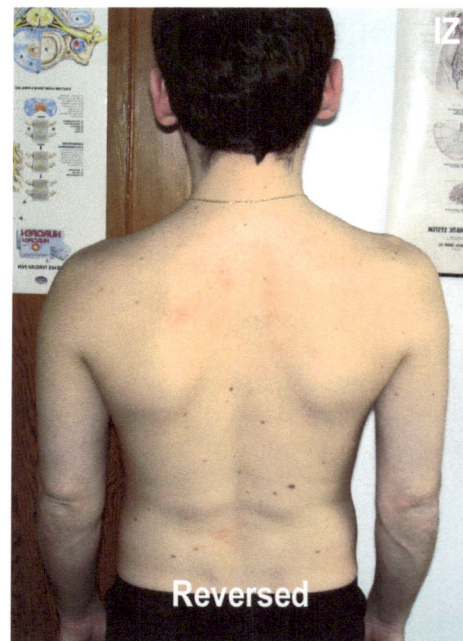

Normal and Reversed

Figures IY and **IZ** show Mathew's back, normally and in reverse, to highlight the opposing shapes and forces at work.

L3-Left-Right:
Plumb Line

Gravity line from below

In **figure IAA** the line of gravity referenced from the midline below has been drawn in against Matthew's back. It can be seen that the line of gravity passes up the left side of his neck.

This is a less lateral line of gravity than that seen in the L3-right-right pattern. For this reason his shoulders are squarer.

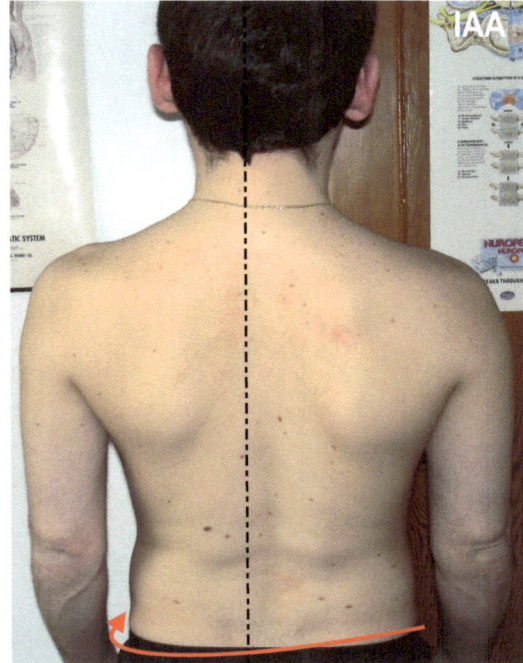

Gravity line from above

Observe the plumb line when it is positioned to pass through the mid-line of his neck, as shown in **figure IAB**. The line of gravity passes down his body and through the left side of his sacroiliac joint. If the photograph carried on downwards, the line of gravity would pass somewhere close to his left medial achilles tendon.

Because the line of gravity does not pass directly through the left ankle joint there is less torsion on the foot than seen in the L3-right-right subluxation pattern. This is why unlike people with the L3-right-right subluxation pattern, people with L3-left-right subluxation pattern are less likely to present with a fallen instep in their left foot.

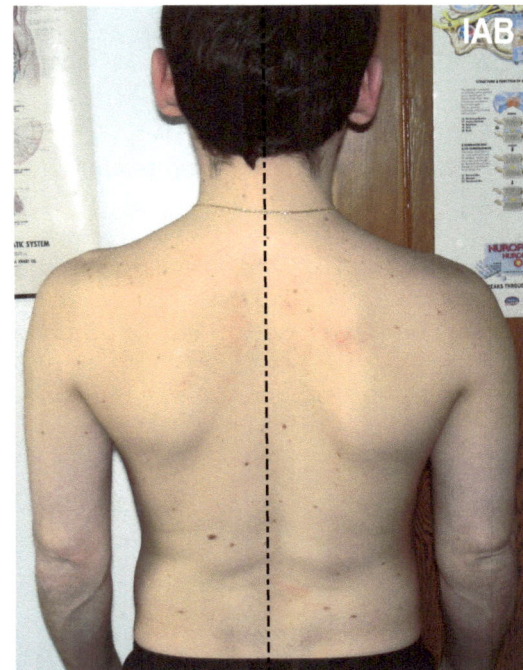

L3-Right-Right and L3-Left-Right: Comparison

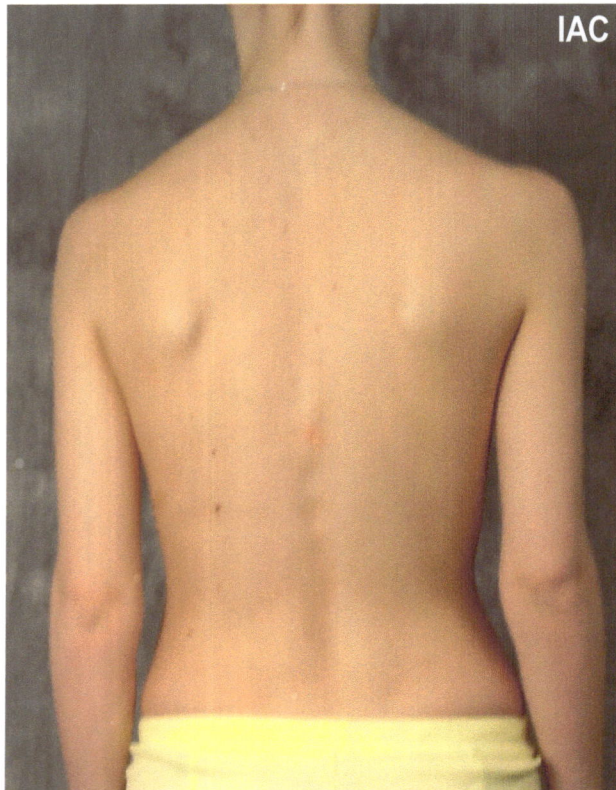

L3-Right-Right
Pelvis side-bent left - rotated left

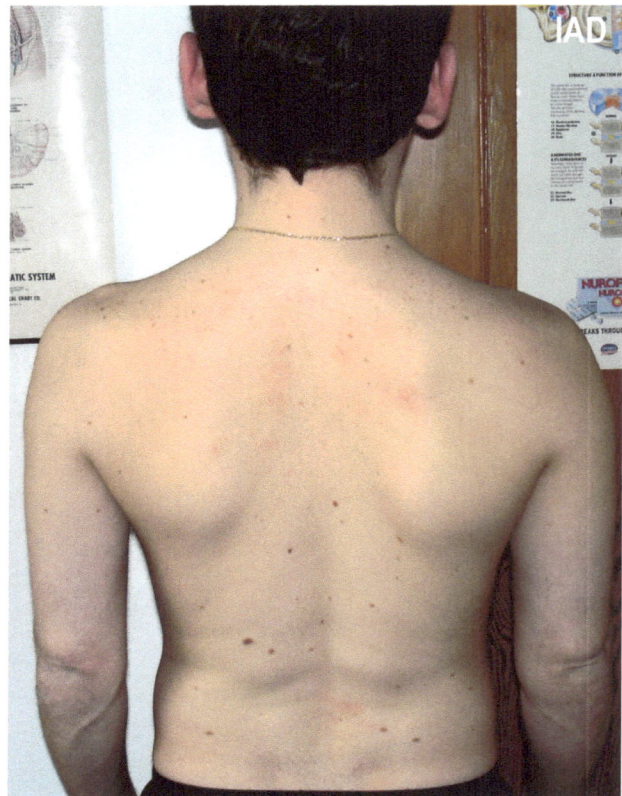

L3-Left-Right
Pelvis side-bent left - rotated right

Figures IAC and **IAD** show the two subluxation pattern models. To find out how these two backs became subluxated like this and created the torsions to their rib cage, shoulders, arms, legs, knees and feet, we need to start at the beginning; the basic anatomy of the facets and their physiology.

Chapter Three
Physiology of the
Sacroiliac Joints

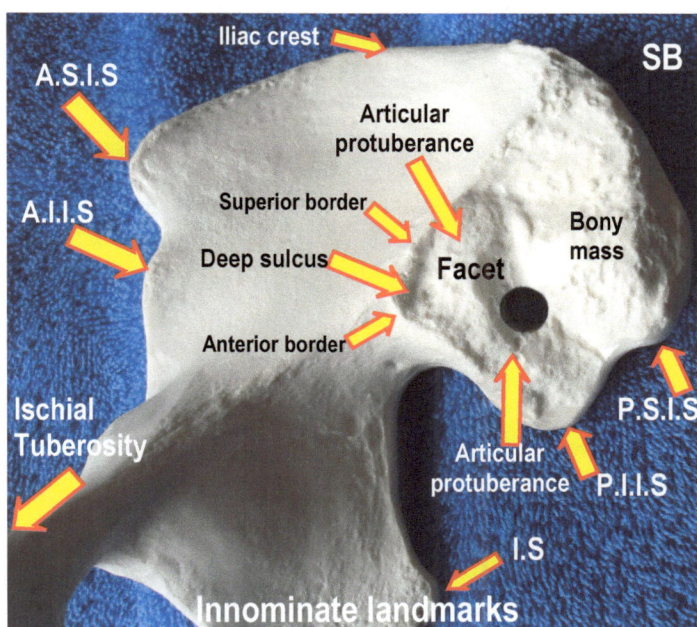

The sacroiliac joint

There are many variations in the shapes and sizes of the sacroiliac articular facets and it is this that seems to have confounded many theorists seeking to discover their secrets in the past. However, all sacroiliac facet shapes share certain common similarities and these are explained in this chapter. **Figure SB** shows a plastic mould of the right ilium detailing the bony architecture.

At the posterior border of the ilium there is a bony mass that stops any posterior shift of the sacrum. Around the border of the facet there are two bony protuberances, one at the superior ridge and one at the lower anterior ridge. There is a deep sulcus at the anterior border on some types of facet that prohibits sacral anterior shift. In other types of facet the anterior ridge of the sulcus is less pronounced. These borders, if crossed, would constitute a form of dislocation.

Bayliss Sacroiliac Theory

Working sacroiliac theory overview

For a theory on the sacroiliac joints to work, it has to fill certain criteria. It has to make due allowance for the action of walking and other methods of motion, together with spinal rotation and side-bending, in both forward and backward bending.

Joints are not designed to semi-dislocate as part of their normal articulation process and the sacroiliac joint is no exception to this rule. We learned from our "rationale" tests, that the sacroiliac joints, via pelvic side-shift and side-bending act as a precursor for spinal rotation to take place. This means that the sacroiliac facets must have been designed to take these movements into account.

The theory that follows, does not rely on dislocation and fulfils all the above criteria.

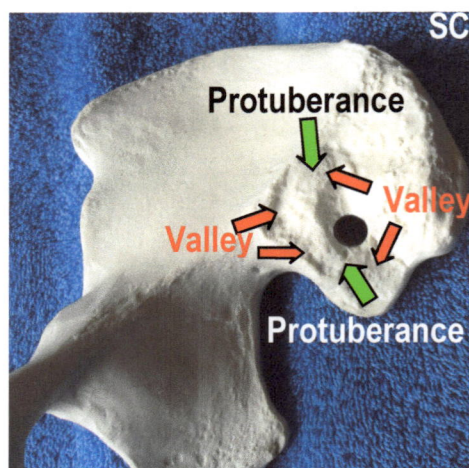

Bayliss sacroiliac theory

To refer to **figure SC,** instead of seeing the sacroiliac joint as an approximate C shape, think of the bony mass running down the vertical length as a pivot for a see-saw action.

At the top there is a protuberance with the bone on either side falling away; below there is another bony protuberance, also with bone on either side falling away.

The valleys that fall away can be divided into two separate facet group surfaces; anterior and posterior.

Figure SD shows the posterior facet group in blue and the anterior facet group in magenta. The posterior facets can be categorized as 'load bearing' and the anterior facets as 'guider facets'.

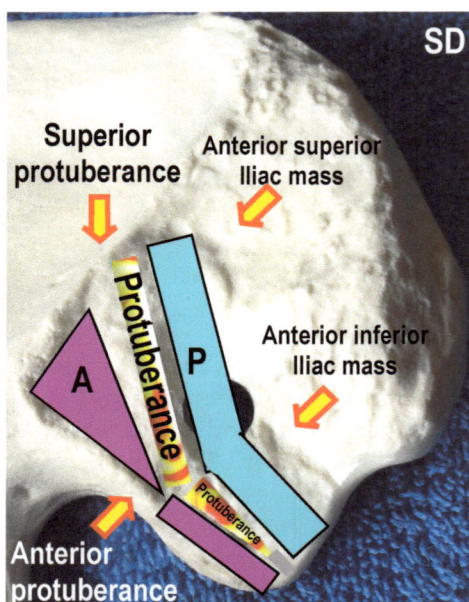

28

Iliac Facet Shape

The four pictures below are exaggerated illustrations of the iliac facet surface contours

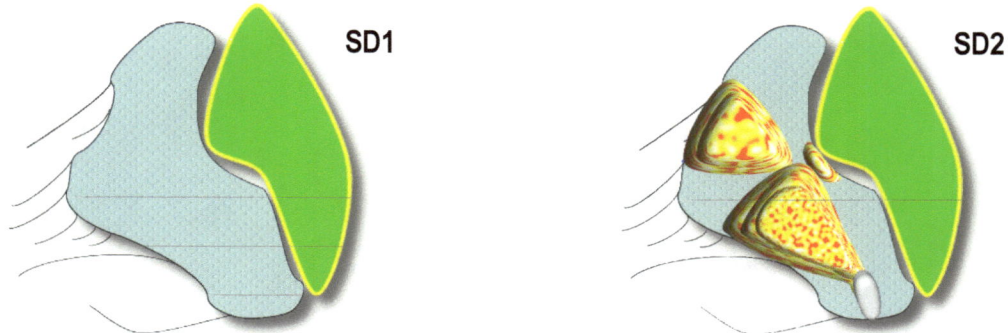

Figure SD1 provides a closer look at an iliac facet without any contours or articular surfaces added. The green colouring is drawn in to represent the bony mass. The bony mass is there to act as a buffer when too much weight is placed on the posterior facets.

In **figure SD2** the bony contours running down the middle have been added in mottled yellow. At first sight the contours look like a design by committee, but nothing could be further from the truth. These contours are designed as part of a complex swivel joint. The light grey contour is a divider.

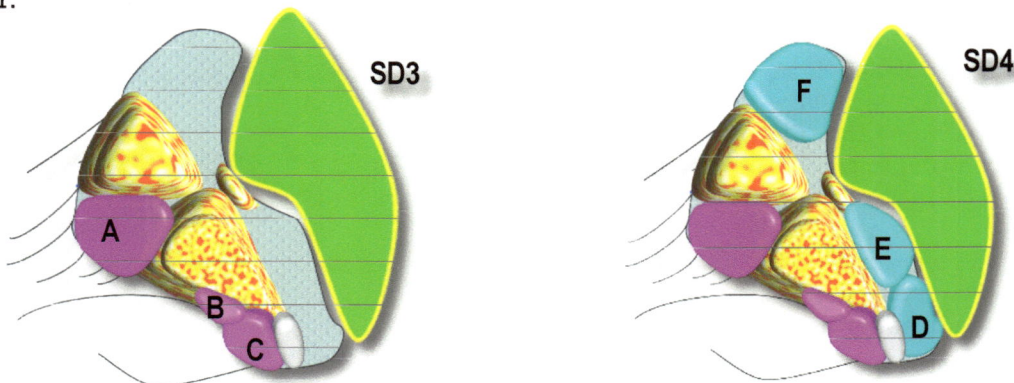

In **figure SD3** the anterior facets have been added. Note that they are not continuous. *Facet A* is the true anterior articular surface and is there to guide the thigh/leg forward, medial and upward in a non weight bearing capacity. *Facet B* has a transitory function and is there to guide the thigh/leg towards the ground. Once the foot touches the ground, the anterior *facet C* acts as a transitory weight bearing cross-over point to the transitory load bearing posterior *facet D*, shown **in figure SD4.** At this point the weight of the body is taken equally on both feet.

As more weight is transferred to the supporting leg, the upward ground-resistance causes the posterior transitory weight bearing *facet E* to engage. Finally when the full weight of the body is taken on the supporting vertical leg, the meeting of the ground-resistance returning up the leg causes the main posterior load bearing *facet F* to engage.

Anatomy of the Sacral Facets

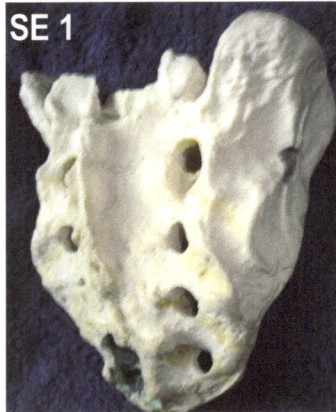

SE 1

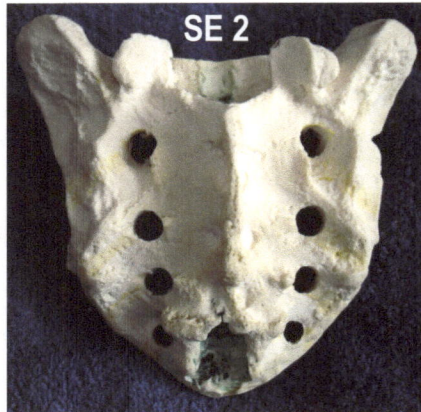

SE 2

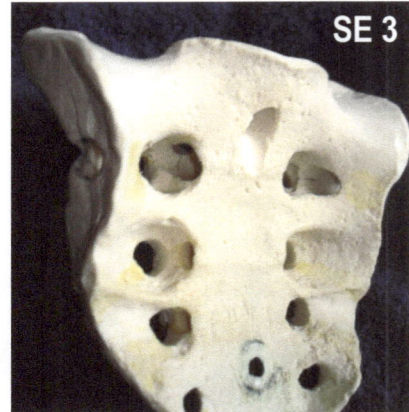

SE 3

Like the innominate's, when you first look at the shape of the sacrum it looks like design by committee. But it is so cleverly designed that even huge variations in the basic shape still work relatively efficiently.

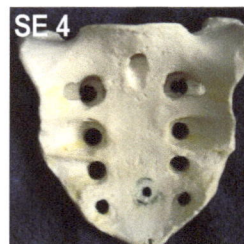

SE 4

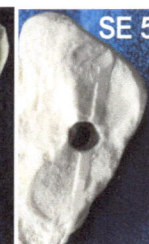

SE 5

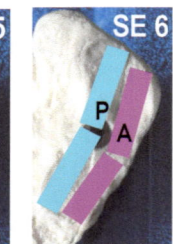

SE 6

The basic shape of the sacral facets is predominantly concave, in contrast to the iliac facets which are predominantly convex. When the articular surfaces of the sacrum and ilium are placed together their complimentary contours form a snug tight fit.

The function of the sacrum is to act as a counter lever between the two innominate bones and form a solid mobile base for the spine.

The complex shape of the sacral facets is not immediately obvious. For simplicity **figure SE6** illustrates how the facets can be divided into two groups; anterior (magenta) and posterior (blue).

These two groups can be further divided into six individual facets. These individual facets are illustrated in **figure SE7.**

(1) represents the convex shape of the posterior splitter protuberance and *(2)* the concave shape of the anterior splitter protuberance.

If you compare these contours with **figures SE1, SE2, SE3** and **SE5** it can be seen how they match.

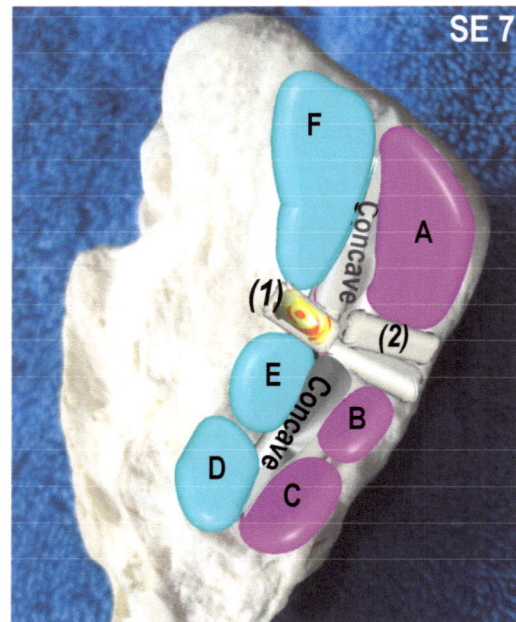

SE 7

30

Sacroiliac Facet Engagement

Figure SF is an aerial view of the right sacroiliac joint. The coloured oblong lines have been drawn in to highlight the shape of the joint.

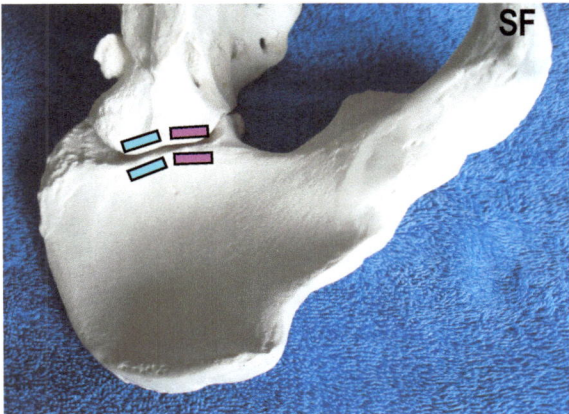

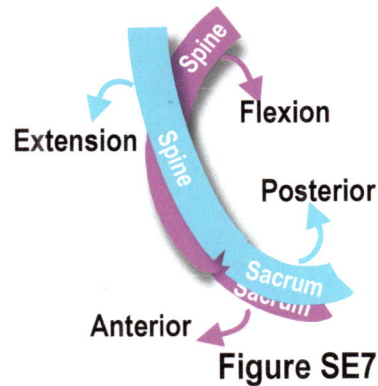

Figure SE7 shows what happens when the lumbar vertebrae flex and extend. When the lumbar flexes the base of the sacrum acts as an extension of the lumbar and moves anteriorly. And when the lumbar extends, the sacral base moves posteriorly.

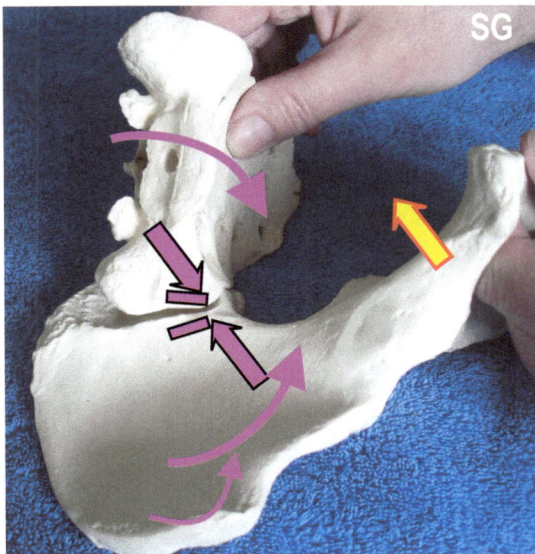

Sacroiliac anterior facets

Figure SG shows the anterior facets of the sacrum and ilium engaged. Note that the pubic crest and anterior superior iliac spine have moved medially.

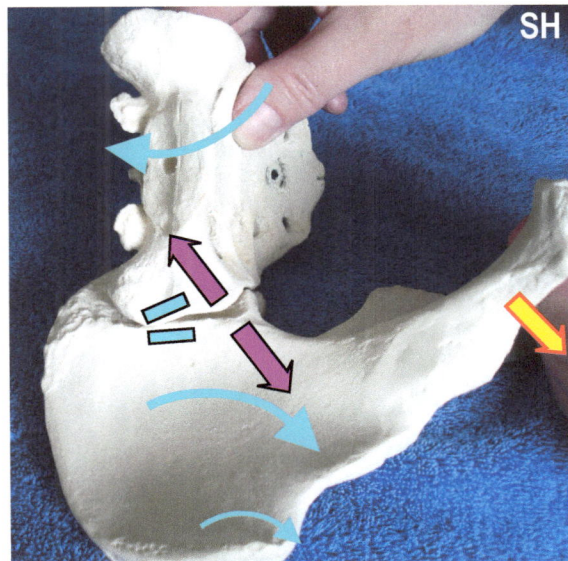

Sacroiliac posterior facets

Figure SH shows the posterior facets of the sacrum and the ilium engaged. Note that the pubic crest and anterior superior iliac spine have moved laterally.

Innominate Movements

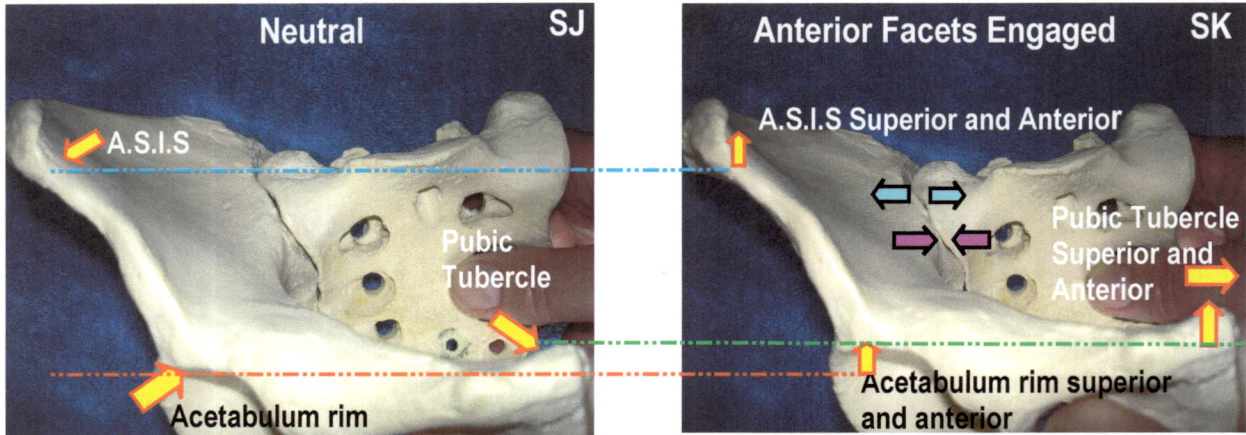

Figure SJ shows the sacroiliac joint in neutral and **figure SK,** with the anterior facets engaged. Lines of reference have been added to highlight the differences between the bony landmarks.

Figure SK shows the positions the right ilium and hip joint take to raise the right leg anteriorly, medially and superiorly.

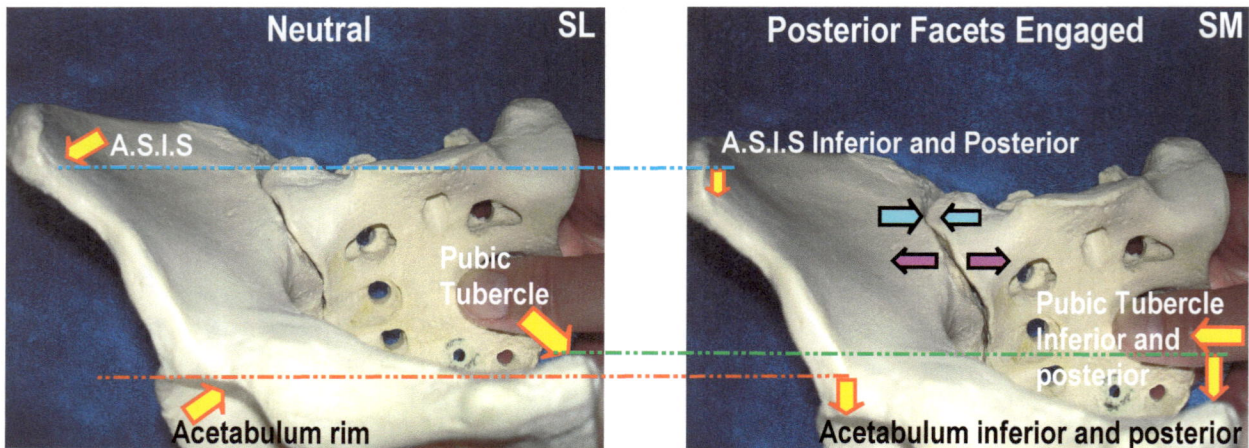

Figure SL shows the sacroiliac joint in neutral and **figure SM,** with the posterior facets engaged. Lines of reference have been added to highlight the differences between the bony landmarks.

Figure SM shows the positions the right ilium and hip joint take to lower the weight bearing right leg posteriorly, laterally and inferiorly.

32

Sacroiliac Principal of Reciprocation

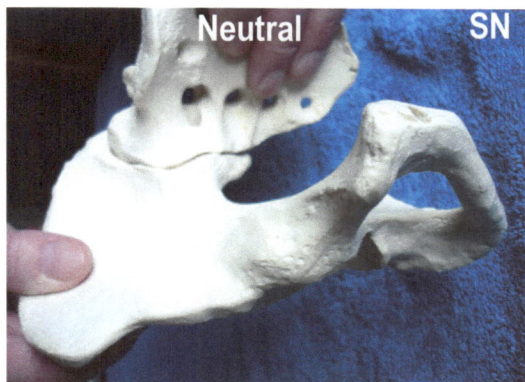

Neutral   SN

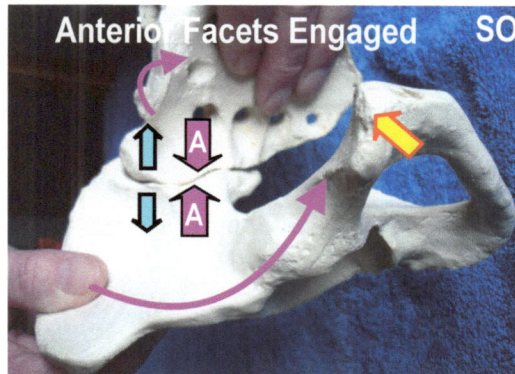

Anterior Facets Engaged   SO

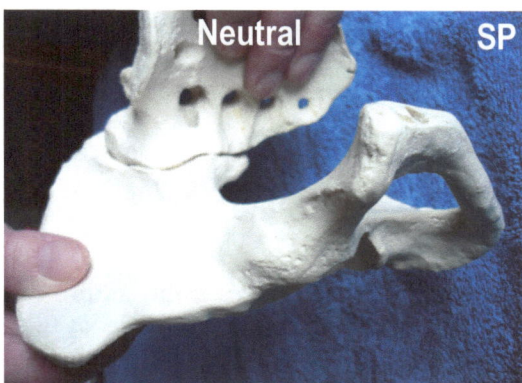

Neutral   SP

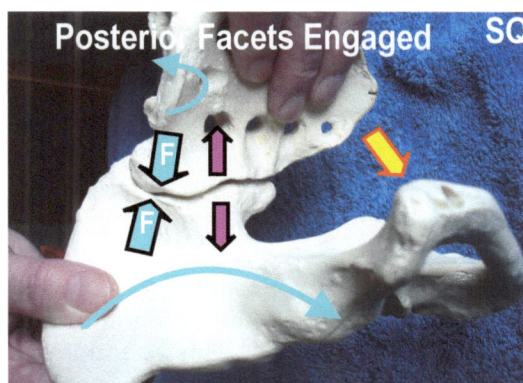

Posterior Facets Engaged   SQ

Above are more comparison photographs. **Figure SO** shows the position of the ilium when the 'A' anterior sacroiliac facets engage. **Figure SQ** shows the position of the ilium when the 'F' posterior facets are engaged.

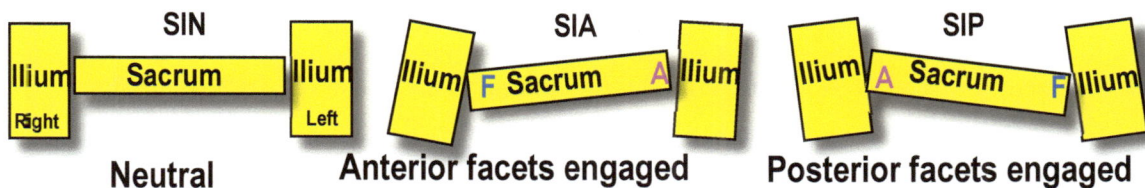

SIN

Ilium Right   Sacrum   Ilium Left

Neutral

SIA

Ilium   F Sacrum A   Ilium

Anterior facets engaged

SIP

Ilium A   Sacrum   F Ilium

Posterior facets engaged

The illustrations above show the reciprocal action of the sacroiliac articulation. **Figure SIN** shows the neutral position.

When the 'A' anterior facets engage on the left, shown in **figure SIA**, the 'F' posterior facets are levered to engage on the right. When the 'F' posterior facets engage on the right, shown in **figure SIP**, the 'A' anterior facets are levered to engage on the left.

33

Pelvic Alignment and Motion

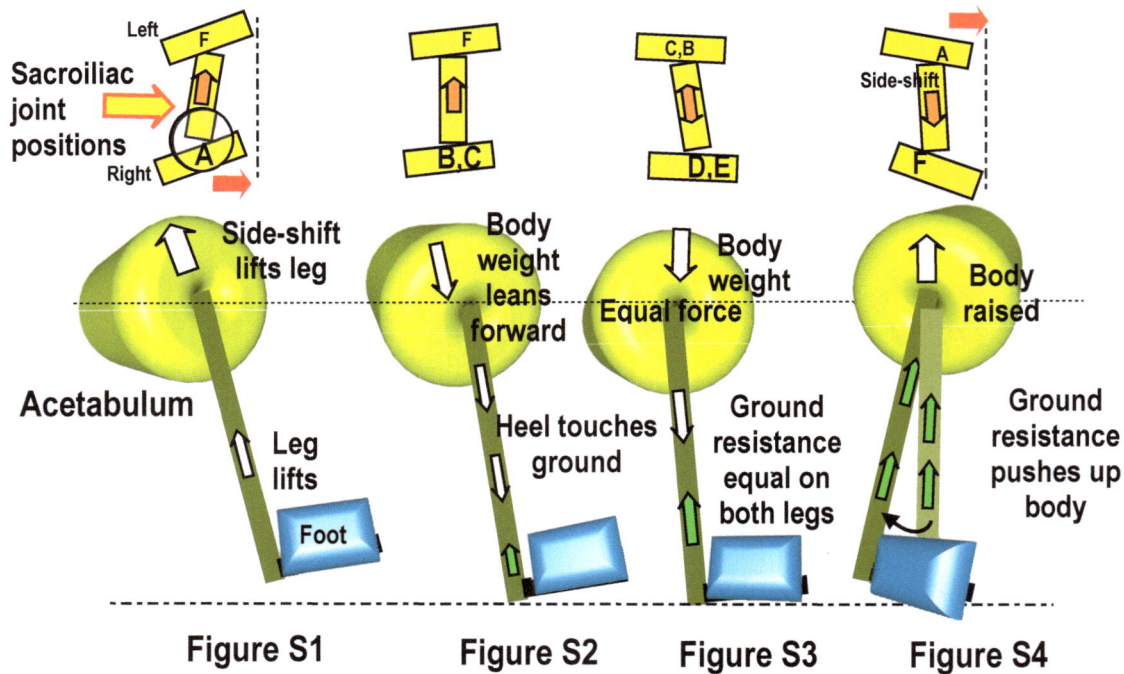

Sacroiliac joint positions

Left / Right

F / A / B,C / C,B / D,E / A / F

Side-shift

Side-shift lifts leg

Acetabulum

Leg lifts

Foot

Body weight leans forward

Heel touches ground

Body weight

Equal force

Ground resistance equal on both legs

Body raised

Ground resistance pushes up body

Figure S1　**Figure S2**　**Figure S3**　**Figure S4**

The illustration above represents the positions the right leg and foot take during the action of walking. **Figure S1** shows the position of the right leg when the weight bearing left side of the pelvis side-shifts to the left. This action levers the right anterior 'A' sacroiliac facets to engage. With the aid of the limb muscles, the right leg moves anteriorly, medially and superiorly.

Figure S2 shows the transitory position of the leg as the upper body weight inclines forward into the direction of motion. *Weight and side-shift are still on the left*. This action causes the right leg to contact the ground and lever the ilium to engage the lower anterior facets 'B' and 'C'.

Figure S3 shows the position of the leg as equal weight is placed on both legs. The position of the leading right leg is anterior and the left, posterior.   This causes the ilium to lever and engage the posterior facets 'D' through to 'E' on the right, and the anterior facets 'C' through to 'B' on the left.

Figure S4 shows the position of the leg in the final stage. Upward ground resistance travels up the right leg and lifts the pelvis on the same side. When weight bearing and side-shift transfer to the right, the right posterior 'F' sacroiliac facets fully engage. When weight bearing and side-shift transfer to the right, the right posterior 'F' sacroiliac facets fully engage.   In turn the articular surface on the left side of the sacrum is levered to engage the 'A' anterior sacroiliac facets.   More about the walking action follows in chapter four.

Sacroiliac Facets when Standing and Sitting

Standing

Figure SQ1 shows the facet engagement when a person stands upright, slightly forward or backward bent. Because there is no side-shift, weight is evenly distributed bi-laterally on the 'F' posterior sacroiliac facets and balanced by the 'A' anterior facets on the same side. The arrow 'a' illustrates how the sacrum is prevented from slipping inferio-posteriorly by the prominent bony mass during weight bearing.

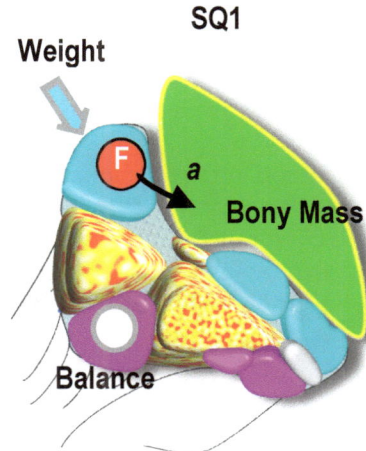

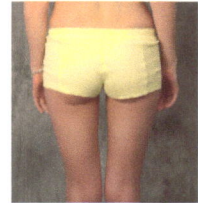

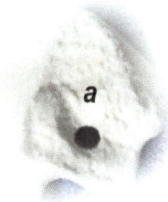

Forward bending and sitting

Figure SQ2 shows the facet engagement when a person bends forward during weight bearing, or is in the sitting position. The forward bending angle of the sacrum brings the centre of pivot lower. Because there is no side-shift, weight is bi-laterally distributed on the 'E' posterior sacroiliac facets. The blue arrow represents the forward direction of the sacrum. The black arrow 'b' shows how the sacrum is prevented from slipping superiorly by the prominent bony mass.

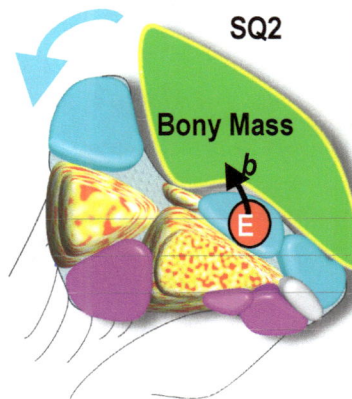

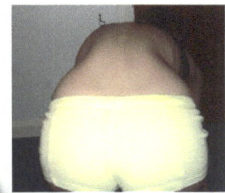

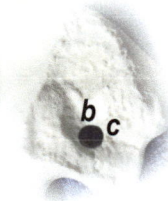

Left leg folded over right

Figure SQ3 shows the facet engagements when a person folds their left leg over the right in the sitting position. Because there is no side-shift, the antero-medial position of the left leg engages the left 'B' anterior facets. Reciprocally the right posterior 'E' facets remain engaged, as described above for the sitting position.

If the left knee moves into a more lateral position, the left thigh is angled further laterally and the left sacroiliac facet engagement changes to 'C'. Reciprocally the right posterior 'D' facets engage.

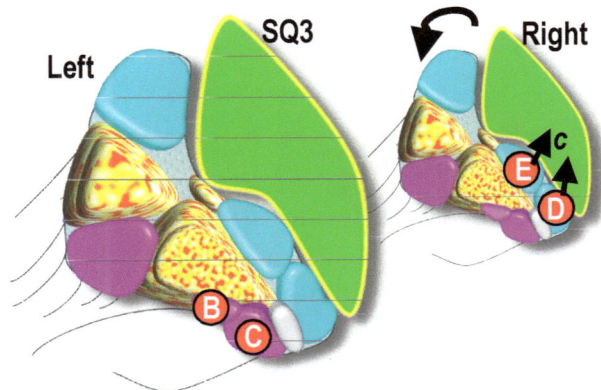

35

Rotation Right in Extension

Rotation right in extension

When the left knee is flexed and body weight is transferred to the right leg as shown in **figure SR**, the posterior 'F' sacroiliac joint facets engage. This action causes the pelvis as a whole to lift on the left and rotate to the right. This introduces general rotation to the right in the lumbar spine.

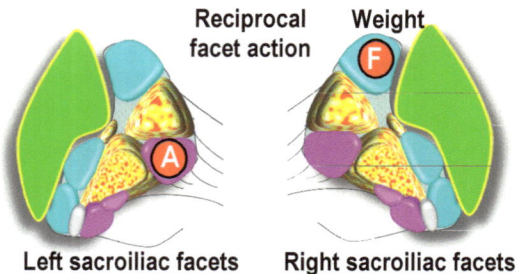

Reciprocal facet action

Weight

A

F

Left sacroiliac facets   Right sacroiliac facets

When the pelvis side-shifts to the right, as shown in **figure SS,** the pelvis becomes more level, whilst the lumbar vertebrae are given the necessary side-shift they need to individually side-bend to the right. This action also increases the rotation to the right.

Key:

TP's   = Transverse processes

⬆   = Upward ground resistance

⮕   = Transverse processes side-bent

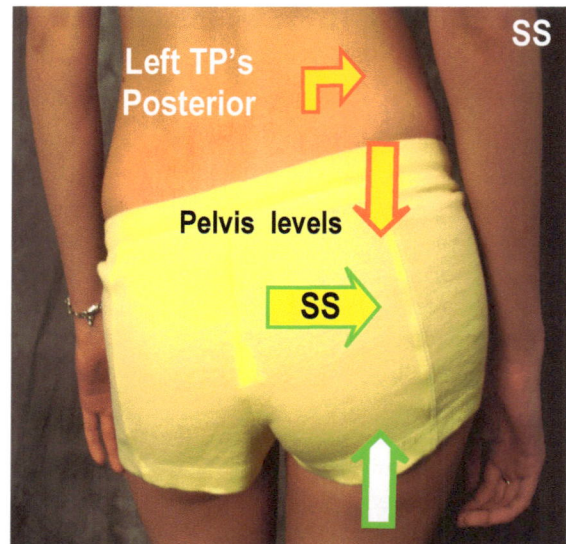

SR

Weight

Posterior

Left knee flexed   Ground resistance

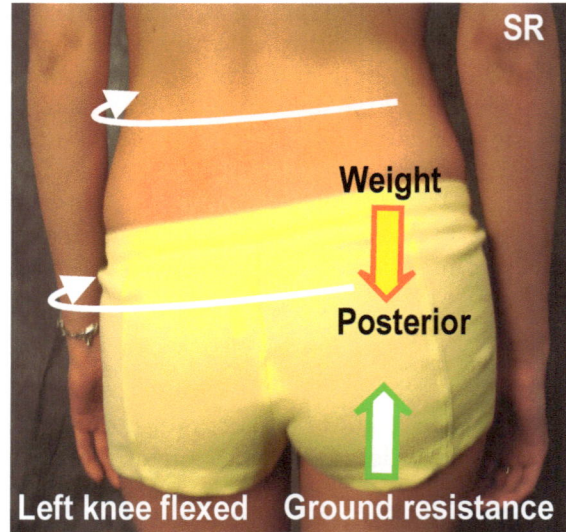

SS

Left TP's Posterior

Pelvis levels

SS

Rotation Right in Flexion

Rotation right in flexion

When the left knee is flexed and body weight is transferred to the left leg, as shown in **figure ST,** the anterior 'A' sacroiliac facets engage. It is this action that causes the pelvis as a whole to side-bend to the left. This makes the right side of the pelvis higher than the left and causes the lumbar spine to side-bend left.

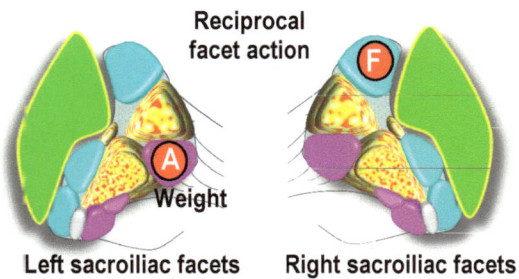

Posterior

ST

Weight

Knee flexed and ground resistance

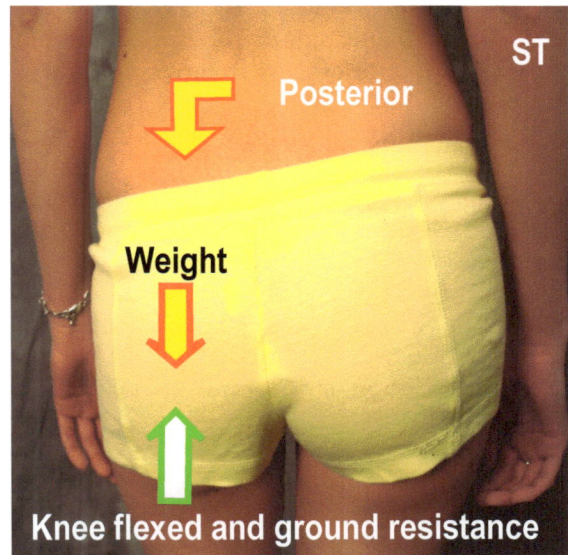

Reciprocal facet action

F

A

Weight

Left sacroiliac facets   Right sacroiliac facets

When the pelvis has side-shifted to the left as shown in **figure SU,** the lumbar vertebrae are given the necessary side-shift they need to individually rotate to the right. This action also increases the side-bending left.

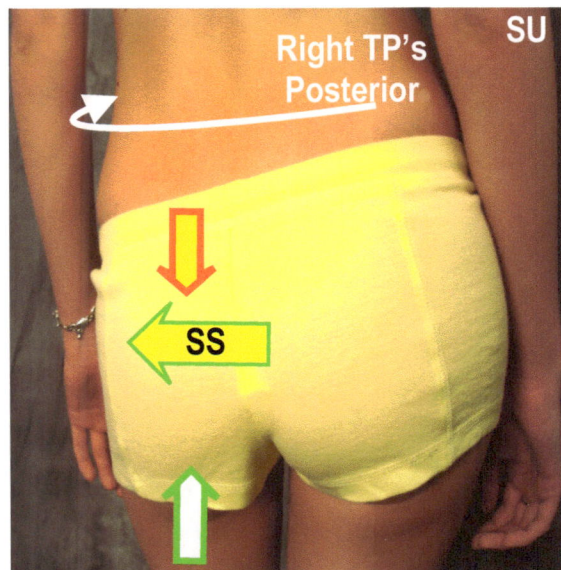

SU

Right TP's Posterior

SS

37

Principles of Pelvic Rotation
and Side-Bending

Throughout the chapters in this book the pelvic movements described in this chapter are constantly being referenced.

Therefore, it is fundamentally important that you understand how pelvic side-bending and rotation take place before you move on.

Take a moment to follow the illustrations and descriptions on pages 36 and 37 and do some experiments with your own body. This will help you understand the rudiments of pelvic side-bending and rotation. Also, with this hands-on approach you should get a better appreciation of the important role, the synchronization of knee flexion, weight bearing and side-shift have on the pelvis.

Try walking whilst blocking all side-shift. If you are truly blocking all side-shift you will not be able to move forward. This simple test provides evidence that muscles are not the sole driving force for ambulation, side-bending and rotation.

Chapter Four
Physiology of the
Lumbar Joints

Terminology

Before we go into any detail about spinal mechanics, we need to co-ordinate our terminology of the lumbar vertebrae.

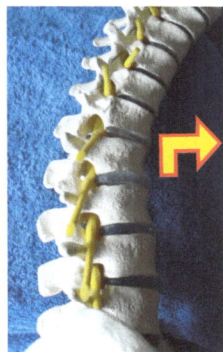

Extension
Forward bending

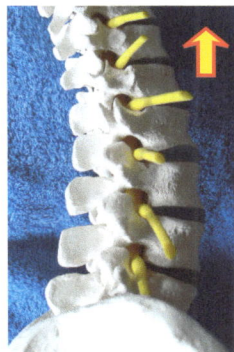

Neutral
Standing vertical

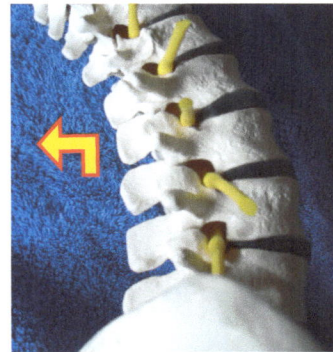

Flexion
Backward bending

Lumbar vertebral function

All the lower vertebrae namely L5, L4, L3 and L2 are designed for weight bearing, flexion, extension, side-bending and rotation. For stability reasons, S1-L5 and L5-4 have less mobility than the lumbar vertebrae above.

The L1 vertebra is designed for flexion, extension and to counter side-bending and rotation in flexion and allow it in extension. L1 also acts as a shock absorber and provides a level plateau for the thoracic vertebrae to sit vertically upon.

We know from our rationale tests that the lumbar will not rotate meaningfully without pelvic side-shift and side-bending. Therefore, side-shift and side-bending must be the driving force that rotates the lumbar vertebrae.

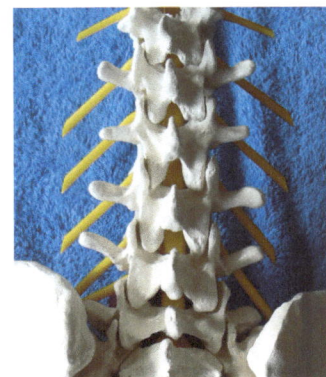

Experiment: Principles of Lumbar Facet Movement

A simple experiment using your hands can be carried out to get a better understanding of how the lumbar joints can sometimes side-bend and rotate to opposite sides and at other times rotate and side-bend to the same side:

1) Starting position

Sit in front of a desk and place a book about 2 inches (5 cm) thick in front of you to your right. Rest your right elbow on the book and your left elbow on the desk. Cup your right hand and make a fist with the left and then place your fist lightly into your cupped hand.

In these experiments the right cupped hand represents L4 and the left fist, L3.

2) Test for side-bending and rotation to opposite sides

We learned in the previous chapter that the pelvis as a whole side-bends in flexion.

If you look at your hands you will notice that due to the thickness of the book, the right elbow has caused both hands to generally side-bend left. Place your weight on the left elbow. If you now side-shift your right elbow towards the left you will observe that your fist rotates naturally to the right.

3) Test for rotation and side-bending to the same side

We learned in the previous chapter that the pelvis as a whole rotates in extension.

If we start from position 1) Place your weight on the right elbow and level the height of your left elbow with the right. Be aware that as you do this your left elbow moves away from you and that both of your hands generally rotate to the right. Now side-shift your left elbow towards the right. If you observe your fist as you do this you will see that it naturally side-bends to the right.

What can be deduced from these experiments?

There are two district movements. the gross movement which comes from the pelvis and the segmental movement which is comes from side-shift.

Lumbar:
L4 Facet Anatomy

L3-4 joint overview

The function of the L4-L3 joint is to be weight bearing. It can move in a vertical plain to compliment flexion and extension movements. It can also rotate and side-bend either in flexion or extension.

The L5-L4 joint has a very similar design and function, though the superior facets are more spade-like and heavy duty.

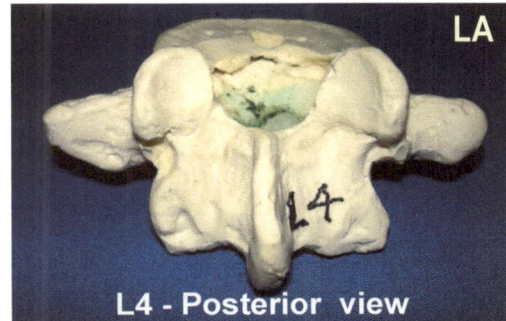

L4 - Posterior view

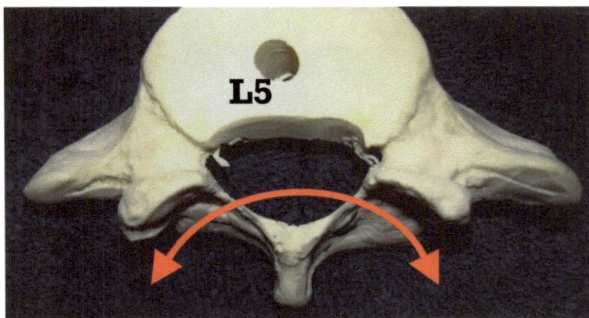

L5

L5 Facet shape for comparison

Figure LA is a typical posterior view of an L4 vertebra. It has two sets of facets; two at the top that face posteriorly and two at the bottom that face anteriorly. We are going to look more closely at the upper facets.

The superior L4 facets are robust and designed with concave banking at either side. This is shown in **figure LB**.

The superior L4 facets shown on their side for clarity in **figure LC**, are convex vertically.

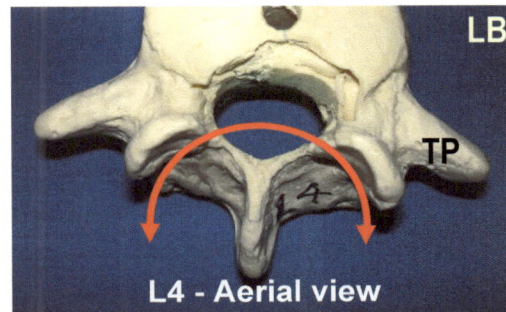

L4 - Aerial view

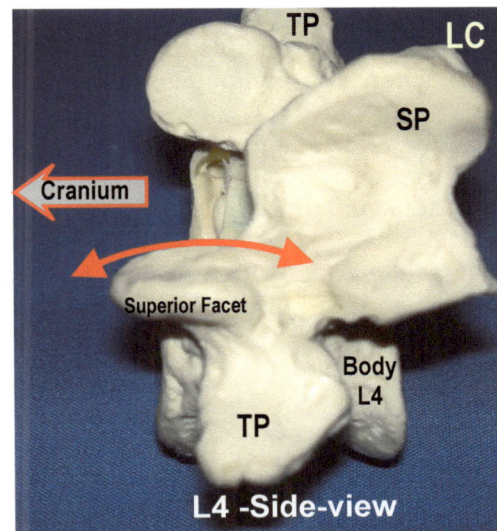

Cranium

TP

SP

Superior Facet

Body L4

TP

L4 -Side-view

Lumbar:
L3 Facet Anatomy Inferior Facets

L3 facet shape

Figure LD is a side-view of the inferior anterior facets of L3. The facets have a design similar to a pair of skis. They are concave vertically, and convex horizontally, as shown in **figure LE**.

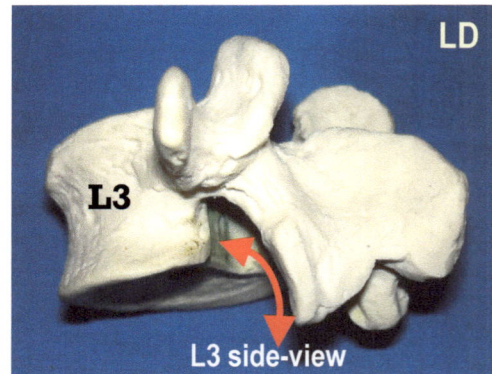
LD

L3

L3 side-view

L4 articulation surface

Each facet has two halves and each a separate purpose; the upper half, shown as two blue dots in **figure LF**, allows the facet of L3 to glide superiorly when a person bends forward.

The lower half of the L4 facet shown in magenta, enables the facets of L3 to glide inferiorly when a person backward leans.

The position between the two halves of the L4 facets, shown as a blue bar, is the neutral position for when a person stands upright.

The L4 facet surface is designed for rotation in flexion and side-bending in neutral and extension.

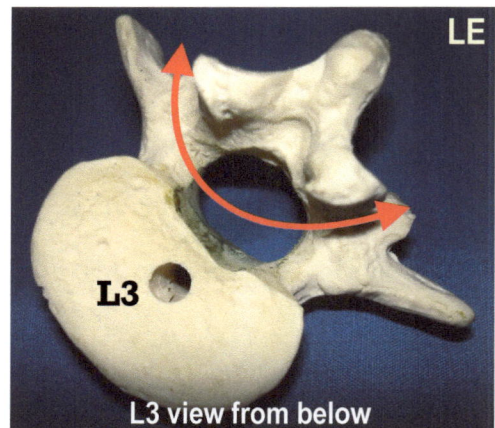
LE

L3

L3 view from below

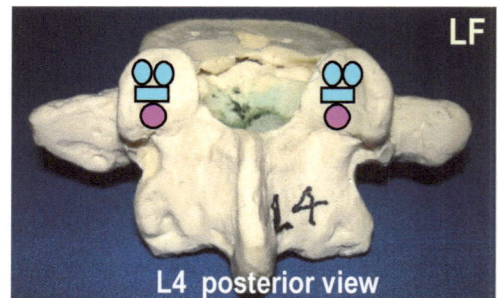
LF

L4

L4 posterior view

The Importance of the Nucleus Pulposus

Before the physiology of the lumbar joints are discussed, a couple of words need to be said about working movements out on a plastic spine. The rubber discs were a real hindrance because they do not simulate the arcing effect of the nucleus pulposus. The nucleus pulposus would appear to be of the utmost importance because it acts as a pivot for vertebral facet movements.

Nucleus Pulposus Shape

Figure LG shows typical medical capsule. It is being used to represent the nucleus pulposus. It is spongy and pliable. The ideal shape would be oval.

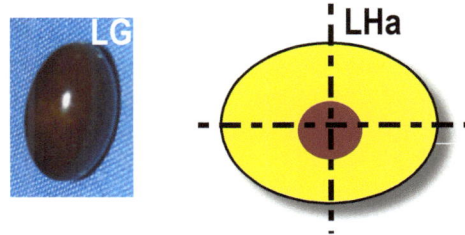

To get the best results, place the nucleus on the body of the lumbar vertebrae, as shown in **figures LHa** and **LHb**. Note that the nucleus pulposus should be positioned towards the posterior half of the body.

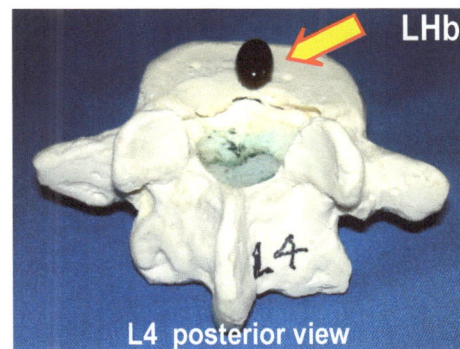

The three drawings below show the horizontal and vertical benefits of a spongy nucleus pulposus, together with the horizontal and vertical orbits that are possible.

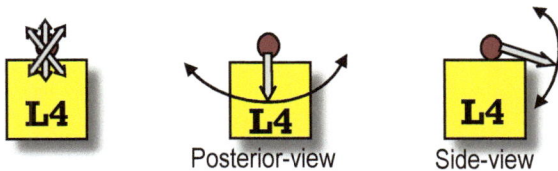

LG

LHa

LHb
L4 posterior view

L4

L4
Posterior-view

L4
Side-view

Extension and flexion of L4-L3

When the nucleus is in place and L3 positioned over L4, the vertical arc of the facets can be illustrated as shown in **figures LHc**, **LHd** and **LHe**.

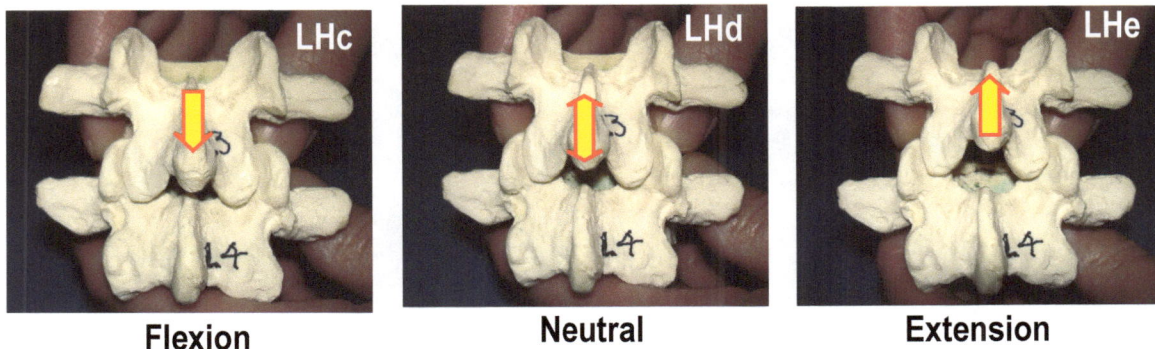

LHc
Flexion

LHd
Neutral

LHe
Extension

L4-L3:
Rotation Right in Flexion

When it is the intention of the person to lean backwards and rotate right the following action takes place:

L3 side-bending in flexion

The lumbar is backward bent as shown in **figure LJ.** Weight bearing is focused on the left leg. The left 'A' anterior sacroiliac facets engage and the weight bearing left knee is flexed. This causes the pelvis to side-bend left. Consequently the left facets of L3 glide down the left facets of L4, as shown in **figure LK,** and side-bend L3 to the left. This is the correct starting position for rotation to the right to follow.

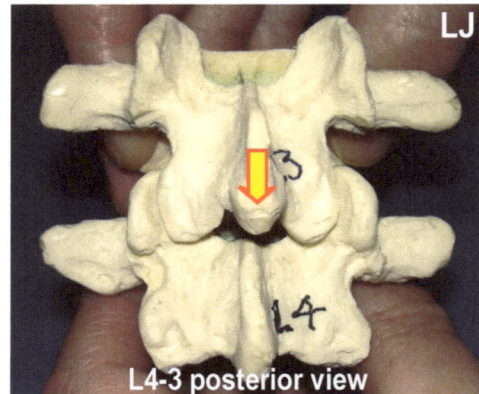

L4-3 posterior view

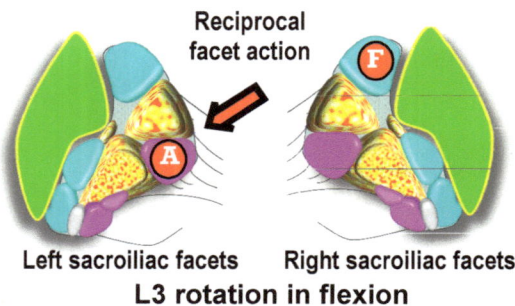

Reciprocal facet action

Left sacroiliac facets   Right sacroiliac facets
L3 rotation in flexion

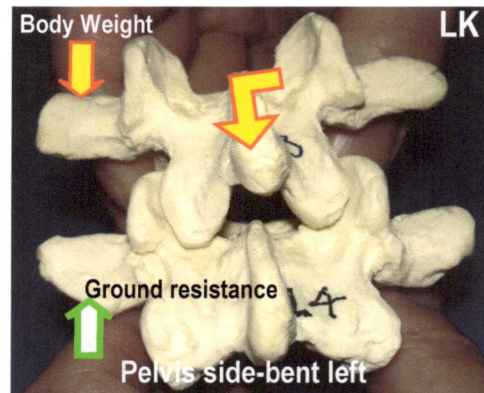

Body Weight

Ground resistance

Pelvis side-bent left

The pelvis then side-shifts to the left. This momentum travels up the spine and forces L4 to side-shift left, as shown in **figure LL**.

The side-shift rotates and banks the right L3 facet up the right L4 facet and rotates it to the right.

It can be seen that the right transverse process of L3 is posterior and superior. Conversely, the left side is anterior and inferior. The spinous process of L3 is approximated and to the right of the L4 spinous process. The concavity is on the left side.

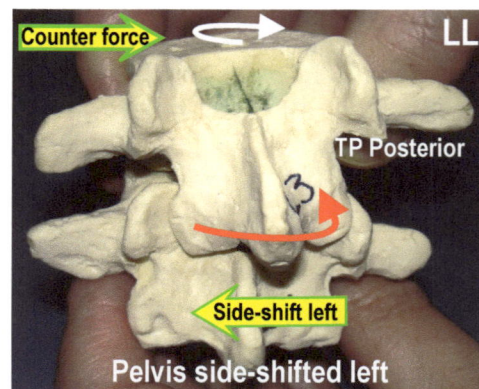

Counter force

TP Posterior

Side-shift left

Pelvis side-shifted left

Why L3 Rotates Right in Flexion and Side-Bends Right in Extension

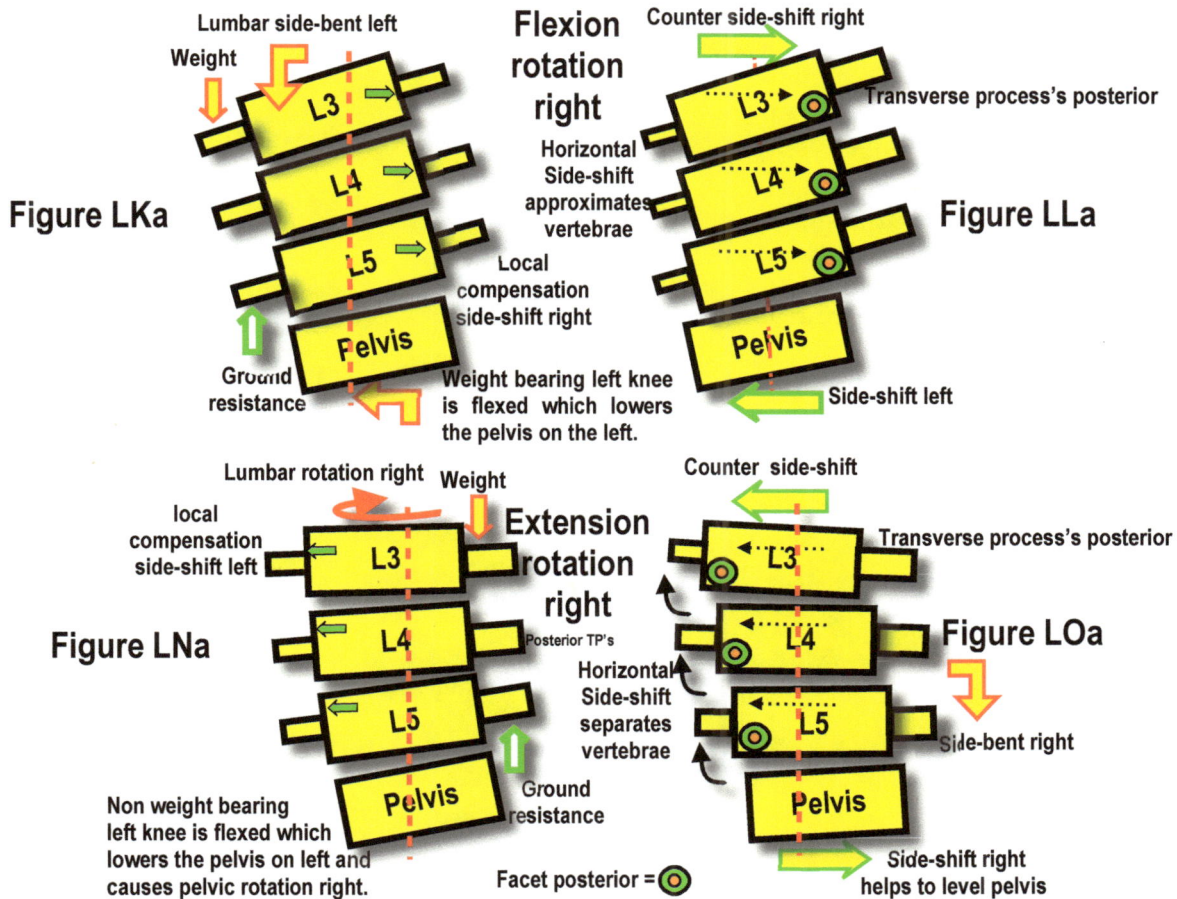

Figure LKa illustrates the effect flexing the left knee on the weight bearing left leg has on the lumbar vertebrae. **Figure LLa** illustrates the next stage. The pelvis side-shifts to the left and stays at the same angle. This has two effects; 1) As the lumbar vertebrae side-shift right the disc spaces approximate on the left, 2) The facets of the vertebrae above bank across the right facet of the vertebrae below and rotate right.

Figure LNa illustrates weight and ground resistance being taken on the right side when the left knee is flexed. This initially side-bends the pelvis left. However, because of the counter force of balance from above the pelvis levels and rotates to the right. Due to the meeting of ground resistance and body weight on the right there is some local lumbar vertebral side-bending to the right. **Figure LOa** is the next stage and illustrates how pelvic side-shift to the right causes the disc spaces between the lumbar vertebrae to separate on the left. It is this that causes the facets of the vertebrae above to bank up the left facets of the vertebrae below and side-bend to the right.

45

L3 Rotation Right in Extension

When it is the intention of the person to either stand in neutral, or lean or bend forward and then rotate right, the following action takes place:

L3 rotation in extension

The lumbar is forward bent a shown in **figure LM**. Weight bearing is focused through the right leg. The right 'F' posterior sacroiliac facets engage and the non weight bearing left knee is flexed. This causes the pelvis to rotate right and guide the lumbar in the same direction. This is shown in **figure LN**. The resistant ground force and opposing body weight on the right approximate the right L4-3 facets, to align the L3 facets for side-bending to follow.

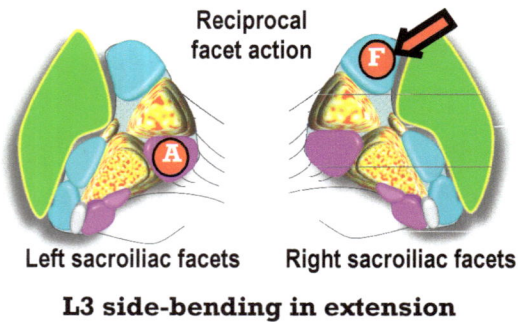

LM

L4-3 posterior view

Reciprocal facet action

F

A

Left sacroiliac facets   Right sacroiliac facets

L3 side-bending in extension

LN

Body weight

Anterior generally

Left knee flexed

Ground resistance

Pelvis rotated right

When the pelvis side-shifts to the right, the side-shift travels up the spine and in turn L4 is forced to side-shift in the direction. This causes the left facet of L3 to arc up the left bank of the left L4 facet and side-bend L3 to the right, as shown in **figure LO**.

The left transverse process of L3 is posterior and superior, while the right side is anterior and inferior. The spinous process of L3 is separated and to the left of the spinous process of L4. The concavity is on the right side.

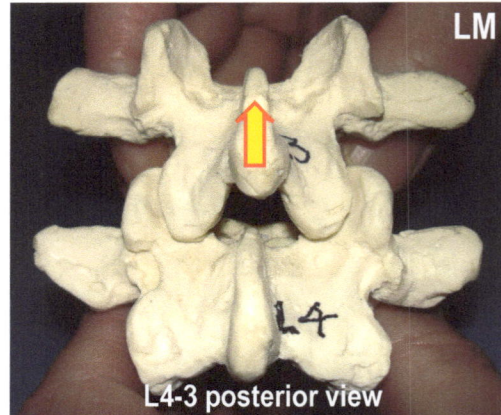

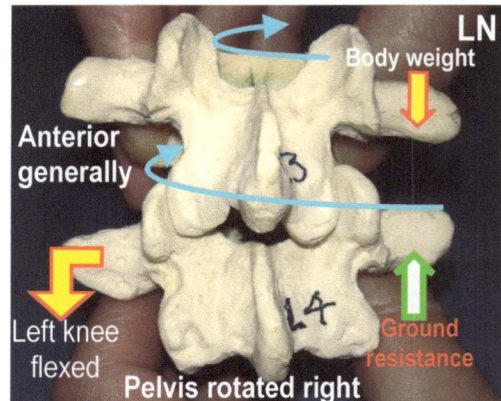

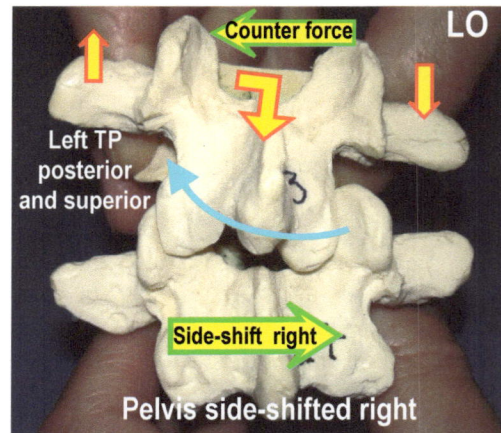

LO

Counter force

Left TP posterior and superior

Side-shift right

Pelvis side-shifted right

L2-L1:
Facet Surface Anatomy

L2 facet shape

Figure LP is a photograph of the upper posterior facets of a typical L2 vertebra. The primary function of the upper facets of L2 is to provide a surface that allows L1 to accommodate lumbar side-bending and rotation. Their vertical facet surface is offset posteriorly, as illustrated in **figure LPa**. The shape of the medial border of the facet surface is convex superiorly and concave inferiorly, as shown in **figure LPb**. From above, the facet shapes appear rounded, as shown in **figure LQ** but they have a flat quality to their surface. **Figure LQa illustrates** this shape in cross section. The L2 facet surface is steeply banked to prevent excessive rotation.

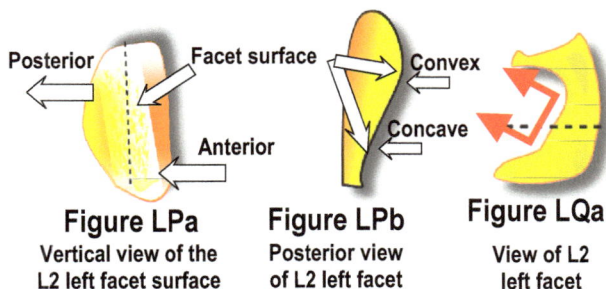

Figure LPa
Vertical view of the
L2 left facet surface

Figure LPb
Posterior view
of L2 left facet

Figure LQa
View of L2
left facet

L1 facet shape

Figures LR and **LS** show the concave and convex facet surface of the L1 vertebra. To make it easier to understand, this shape has been exaggerated and illustrated in **figure LRa**.

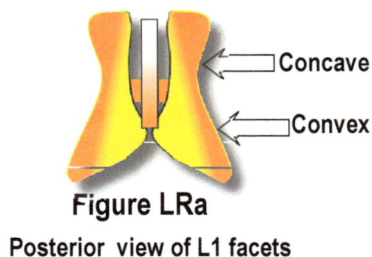

Figure LRa
Posterior view of L1 facets

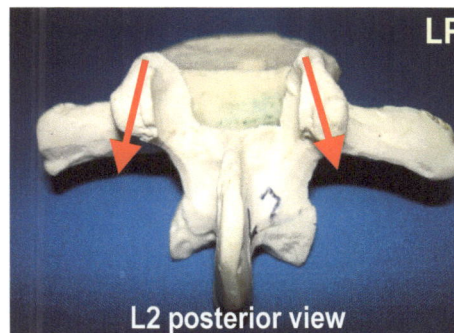

L2 posterior view

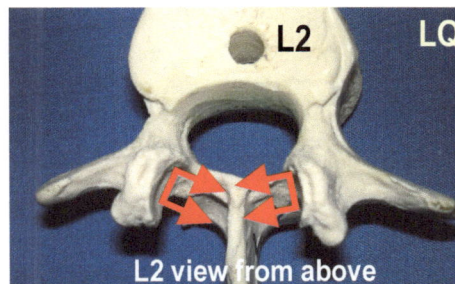

L2 view from above

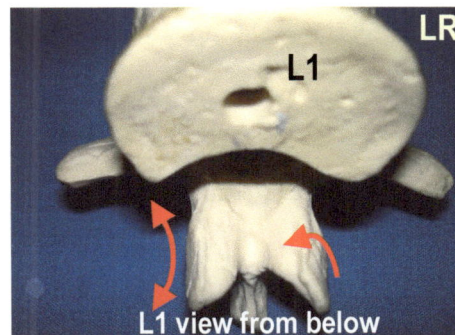

L1 view from below

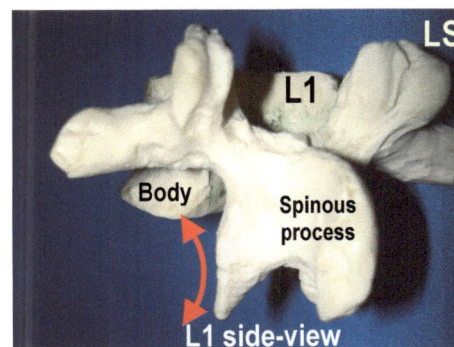

L1 side-view

L1:
The Plateau Base

Figure LT shows the position of the nucleus pulposus on the body of L2. **Figure LUa** is a cross section, illustrating how the facet surfaces of the L1 and L2 vertebrae engage. **Figure LUb** is an illustration of the joint in neutral

L1 the plateau base overview

The purpose of the L1 vertebra is to create a stable and level base for the thoracic column. L1 acts as a shock absorber that shields the thoracic column from the lumbar side-bending and rotation that takes place during walking. L1 also creates a level base for the thoracic column during rotation. L1 is also capable of making flexion and extension movements as illustrated in **figures LUc** and **LUd** when rotation is not present.

L2 side-bending and rotation

When L1 and L2 are placed together the first thing to notice is the amount of 'play' in the joint. This is illustrated in **figures LV** and **LW**. This amount of 'play' would appear to be a deliberate design feature because it allows L1 to efficiently absorb small amounts of side-bending and rotation without touching the facets of L2.

Due to the oblique angle of the L2 facet shape, see **figure LPa**, rotation from the lumbar vertebrae below is dissipated when the L1 facets travel this line.

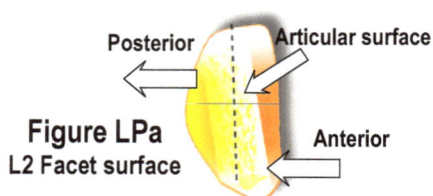

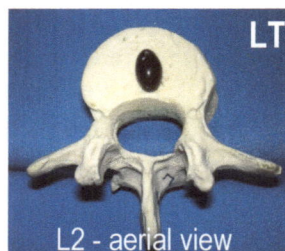

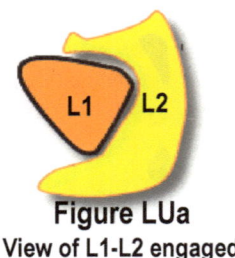

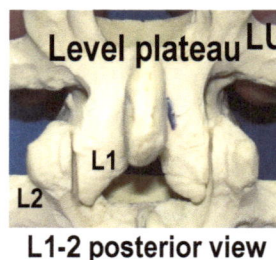

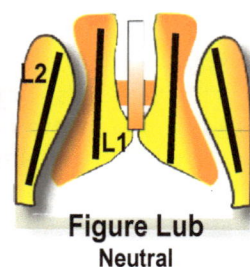

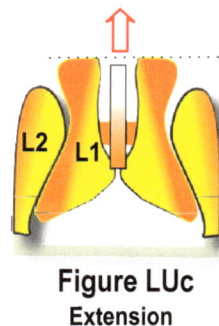

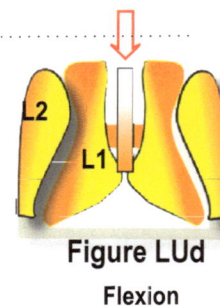

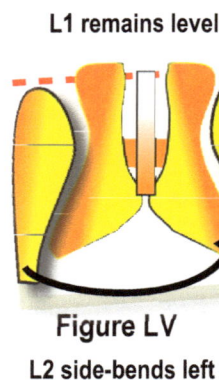

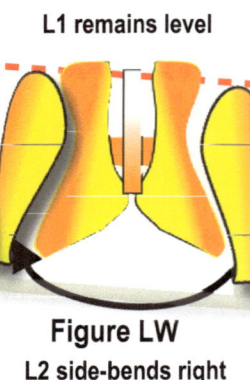

Figure LUa
View of L1-L2 engaged

Level plateau LU

L1-2 posterior view

Figure Lub
Neutral

Figure LUc
Extension

Figure LUd
Flexion

L1 remains level

L1 remains level

Figure LPa
L2 Facet surface

Posterior

Articular surface

Anterior

Figure LV
L2 side-bends left

Figure LW
L2 side-bends right

L1:
Rotation Right in Flexion

L1 flexion-rotation right

When the intention of a vertical person is to rotate to the right whilst leaning backwards, the following movements take place:

Figure LU on the previous page shows the L1-L2 joint in the neutral starting point for the attempted flexion rotation to follow. *(Be aware that the facets of the L1 mould are asymmetrical, which is what you would find in real human bones).*

Weight bearing is taken on the left flexed knee through the anterior left 'A' sacroiliac facets. This causes L2, along with the lumbar vertebrae below, to side-bend to the left. **Figures LY** and **LYa** show the left L2 facet side-bending against the left L1 facet.

Side-shift left in lumbar flexion is deliberately cancelled out for logistical reasons at L1. The mechanism of cancellation is illustrated in figure 1 on page 50, and figures LZ and LZa.

When pelvic side-shift to the left takes place, the lumbar vertebrae including L2 are forced to the right. This causes L2 to cross over and engage against the right L1 facet, as shown in **figure LZa.**

Due to the vertical offset angle of the L1-L2 facets, as shown in **figure LZb,** the posterior aspect of the rotation of L2 is blocked.

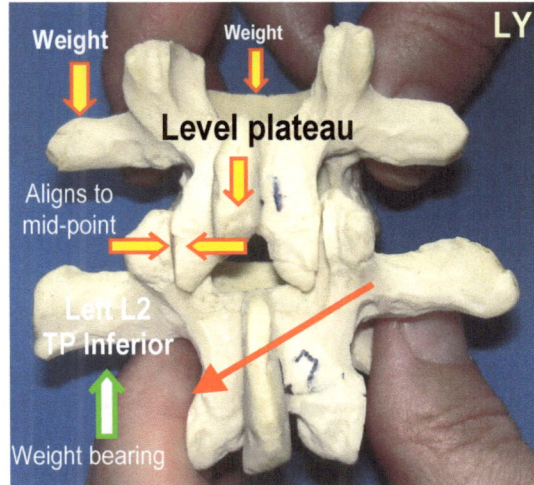
LY

Weight — Weight
Level plateau
Aligns to mid-point
Left L2 TP Inferior
Weight bearing

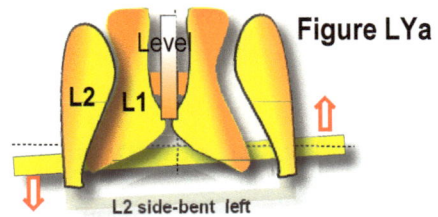
Figure LYa
Level
L2 — L1
L2 side-bent left

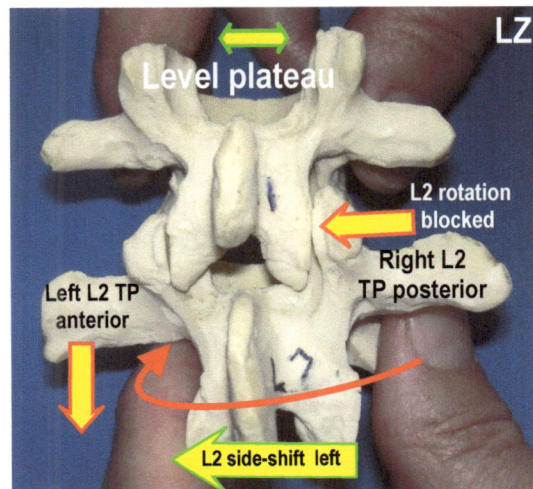
LZ
Level plateau
L2 rotation blocked
Right L2 TP posterior
Left L2 TP anterior
L2 side-shift left

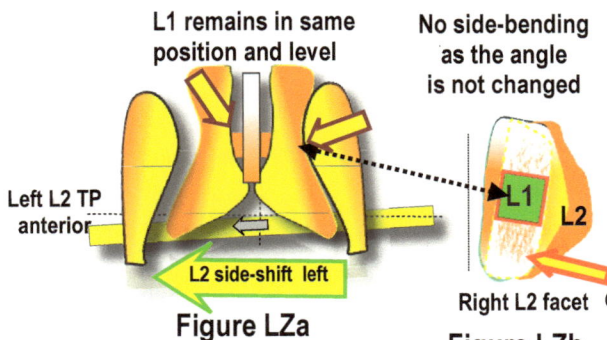

L1 remains in same position and level

No side-bending as the angle is not changed

Left L2 TP anterior

L2 side-shift left

Figure LZa

L1 — L2

Right L2 facet

Figure LZb

Lumbar rotation is absorbed by the offset vertical angle of the L2-L1 joint.

L3-Left-Right and L3-Right-Right: Lines of Gravity

L1, the flexion gravity blocker

Figure 1 is a drawing of the gravity line when L1 attempts rotation right in lumbar flexion. Notice that the gravity passes directly through L1. This is not accidental, it is designed this way to block the pelvic side-shift driving force, from passing up the left side of the thoracic column. With no side-shift taking place above L1, the extended thoracic vertebrae are deprived of the necessary side-shift they require to make rotational movements. The mechanics of this are explained in chapter 6.

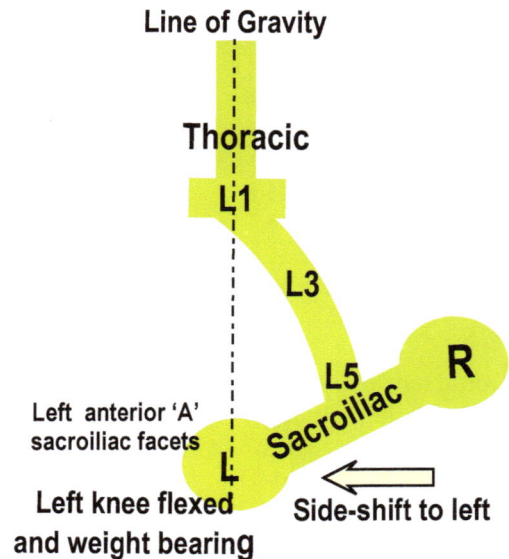

Figure 1

L1, the extension gravity gateway

Figure 2 is a drawing of the gravity line when L1 attempts rotation right in extension.

When pelvic side shift takes place to the right, the line of gravity passes to the right of L1. In passing to the right, the side-shift driving force is allowed to continue upwards to the thoracic vertebrae. It is this side-shift that becomes the driving force the thoracic vertebrae require to physiologically rotate right in thoracic flexion.

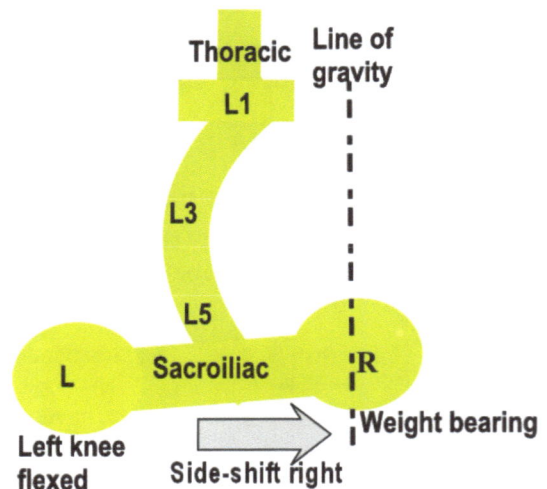

Figure 2

L1:
Rotation Right in Lumbar Extension

L1 extension, rotation right

Wher. the intention of a vertical person is to rotate to the right whilst leaning forwards, the following movements take place.

Figure LU shown on page 48 is the neutral starting point for this movement.

Figures LBB and **LBBa** show L2 and L1 rotating to the right. To cause this to happen, the left knee is flexed with the body weight taken on the right leg through the right sacroiliac 'F' facets. This action causes the pelvis and all the lumbar vertebrae, including L2-L1 to rotate right. The side-bending of the pelvis causes L2 to side-bend left fractionally, though the counter bodyweight and ground resistance on the right side make the side-bending considerably less than that caused in the flexion movement. L1 remains vertical throughout.

The pelvis then side-shifts right and in turn all the lumbar vertebrae along with L2 side-shift right. In doing this the middle of the L2 facet engages with the middle of the left L1 facet, as shown in **figure LCCa.**

The side-bending to the right that takes place in the lumbar vertebrae below causes the left facet of L2 to move up the left L1 facet, as shown in **figure LCCb**. In doing this L1 remains vertical as L2 side-bends right. In relation to L2, L1 is rotated right and side-bent left.

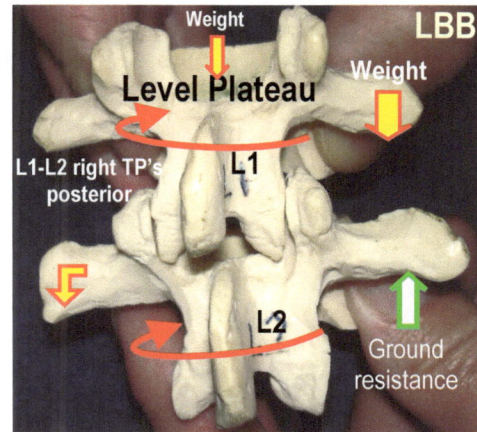

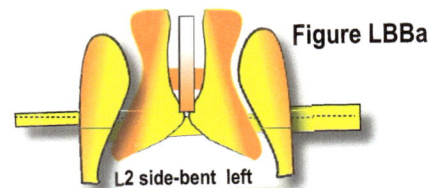

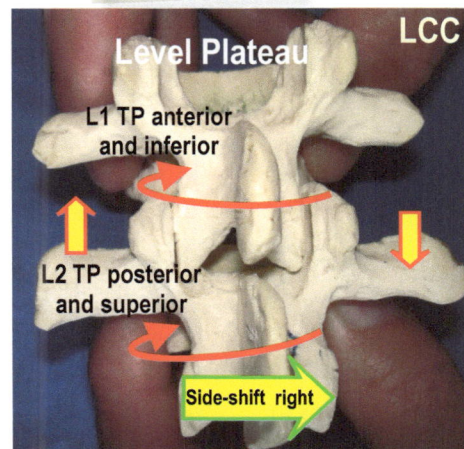

Figure LBBa

With. continued contact on the left facets of L1, pelvic side-shift can be passed upwards.

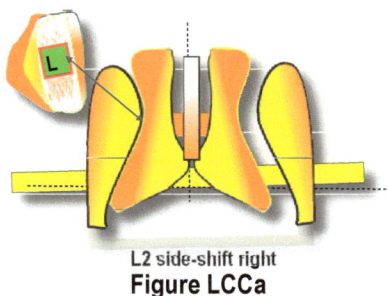

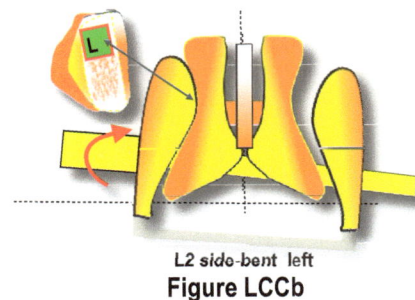

L2 side-shift right
Figure LCCa

L2 side-bent left
Figure LCCb

L1-T12:
Anatomy

As was shown in the L2-L1 joint, rotation is limited. This shortcoming is corrected in the L1-T12 joint, where together with providing additional side-bending, rotation is the main purpose.

L1 facet shape

Figures **LCD** and **LCDa** show the upper posterior L1 facets of a typical L1 vertebra. The upper facets of L1 are parallel vertically and very marginally concave.

Figure **LCE** and **LCEa** show the concave and rounded shape of the upper L1 facets.

Figure **LCEb** illustrates the angle of the facet trajectory.

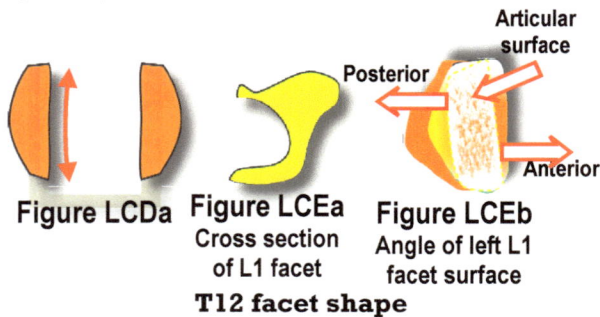

Figure LCDa

Figure LCEa
Cross section of L1 facet

Figure LCEb
Angle of left L1 facet surface

T12 facet shape

Figure **LCF** and **LCG** show the long marginally rounded shape of the inferior posterior facets of T12.

These shapes are made clearer by the illustrations shown in figures **LCFa** and **LCGa**.

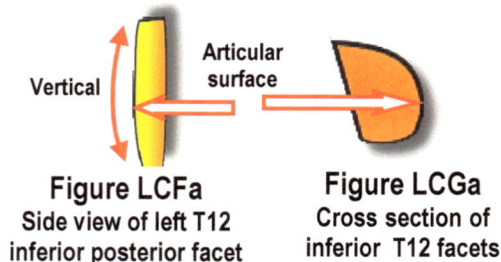

Figure LCFa
Side view of left T12 inferior posterior facet

Figure LCGa
Cross section of inferior T12 facets

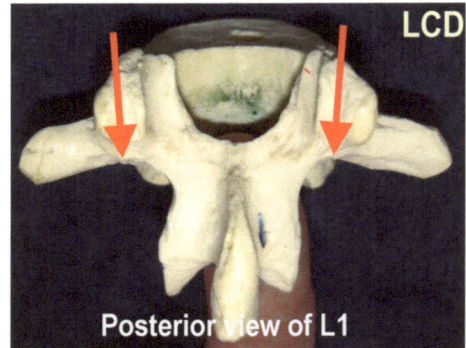
LCD
Posterior view of L1

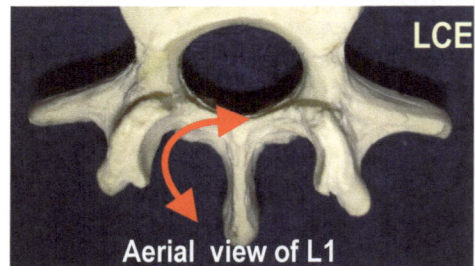
LCE
Aerial view of L1

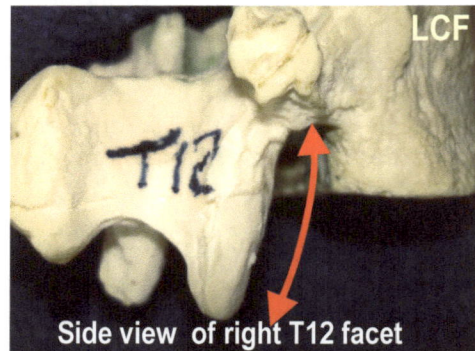
LCF
Side view of right T12 facet

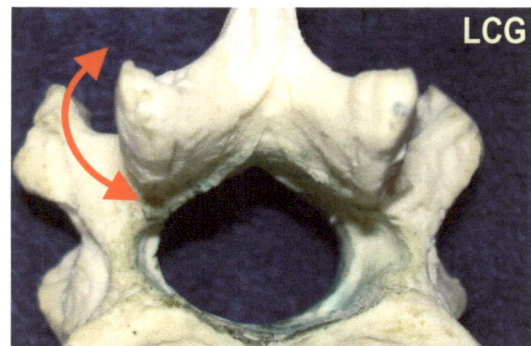
LCG
View from below of T12 facet

L1-T12: Physiology

Like the L2-L1 joint the first thing to notice when the L1-T12 facets are placed together is the amount of 'play' in the joint. This is illustrated in **figures LCH** and **LCHa.** The rounded facet shapes and the amount of play in the joint, are illustrated in the cross section **figure LCHf.**

Due to the amount of 'play' in the joint, L1 has the ability to side-bend left and right without making contact with the sides of the T12 facets. This is illustrated in **figures LCHb** and **LCHc.** The 'play' in the L1-T12 joint and that found in the L2-L1 joint, act synergetically as a shock absorber during walking. Their purpose is to shield the thoracic column, neck and head from jerks, rotation and side-bending with minimal effort.

To further illustrate the versatility of the way the L1 facets move around the T12 facets **figure LCHbb** illustrates rotation singularly, and **figure LCHcc,** when rotation and side-bending are combined. Notice again that the sides of the L1 facets do not touch the sides of the T12 facets. **Figures LCHg** and **LCHh** illustrate this in cross section and show the way L1 rotates around T12 to take up the side-bending and rotation caused by the walking action without contact.

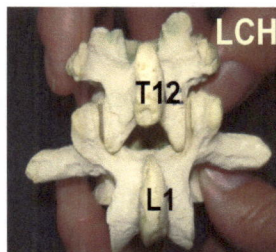

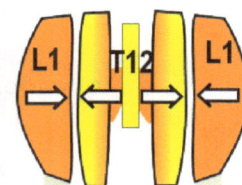

Figure LCHa
Neutral L1-T12 joint

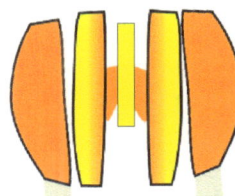

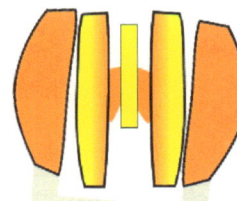

Figure LCHb	Figure LCHc
L1 side-bending left against T12	L1 side-bending right against T12

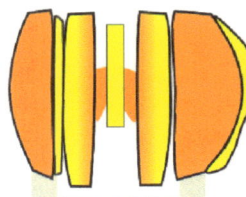

Figure LCHbb	Figure LCHcc
L1 rotating right against T12	L1 rotating and side-bending right against T12

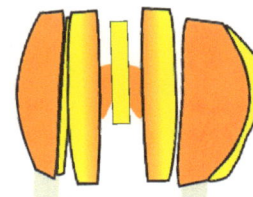

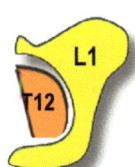

Figure LCHf
Cross section facets in neutral

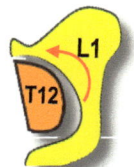

Figure LCHg
Cross section L1 rotation

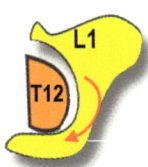

Figure LCHh
Cross section L1 rotation

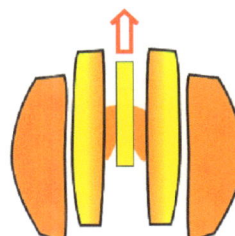

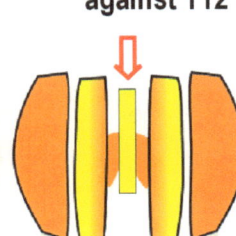

Figure LCHd	Figure LCHe
Thoracic flexion	Thoracic extension

The joint is also able to flex and extend as shown in **figures LCHd** and **LCHe.**

T12 when Side-Shift is to the Right

Rotation left in thoracic flexion

When the L2-L1 joint rotates right as described on the previous pages, L1 should be level and rotating right in relation to L2. With side-shift and weight to the right, the gravity line will pass to the right of L1 and the thoracic column. This was shown in **figure 2** on page 50.

At the joint of L1-T12, two possible actions take place. **Figures LCHa** and **LCJ** show neutral.

Thoracic rotation right

1) When the intention is for the thoracic vertebrae to rotate right, the right side facets of L1 side-shift right and engage squarely against the left T12 facets. In doing this T12 follows the general pelvic rotation to the right. This is illustrated in **figures LCK** and **LCL**.

T12 rotation left

2) If side-shift is taken further to the right, along with increased left knee flexion, there would be an excessive amount of rotation to the right in the upper torso. This would cause de-stabilization.

To compensate for this, T12 limits the amount of rotation right originating from the pelvis by rotating left. The mechanics of this are that when excessive side-shift to the right continues unchecked, as shown in **figures LCM** and **LCN**, the left T12 facet banks up the left L1 facet and causes T12 vertebra to rotate left.

This brings back stability to the spine and limits thoracic rotation right. This is illustrated in **figures LCO** and **LCP.**

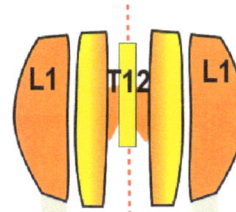

Figure LCHa
Posterior view
L1-T12 facets in neutral

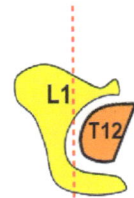

Figure LCJ
Cross section
left facets in neutral

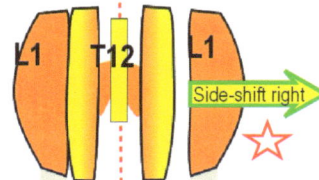

Figure LCK
L1 side-shift right

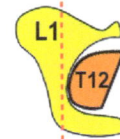

Figure LCL
L1 side-shift right

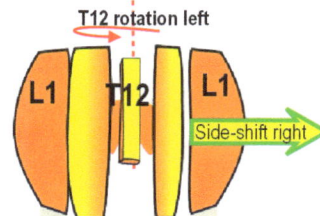

T12 rotation left

Figure LCM
L1 continues to side-shift right

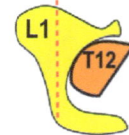

Figure LCN
T12 rotates up L1 facet

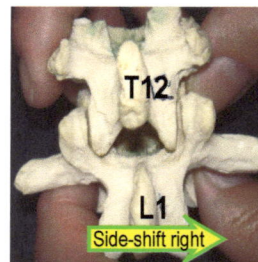

Figure LCO
L1 continues to side-shift right

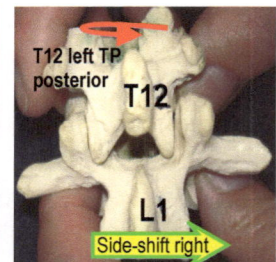

Figure LCP
T12 rotates up L1 facet

Chapter Five
Physiology of Walking

For a sacroiliac theory to be proved, it must satisfy working criteria. It must be capable of applying forward and backward bending, side-bending, rotation and most important of all, locomotion.

Ambulation overview

The **photograph WA** shows Lisa demonstrating the first stage of the walking action.

It can be seen that her pelvis has side-shifted to the right and that her right leg is posterior, lateral and weight bearing.

Reciprocally her left leg is lifted medially, superiorly and anteriorly.

From above, the sacroiliac joints would look like the illustration in **figure WAa**.

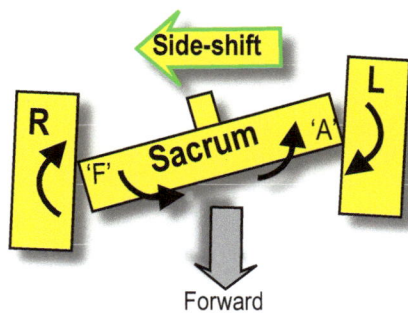

Figure WAa

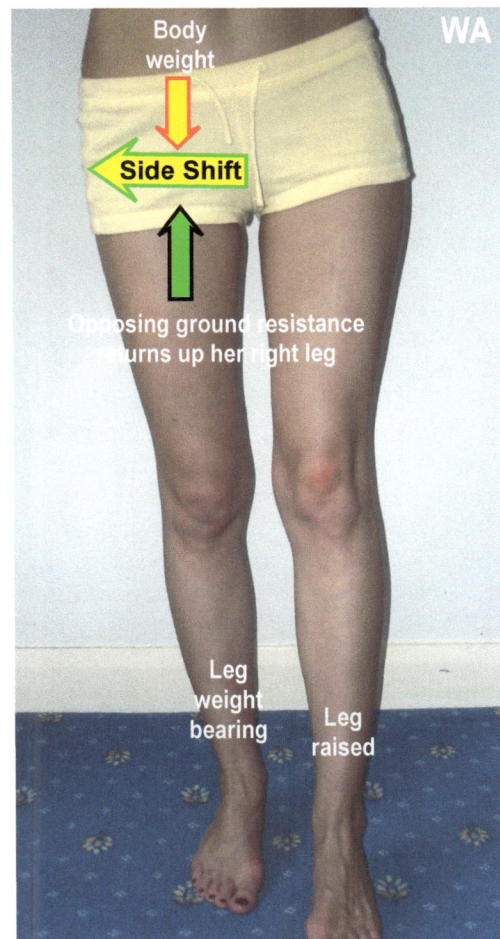

Walking: Stage One: Weight Bearing

To initiate the walking action, body weight must be directed to one leg. In our example, the right leg is being demonstrated.

Figure WB shows the weight bearing right sacroiliac joint. The left knee would be non-weight-bearing and fractionally flexed. This lifts and rotates the pelvis as a whole to the right. (The greater the knee flexion, the greater is the pelvic rotation).

The resistant ground counter force passes up through the right acetabulum and levers the right 'F' posterior facet of the ilium to engage against the 'F' posterior facet of the sacrum. The mating of the 'F' facets rotates the right ilium to the right and the sacrum to the left.

The engaged 'F' posterior sacroiliac facets lever the right acetabulum posteriorly, laterally and inferiorly.   This downward inclination of the acetabulum, described in more detail in **figure SM** on page 32, is met by the counter force of the ground returning up the right leg. The merging of these two forces lifts the right side of the pelvis and rotates it right.

With the 'F' facets engaged and weight bearing, the lumbar vertebrae (using L4-L3 as an example) follow the general rotation of the pelvis and rotate to the right.

The body weight and opposing ground counter force on the right side approximate the right L3-L4 facets. This aligns the left facets of L3 in the correct starting position for side-bending to the right to follow when side-shift right is applied, as shown in **figure WC.**

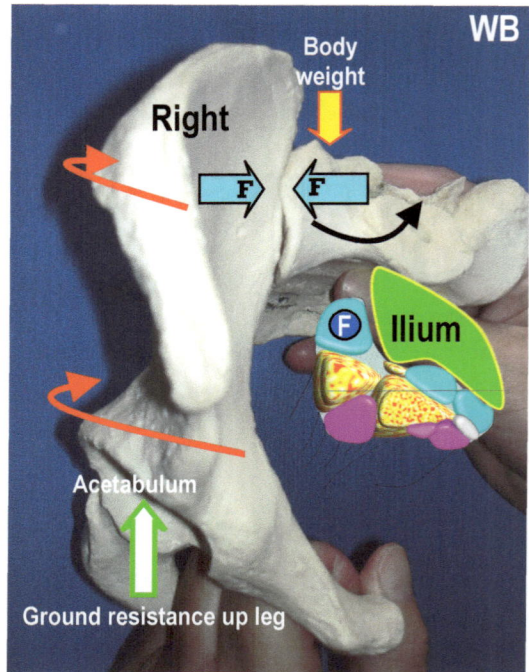

Anterior view of right sacroiliac 'F' posterior facets engaged

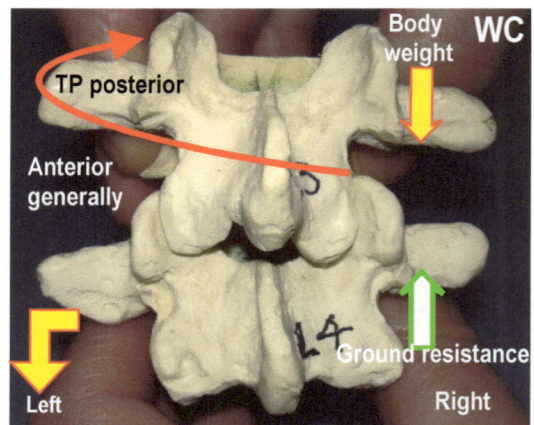

Posterior view of L4-L3 rotation right from pelvis

56

Walking: Stage Two: Side-Shift

When pelvic side-shift to the right is applied as shown in **figure WD,** the right 'A' anterior facets are forced apart still further and the sacrum rotates left, as shown in **figure WAa** on page 55.

The side-shift to the right levers the right acetabulum with sufficient force to lift the left side of the pelvis, as shown in **figure WDa**.

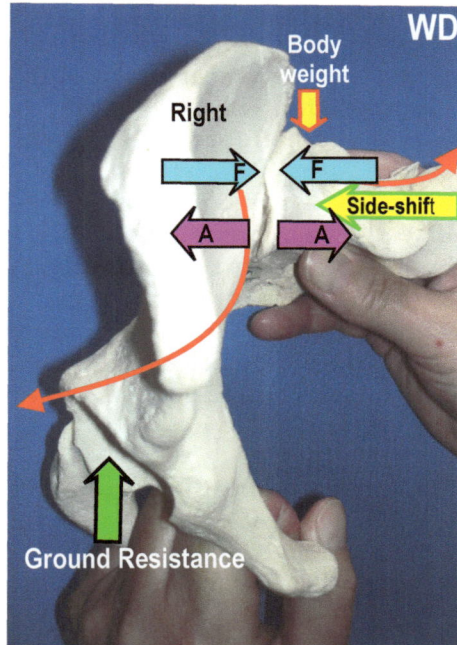

WD

Body weight

Right

Side-shift

Ground Resistance

Anterior view of right innominate

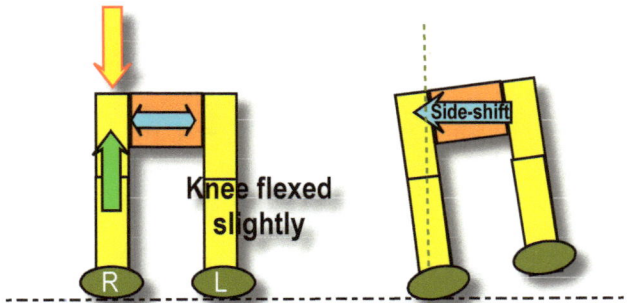

Knee flexed slightly

Side-shift

R   L

Figure WDa
Anterior View

The pelvic side-shift continues up the spine and in turn L4 side-shifts to the right. With counter resistance to the left from above, the left facet of L3 banks up the left facet of L4. In doing this L3 becomes side-bent to the right, as shown in **figure WE.**

Therefore, in the walking lumbar movement, rotation and side-bending are to the same side, which is extension.

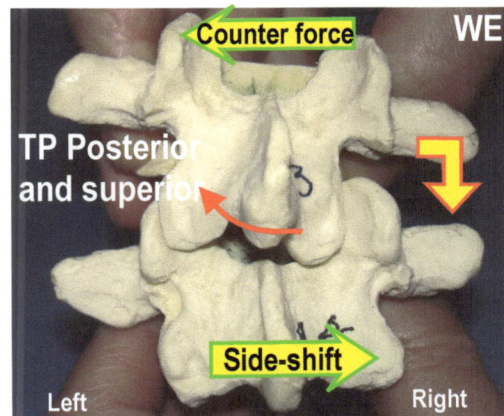

Counter force   WE

TP Posterior and superior

Side-shift

Left   Right

Posterior view of L4-L3
L3 side-bending right

Walking: Stage Three: Reciprocal Facet Action

When the weight bearing 'F' right posterior sacroiliac facets are engaged and side-shift is to the right the reciprocal action of the sacrum is to engage the left 'A' anterior sacroiliac facets; as shown in **figures WF and WFA**.

When the left non-weight-bearing 'A' anterior sacroiliac facets are engaged, the left acetabulum is levered anteriorly, medially and superiorly. This is described in more detail in **figure SK** on page 32. This force, with the aid of the left leg muscles, lifts the left leg forward as shown in **figure WA** on page 55 and **illustration A** below.

The right leg shown in **illustration B** is straight and weight bearing. The line of the body weight is taken through the load bearing 'F' posterior sacroiliac facet.

If you watch an athlete run you will see that their left shoulder and arm move anteriorly when their body weight is to be taken on their right leg. This is an efficient way of transferring body weight without having to lean forwards and backwards.

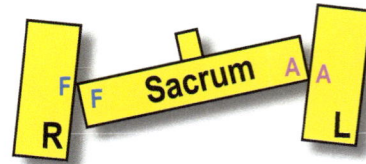

Figure WF
Anterior left facets engaged

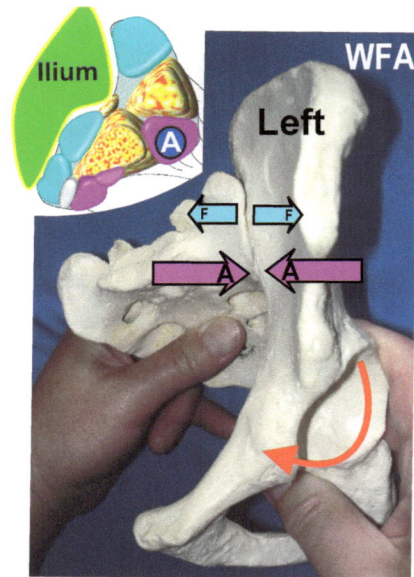

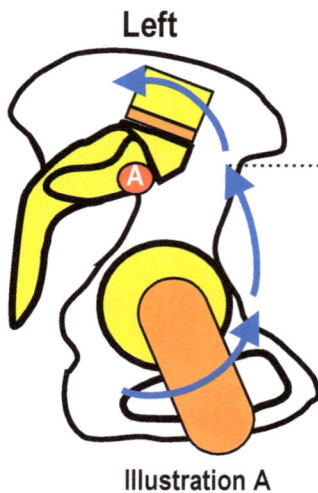

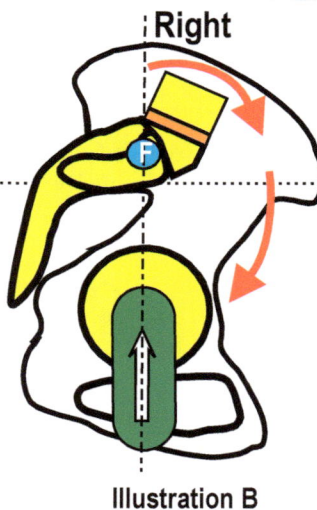

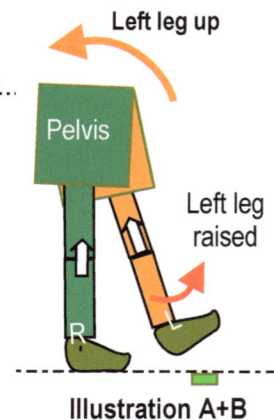

Illustration A

Illustration B

Illustration A+B

58

Walking:
Reciprocal Facet Action

To move forward the upper body inclines anteriorly on the left. This changes the weight focus and pushes the left leg downwards and levers the transitory 'B' anterior sacroiliac facets on the left to engage and guide the left leg laterally. The heel of the left foot is the first to touch the ground. However, at this point the leg is still not fully weight bearing. Body weight is still taken on the right leg, though at this point, through the transitory right 'E' facets.

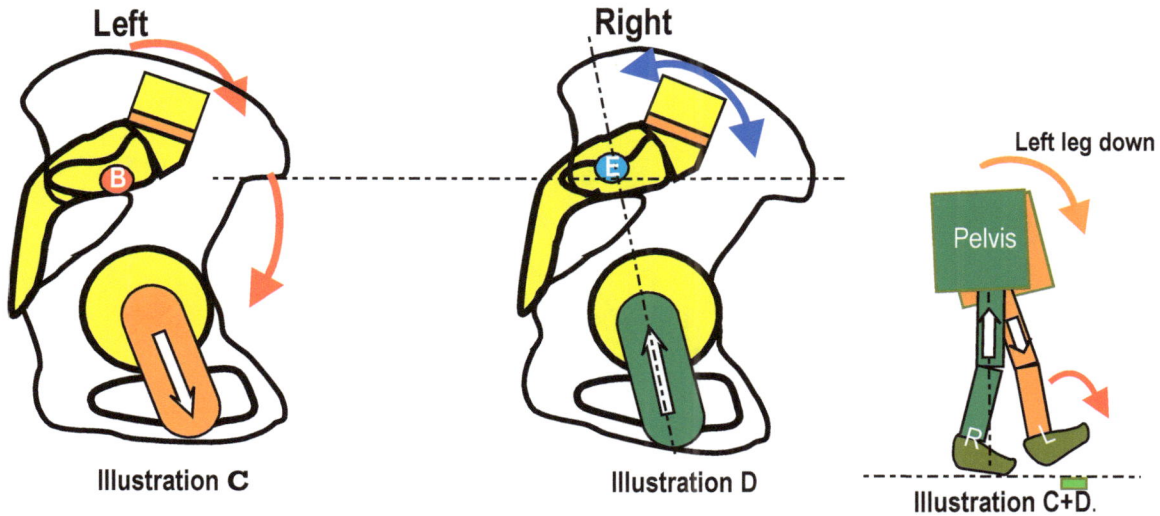

Left   **Right**

Left leg down

Pelvis

B   E

Illustration **C**   Illustration D   Illustration C+D.

As the body weight continues to focus down on the left leg, the sacroiliac fulcrum changes from the left 'B' sacroiliac facets to the transitory 'C' anterior sacroiliac facets, as shown in **illustration E.** Reciprocally, the right sacroiliac 'E' facets transfer to the right transitory 'D' posterior sacroiliac facets, as shown in **illustration F.** At this transitory point, weight is evenly distributed down both legs, as shown in **illustrations E** and **F.** Side-shift is marginally to the left.

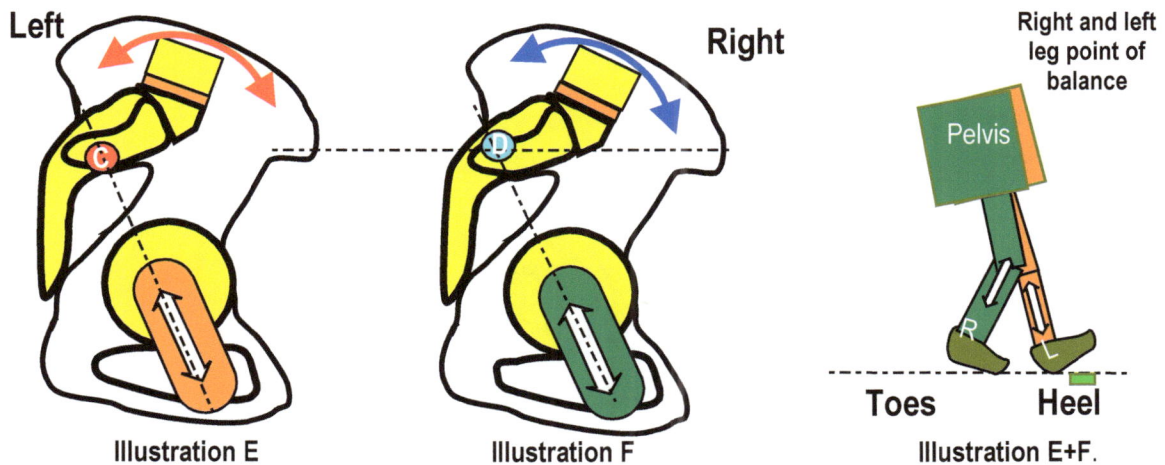

Left   **Right**

Right and left leg point of balance

Pelvis

C   D

Toes   Heel

Illustration E   Illustration F   Illustration E+F.

Walking:
Reciprocal Facet Action

As the upper body weight continues to bear down on the left leg, the fulcrum applied to the left sacroiliac facet transfers to the opposite side against the weight bearing 'E' sacroiliac facets, as shown in **illustration E**. Reciprocally on the right, the facets transfer to the transitory non-weight-bearing 'B' sacroiliac facets, shown in **illustration F**. The left knee flex's to accommodate the transfer of body weight onto the left leg, shown in **illustrations E** and **F.**

Left **Right**

Left leg becomes fully weight-bearing

Pelvis

Illustration E Illustration F Illustration E+F

And finally we have come full circle. The left leg becomes the true weight bearing leg with the weight taken through the left posterior 'F' facet. When pelvic side-shift to the left takes place, the right 'A' facets engage and the right leg is levered forward.

Left **Right**

Left leg up

Pelvis

Illustration G Illustration H Illustration G+H

60

Walking: Backwards

The principles shown previously within this chapter refer specifically to walking forward. These principles can be equally applied to the actions of running or climbing stairs. Forward motion is mainly governed by the lower limbs of the body interacting on the ilia. Within this action the sacrum plays a secondary role. Therefore, **walking forward is an iliosacral movement**.

These principles however, cannot be applied to the action of walking backwards. This involves a much less complicated procedure and is described next. Backward motion is governed by the top half of the body placing a rotational force on the sacrum. Within this action the ilia play a secondary role. Therefore, **walking backwards is a sacroiliac movement**.

Figure WQ shows Sam taking a step backwards with her right leg. In order to complete this movement she had to focus her body weight through her left sacroiliac joint and leg.

Her torso had to be inclined forward with her muscles braced, so as to act as a long lever. Her pelvis then had to be side-shifted to the left to engage the 'F' posterior sacroiliac facets.

The combination of the side-shift and weight focus on the left side of her pelvis and leg caused her right leg to lift. The side-shift also caused her sacrum and therefore her torso to rotate to the right and thereby guide her right leg backwards, with minimal effort.

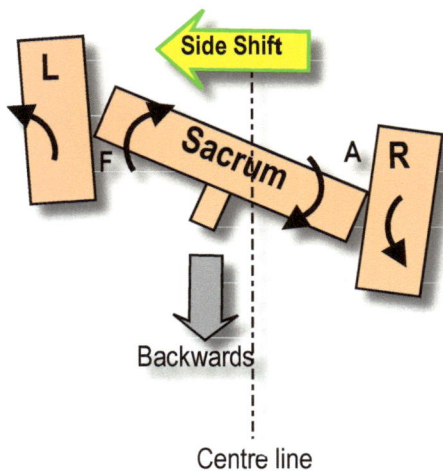

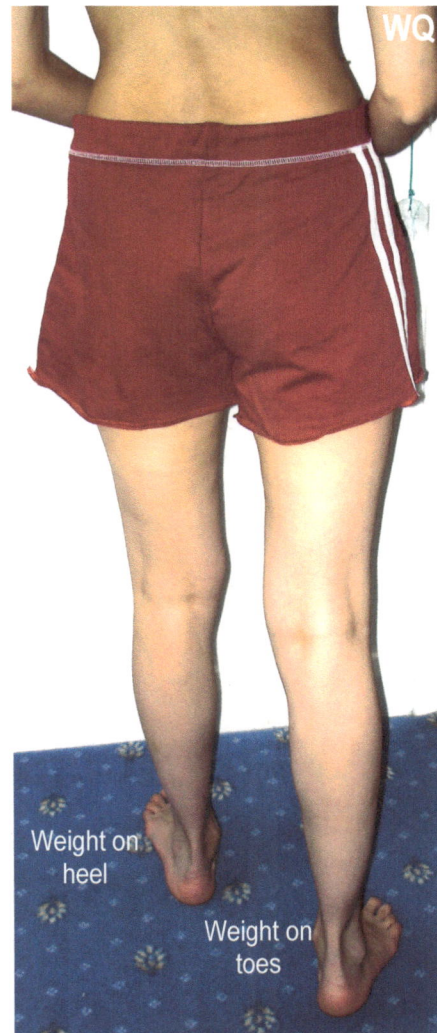

Walking:
Backwards Left Side Facet Action

Figure WO shows the left side of the sacroiliac joint when weight bearing is on the left. The sacrum is rotated to the right by the engagement of the left posterior 'F' sacroiliac facets.

It is important to remember that the sacrum is moving against the ilium.

Figure WM is a picture of the L4-L3 joint. With body weight pivoting through the left leg, the levering lumbar vertebrae work as one with the sacrum and rotate to the right.

When pelvic side-shift takes place to the left and compress the posterior 'F' sacroiliac facets, L3 as shown in **figure WP**, side-bends to the left.

This means that when walking backwards, lumbar rotation and side-bending are to opposite sides.

Below for information, **figure WPa** shows the line of gravity passing to the left of L1. This line of gravity causes the thoracic vertebrae which will be in thoracic flexion, due to the leaning forward, to rotate to the left.

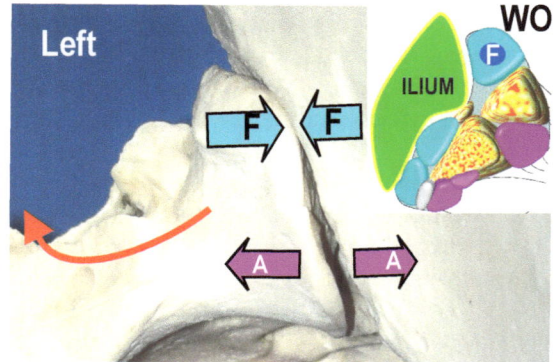

WO

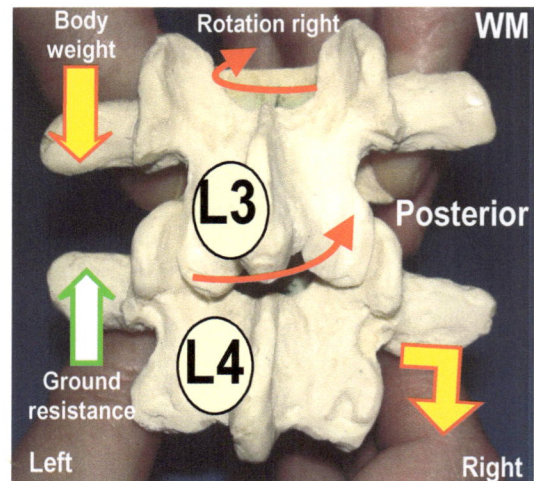

WM

Body weight — Rotation right
L3
L4
Ground resistance
Posterior
Left — Right

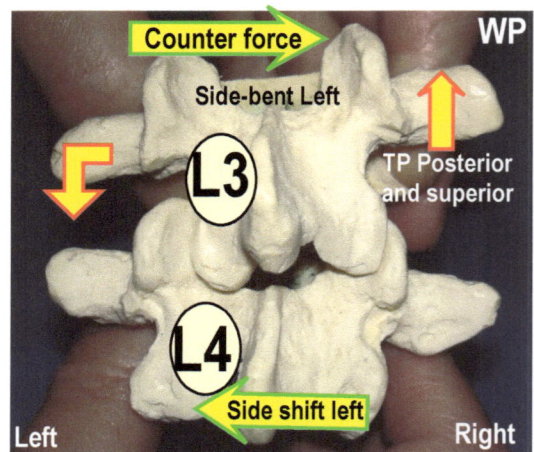

Figure WPa

Thoracic
L1
L3
Lifted and rotated right
L5
L   Sacrum   R
Side-shift
Left leg weight bearing

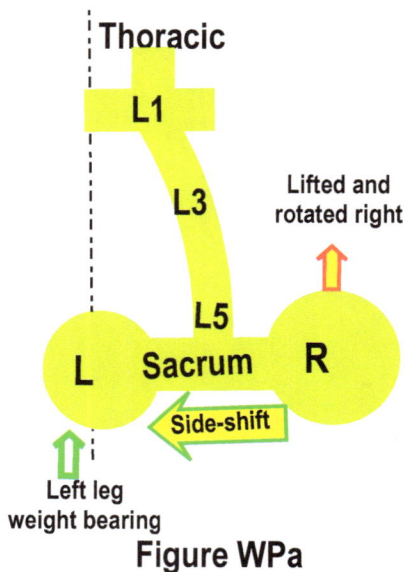

WP

Counter force
Side-bent Left
L3
TP Posterior and superior
L4
Side shift left
Left — Right

Walking:
Backwards Right

When the right leg rotates backwards, the right 'A' sacroiliac facets engage, as shown in **illustration WR**.

To continue moving backwards, side-shift transfers to the right and the torso rotates to the left. This causes the weight bearing 'F' posterior sacroiliac facets on the right to engage and reciprocally, the guider 'A' facets to engage on the left. This is shown in **figure WRa**.

Because the guiding rotation originates from the torso/vertebrae, the torso rotates from side to side as the person walks backwards.

This is because backward walking is governed by the forward bent rotation of the torso acting on the sacrum. This limits the articulation of the sacrum to two facets of the ilia only; the posterior 'F' facets on one side and the anterior 'A' facets on the other.

With only two facet engagements, walking backwards is uneven and jerky when compared to the smooth motion of walking forward.

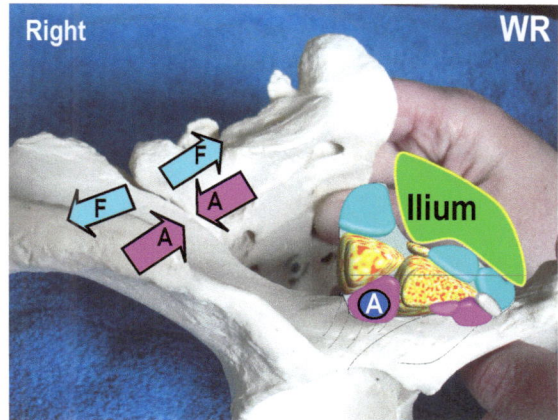

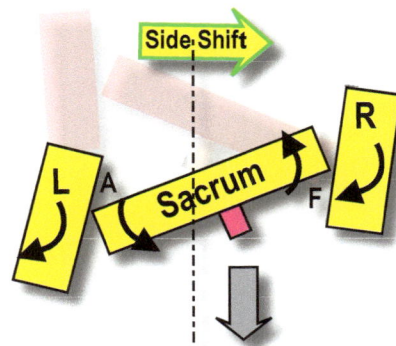

Direction of Rotation

During backward walking, when backward rotation to the left takes place, the torso rotates along with the sacrum to the right. This is illustrated in **figure WRb**.

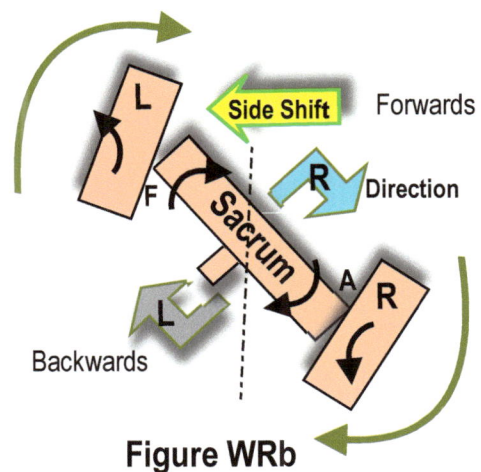

Figure WRa

Figure WRb

Chapter Six
Physiology of the
Thoracic Joints

Overview

Attached to the thoracic vertebrae are ribs. The main functions of the ribs are to:

- 1) Protect the heart and lungs;

- 2) To provide a mechanism that enhances inhalation and exhalation;

For the rib bucket handle mechanism, shown on pages 69 and 192, to work efficiently the ribs need to be kept parallel at all times. To take account of this, nature has developed a facet shape for the thoracic vertebrae that not only enables this to happen when the thoracic vertebrae are vertical, but when rotation and side-bending takes place.

The overall shape of the thoracic spine is convex posteriorly, which is an opposite curve to that seen in the lumbar.

We know from our rationale tests in chapter one that the thoracic vertebrae will not rotate without pelvic side-shift. Therefore, it can be concluded that side-shift is the most likely precursor to side-bending and rotation in the thoracic vertebrae.

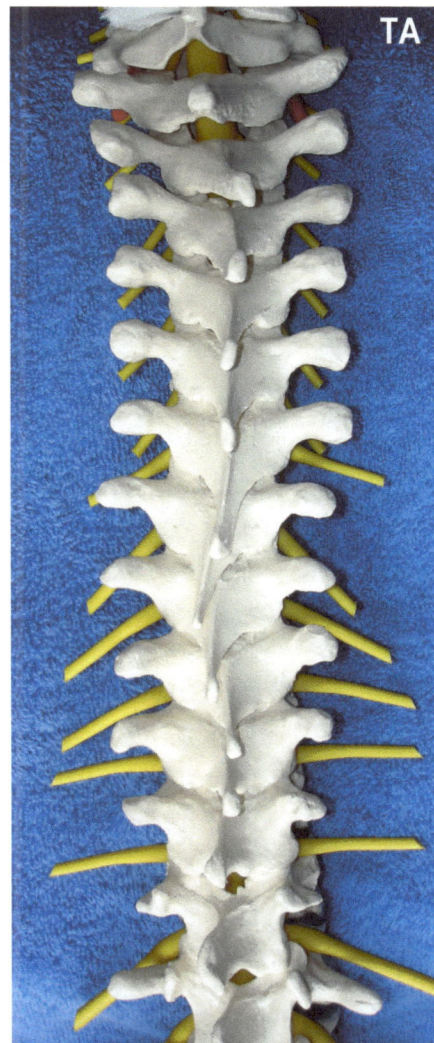

TA

Thoracic Reference

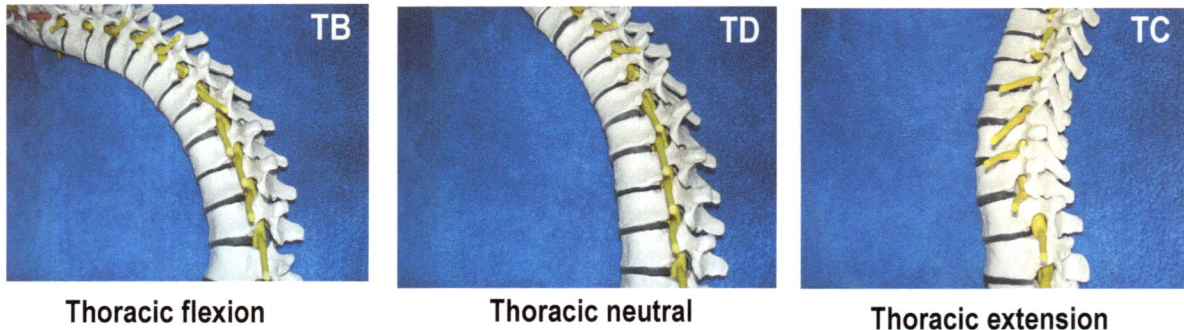

Thoracic flexion   Thoracic neutral   Thoracic extension

Figure TB shows the thoracic spine in flexion. Flexion is forward bending.

Figure TC shows the thoracic spine in extension. Extension is backward bending.

When neither flexion or extension is present, the thoracic spine is in neutral, as shown in **figure TD**.

There are twelve thoracic vertebrae. The facet shapes are not all the same. Some of the facets look obviously rounded in their horizontal plane and others flat. However, they are all rounded in such a way as to allow the joint above some degree of rotation. The T2-T1 joint facets are concave and work in a vaguely similar way to the lower lumbar facets. The list below compares the facet shapes of my plastic bones with real bones:

Thoracic Vertebrae	Plastic Bones Facet shape	Real Bones* Facet shape
T1	Convex	Convex
T2	Concave***	Concave***
T3	Convex	Convex
T4	Convex	Convex
T5	Convex	Convex
T6	Convex	Convex
T7	Flat -Convex**	Convex
T8	Flat -Convex**	Convex
T9	Flat-Convex**	Convex
T10	Flat -Convex**	Convex
T11	Flat -Convex**	Convex
T12	Flat -Convex**	Spacer

* The real bones originate from Asia. I think the skeleton is that of a boy who must have unfortunately died somewhere between the age of ten to thirteen years of age.

** Flat-Convex, is shown on the next page. Convex facets would provide greater rotation than those that are flatter yet angle convexly in relation to each other.

*** At T2-T1 there is a change in the thoracic curve from flexion to extension.

66

Thoracic:
T7 Facet Anatomy

Thoracic joints.

Figures TE and **TEa** show the posterior superior facets of T7 and T4 in overview. T4 has been added for facet comparison purposes.

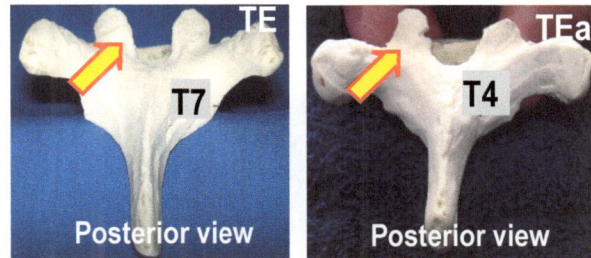

TE — T7 — Posterior view

TEa — T4 — Posterior view

Figures TF and **TFa** show side views of the T7 and T4 facets. Both are marginally convex along their vertical plane. Note that the T7 facets are more upright and less convex vertically.

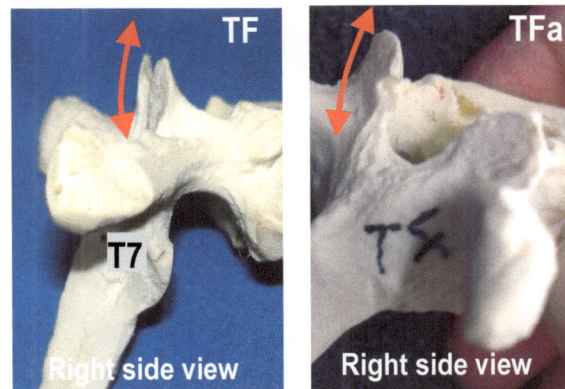

TF — T7 — Right side view

TFa — Right side view

Figures TG and **TGa** show aerial views of the T7 and T4 facets. It can be seen that both are convex horizontally. The T4 facets form a more rounded circumference. This is illustrated more clearly in **figures TGb** and **TGc**.

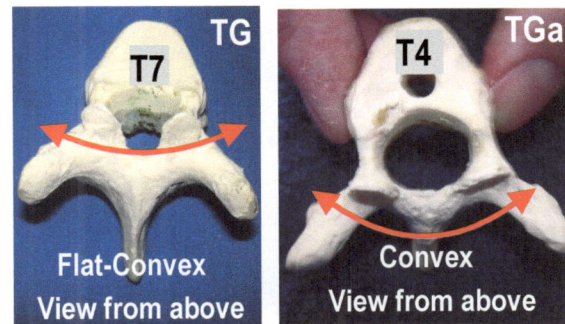

TG — T7 — Flat-Convex — View from above

TGa — T4 — Convex — View from above

Figure TGb
Flat-Convex

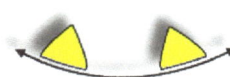

Figure TGc
Convex

Thoracic:
T6 Facet Anatomy

Figures TH and **THa** show for reference the T6 and T3 vertebrae in overview. Again, T3 has been added for facet comparison.

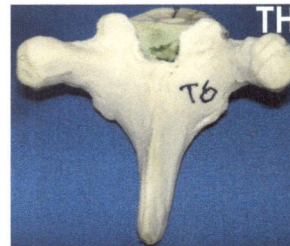

Posterior view of T6

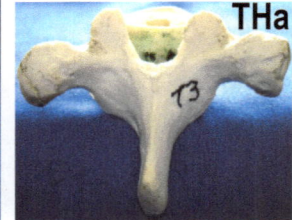

Posterior view of T3

Figures TJ and **TJa** show views from below of the T6 and T3 facets. It can be seen that both sets of facets are concave horizontally. The T4 facets are more rounded.

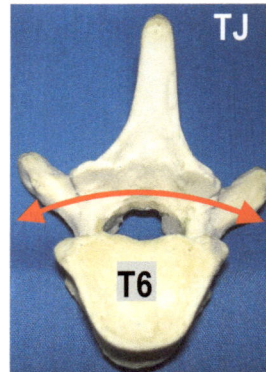

View from below of T6 facets

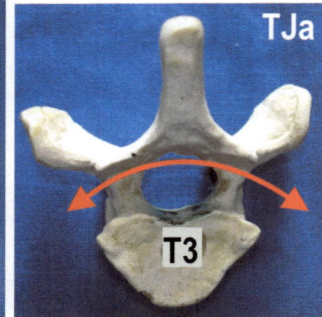

View from below of T3 facets

Figures TK and **TKa** show side-views from below of the T6 and T3 inferior facets. It can be seen that both sets of facets are marginally concave in their horizontal axes. The vertical concavity provides the facets with the ability to flex and extend.

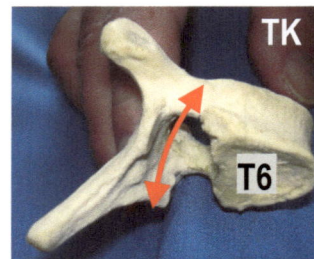

Right side view from below of T6

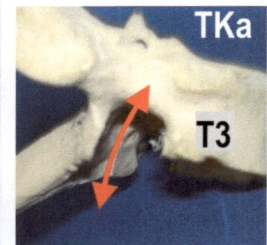

Right side view from below of T3

Thoracic Flexion and Extension

There are two reasons why thoracic vertebrae flex and extend:

•**1**. To aid the rib breathing mechanism with very small amounts of flexion and extension.

•**2**. To achieve forward and backward bending of the thoracic spine.

Figure TL shows the position of the facets when the T7-T6 joint is in neutral.

Figure TM shows the position of the facets when the T7-T6 joint is placed in flexion or when breathing out; expiration.

Figure TN shows the position of the facets when the T7-T6 is placed in extension or breathing in; inspiration.

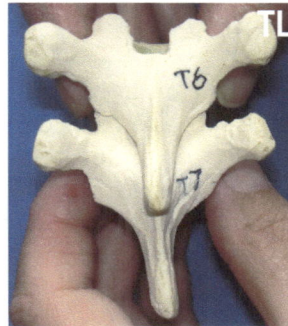

Posterior view Neutral

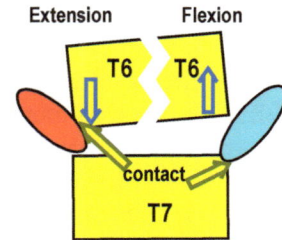

Figure TOc
Exaggerated side-views showing how each side of the demi-facets connect with the ribs

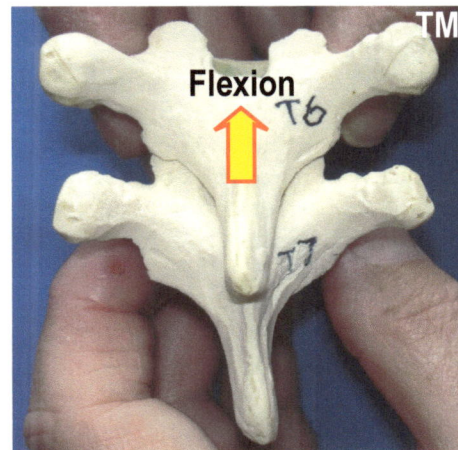

Figure TOa
Anterior view of left side of T6-T7 joint

Refer to **figures TOa** and **TOc**.

Extension: During inspiration the inferior demi-facets of T6 travel inferiorly where they engage against the superior facets at the heads of the T6 ribs.

Flexion: During expiration the superior demi-facets of T6 travel superiorly leaving the inferior facets at the heads of the T6 ribs to engage against superior demi-facets of T7.

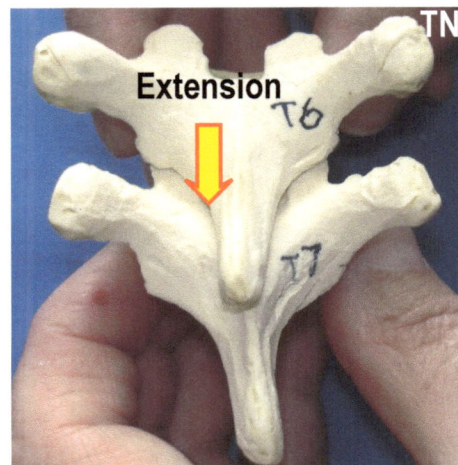

Expiration

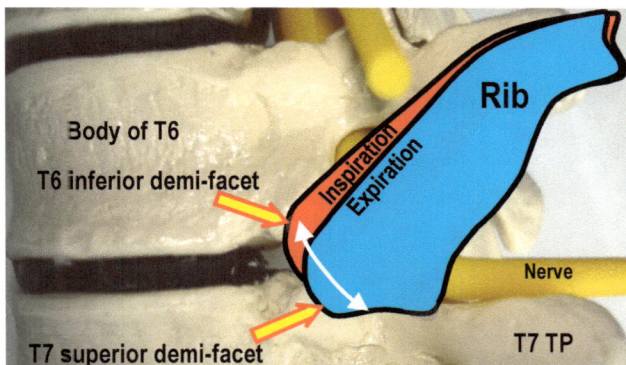

Inspiration

69

Thoracic Rotation and Side-bending Problems

Working rib theory overview

For a rib theory to be proved, it must satisfy working criteria. It has to make due allowance for keeping the ribs level at all times for efficient breathing, whilst also making allowance for movements in flexion, extension, side-bending and rotation.

The thoracic joints **do not** rotate and side-bend, as shown in **figure TOb.** This is because if they moved like this, the ribs which need to be kept in parallel at either side to function efficiently, would be compromised.

For arguments sake, if the side-bending shown in **figure TOb** were to occur, the left transverse process of T6 would be raised superiorly. This would angle the conical apex of the attaching 6th rib superiorly by several degrees and thereby seriously hinder the ribs ability to function normally. See page 11.

Side-bending followed by rotation are necessary for the normal physiological movement of the thoracic vertebrae. Via moving X-rays, I was able to observe how the thoracic spine side-bent and rotated in a way that kept the ribs parallel. The method is very simple and is demonstrated below.

Imagine the line of cards shown in **figure TP** represents the thoracic column and each card an individual vertebra.

If the cards are moved into a stepping sequence, as shown in **figure TQ,** it can be seen that a general side-bending pattern emerges that keeps the cards in horizontal alignment.

It is this principle that the thoracic vertebrae use when side-bending is required.

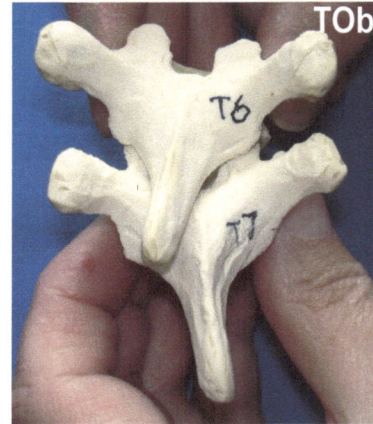

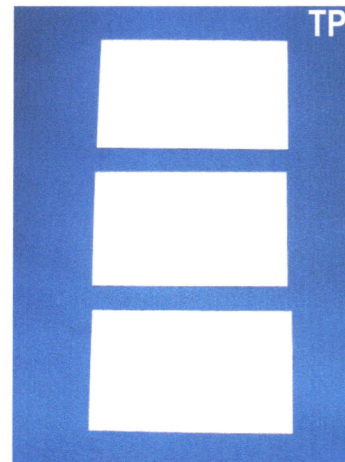

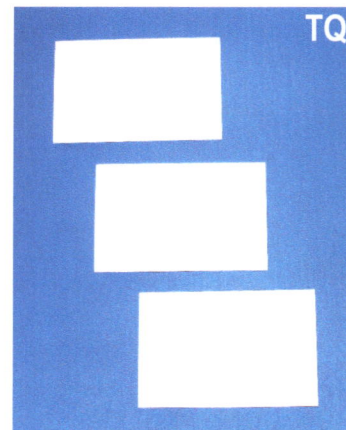

Thoracic:
Nucleus Pulposus Placing

To allow the thoracic joints to articulate efficiently the nucleus pulposus needs to be positioned towards the anterior half of the T7 body, as shown in **figure TR.**

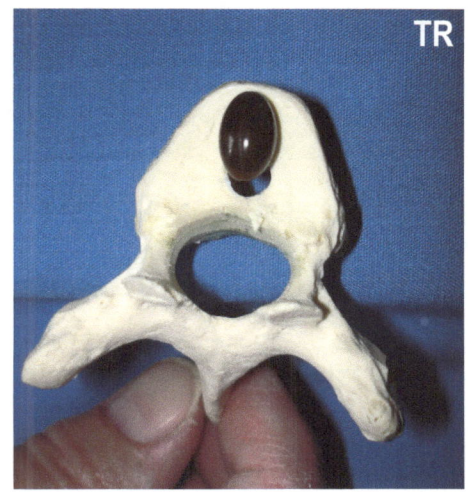

Figure 2b is an approximation of the arc taken by the T6 facets.

This convex arc is in contrast to the concave arc produced by the more posteriorly positioned nucleus, found in the lumbar discs. **Figure 2a** shows for comparison an approximation of the more rounded arc taken by the L3 facets.

The anterior placement of the nucleus pulposus in the thoracic vertebrae probably explains why disc related problems are rare in the thoracic vertebrae.

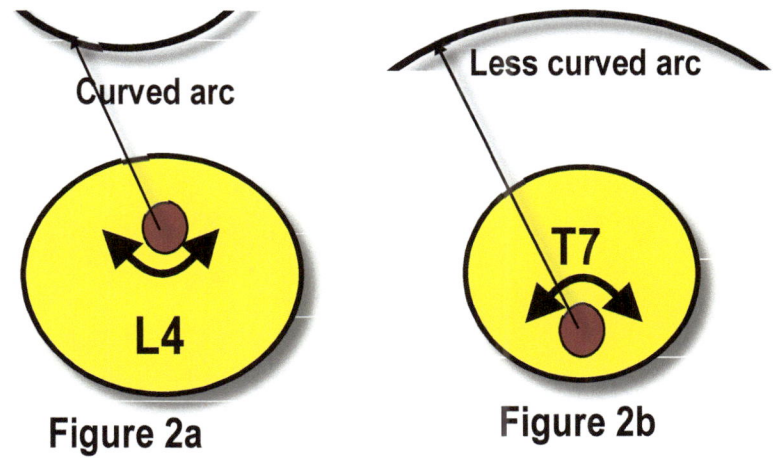

Figure 2a

Figure 2b

Thoracic Rotation Right: Flexion

Figure TS shows what happens when T7 is side-shifted to the right in neutral or flexion. The nucleus pulposus arcs the facets of T6 like a pendulum to the left. This swings the facets superiorly and laterally to the left and creates side-bending and rotation to the right. That is side-bending and rotation to the same side in thoracic flexion?

If we analyse this further, it can be seen that the left transverse processes have separated and the right approximated. This means that the transverse processes are no longer parallel and therefore not achieving the side stepping action required to keep the ribs parallel.

Figure TT is an aerial view showing the rib attachments either side of the thoracic vertebrae. It shows the stabilizing effect the ribs have on either side.

Articular surfaces for rib attachment

Figure TU is a side-view of T6 and shows the articular surfaces where the sixth and fifth ribs attach to the T6 vertebra.

The inferior head of the fifth rib articulates with the T6 body at the superior demi facet, shown by arrow A.

The articular facet of the sixth rib tubercle attaches to the costo-transverse facet. Shown by arrow B.

The superior head facet of the sixth rib attaches to the inferior demi-facet of T6. Shown by arrow C.

More detailed information on how the ribs articulate with the thoracic vertebrae can be found in Chapter 16.

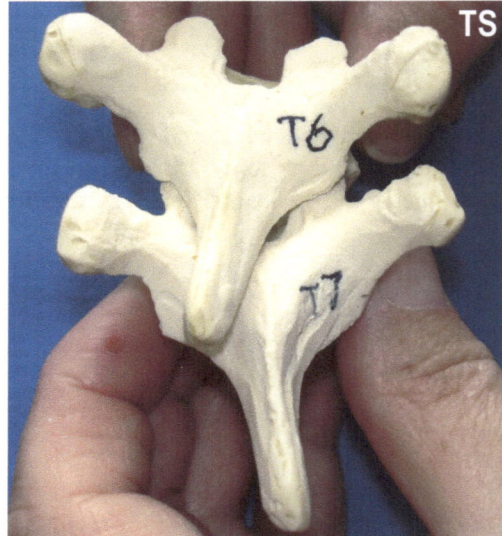

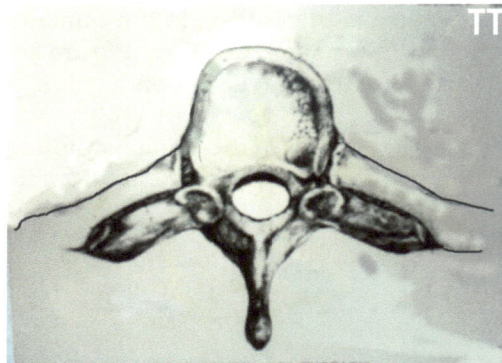

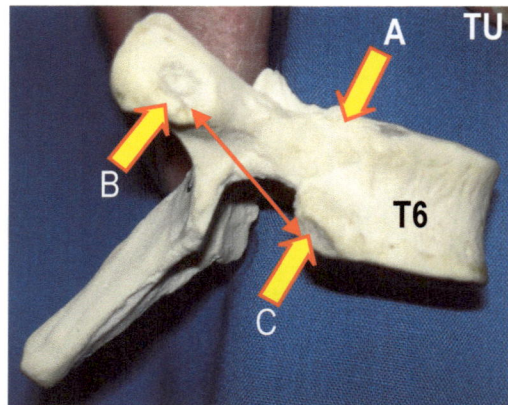

Side-view of T6 thoracic vertebra

Thoracic Rotation Right: Stepping Action

When T7 follows the pelvic side-shift to the right, the movement of T6 is not only governed by the shape of the facets and nucleus pulposus, it has the additional stabilizing influence of the attached ribs.

In **figure TV** the action of rotating to the right is shown again, only this time T6 is held in parallel to simulate the counter force of the ribs on either side. The facets still engage, provided that the nucleus pulposus has the ability to side-shift.

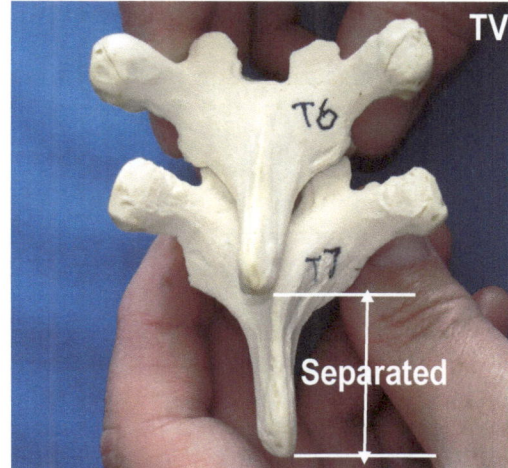

By observing the shape of the upper body of T7 it can be concluded that the thoracic nuclei pulposi have the ability to side-shift. This is because the side-shift can be kept in check by a purpose built scooped design. This scooped shape is shown in **figure TW.**

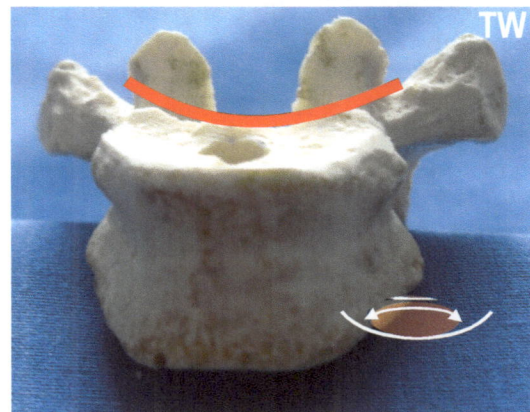

With T7 and T6 held in parallel, the left lateral shift of T6 has no choice other than to conform to a stepping sequence. Shown in **figure TQ** on page 70.

If the completed side-shift movement is examined, using **figures TV** and **TX** for reference, it can be seen that the left transverse process of T6 is marginally anterior and that the spinous process of T6 is separated and to the right of the T7 spinous process. This means that rotation to the right has also taken place.

This is thoracic flexion with side-bending and rotation to opposite sides.

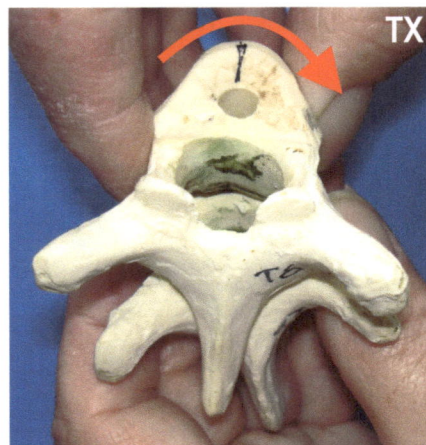

Rotation Right, Side-Bending Left in Thoracic Flexion

Recap on the complete movement.

In the case of thoracic flexion (forward bending), side-shift continues up the spine past L1, as shown in **figure 2.**

T6 is being used as an example. Flexion-rotation movements start with the T6 facets sliding up the T7 facets as shown in **figure TM.**

The left knee is then flexed as weight is directed to the right leg. This causes the pelvis to rise up and engage the right 'F' posterior sacroiliac facets and rotate the pelvis to the right. If the intention is for the thoracic spine to rotate right, the thoracic column will generally follow the pelvic rotation.

The side-bending caused by the raising of the pelvis on the right is blocked at L1 and T12, as shown in **figure 2.**

When pelvic side-shift to the right takes place it passes to the right of L1. The pelvic side-shift causes the T7 facets to side-shift to the right. As can be seen from **figure TO**, the counter force of balance emanating from above causes the facets of T6 to slide left across the convex T7 facets. In doing this the body of T6 is forced to rotate to the right. This is shown from above in **figure TX**.

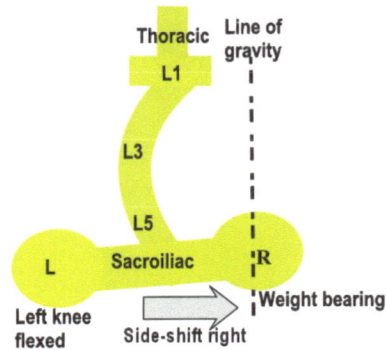

Figure 2

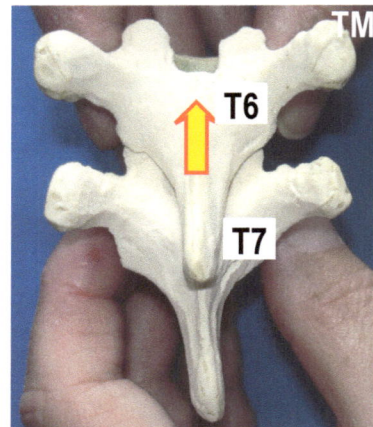

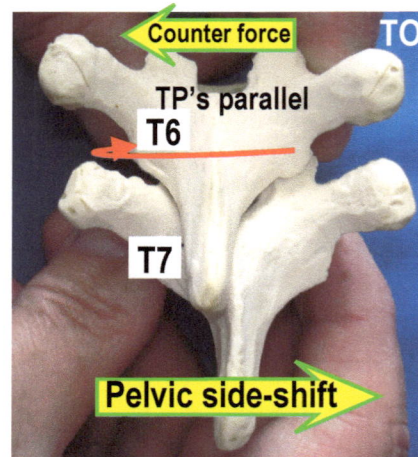

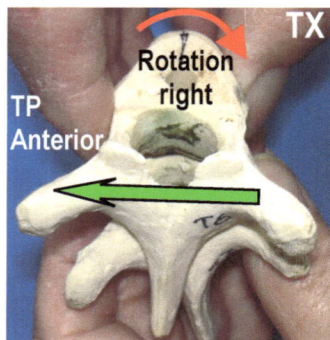

Blocked: Rotation in Thoracic Extension

All side-shift is initiated by the pelvis. Without side-shift, rotation in the thoracic vertebrae cannot take place. This was confirmed in the rationale tests.

It can be seen from **Figure 1** that L1 blocks the lumbar side-bending and side-shift reaching the thoracic vertebrae.

Since there is no side-shift to the left above L1, T6 has no driving force to rotate right in thoracic extension.

But, for the sake of argument, if T6 was placed in thoracic extension, as shown in **figure TY** and pelvic side-shift continued upward to the left of L1, **figure TZ** shows what would happen when the side-shift reached T7. The T7 facets would side-shift to the left and the counter force emanating from the sense of balance from above, would cause the T6 facets to side-shift across the T7 facets to the right. The consequence of this is that the body of T6 would be forced to rotate to the left, as shown in **figure TAA**. This is the completely opposite direction to that intended. This is why L1 blocks the movement.

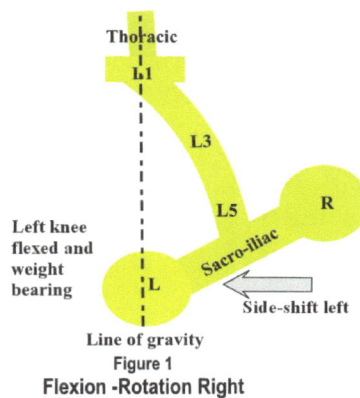

Figure 1
Flexion -Rotation Right

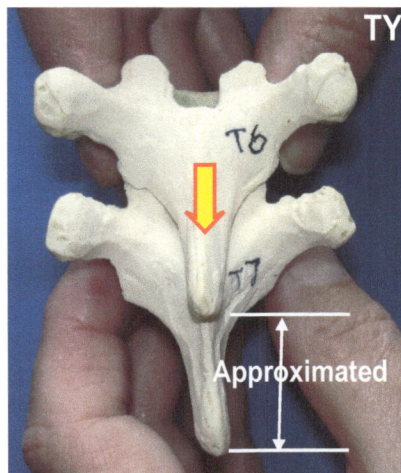

TY

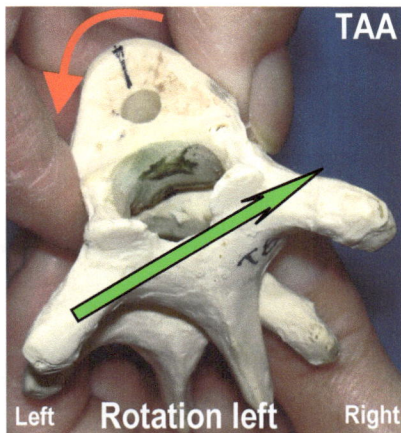

TAA
Rotation left

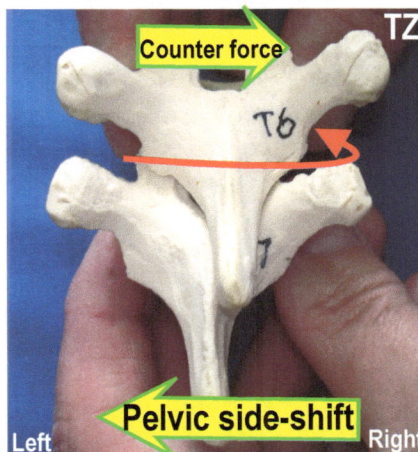

TZ

Thoracic Anatomy: T1 and T2

The T2-T1 joint is unique from the thoracic joints below, because they link the thoracic vertebrae with the cervical vertebrae and form a reverse change in the vertical curve.

Figure TAB shows the superior posterior facets of a typical T2 vertebra. The facets of T2 follow the line of a swinging pendulum.

Figure TAC shows an inferior anterior view of the facets of a typical T1 vertebra. Like the T2 facets the T1 facets follow the line of a swinging pendulum.

Figure TAD shows the T2 superior posterior facets from above. The red arrow highlights the convex shape of the facets.

Figure TAE shows the inferior anterior facets of T1 from below. The red arrow highlights the concave shape of the facets.

Figure TAF shows the vertical slightly convex shape of the T2 superior facets from the right side.

Figure TAG shows the vertical slightly concave shape of the inferior T1 facets.

Figure TAH is a side view from the right of the T2-T1 joint in neutral. Notice that when the facets meet, T1 becomes backward leaning.

Figure TAJ is a posterior view of the T2-T1 joint in neutral. Again notice the backward leaning position of T1. Again note the scooped line of the facets, indicated in red. This would mean that the joint is capable of small amounts of pendulum swing.

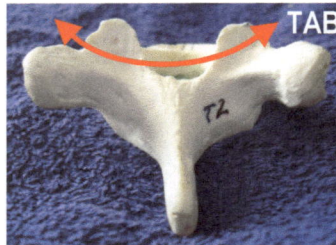
Posterior view of T2

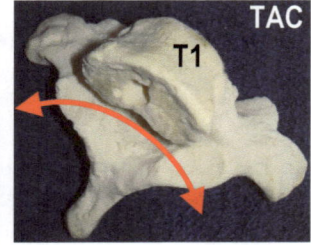
Anterior inferior view

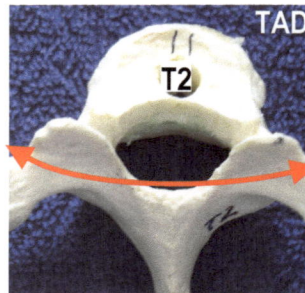
Posterior aerial view of T2 superior facets

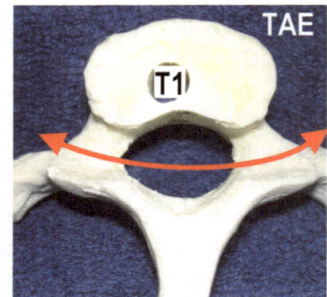
View from below of T1 inferior facets

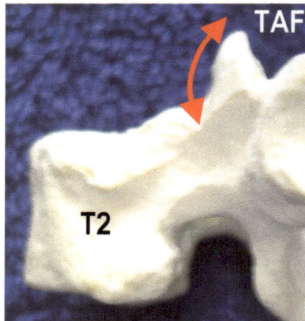
Right side- view of T2 superior facets

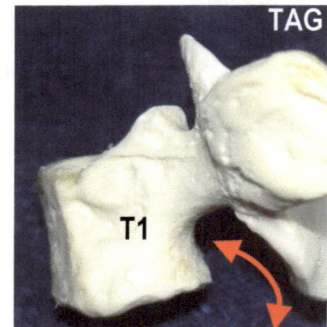
Right side- view of T1 inferior facets

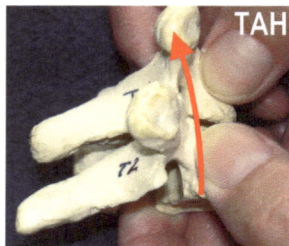
Right side- view of T1-T2

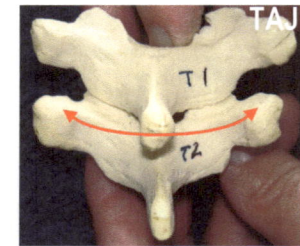
Posterior view of T1-T2

Thoracic Physiology:
T1 and T2

Figure TAK is a posterior view of T2-T1 in thoracic extension (backward bending). T1 has approximated with T2. Because of the close proximity of the T1 and T2 facets, **no** rotation can take place.

Figure TAL is a posterior view of T2-T1 in thoracic flexion (forward bending). T1 has separated from T2.

Figure TAM shows T1 rotating right in thoracic flexion. T2-T1 rotation to the right works on a similar principle to the vertebrae below. Pelvic side-shift causes T2 to side-shift right. Whilst the counter balance from above causes T1, steadied by the ribs at either side to side-shift to the left. In doing this the T1 facets slide over the convex T2 facets and rotate right in a small pendulum arc that keeps T1 level. See illustration 'A' below.

There is probably slightly more allowable side-shift in this joint in neutral and extension than the other thoracic joints. This is because T1 has to counter the side-shifting of the joints below.

The T2 -T1 joint has two main functions:

1) To change the direction of the anterior-posterior curve of the thoracic spine in order to align the neck in a upright and vertical position. See 'B' below.

2) To keep the neck vertical by countering the side-bending (side-shifting) of the thoracic vertebrae below. See **figure TAM** and 'A' below.

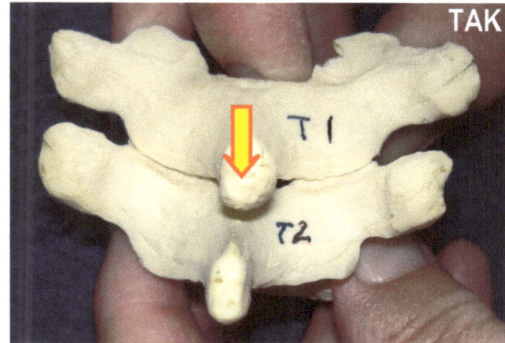

Posterior view of T1-T2
Thoracic extension

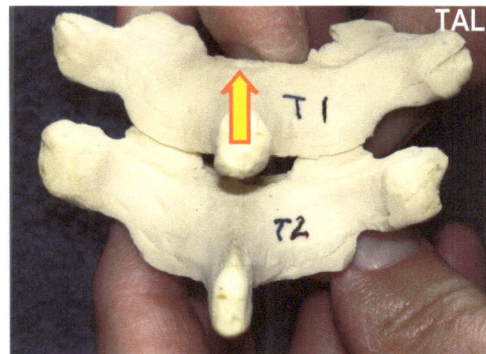

Posterior view of T1-T2
Thoracic flexion

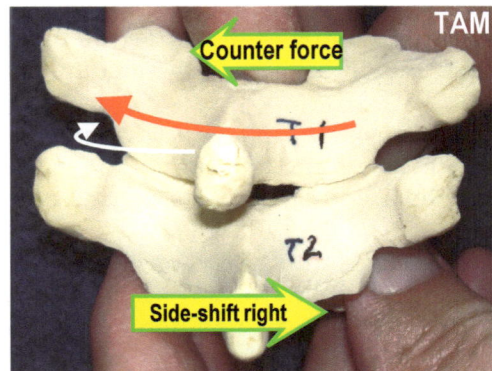

Posterior view of T1-T2
T1 rotating right

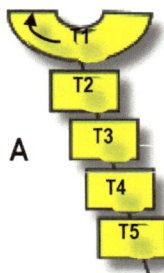

A

Posterior view showing how T1 compensates for side-bending

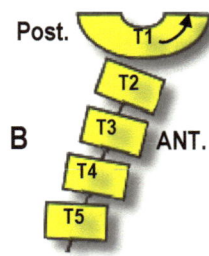

B

Side-view showing change of A-P curve

77

Thoracic Physiology: Rotation and Side-Shift

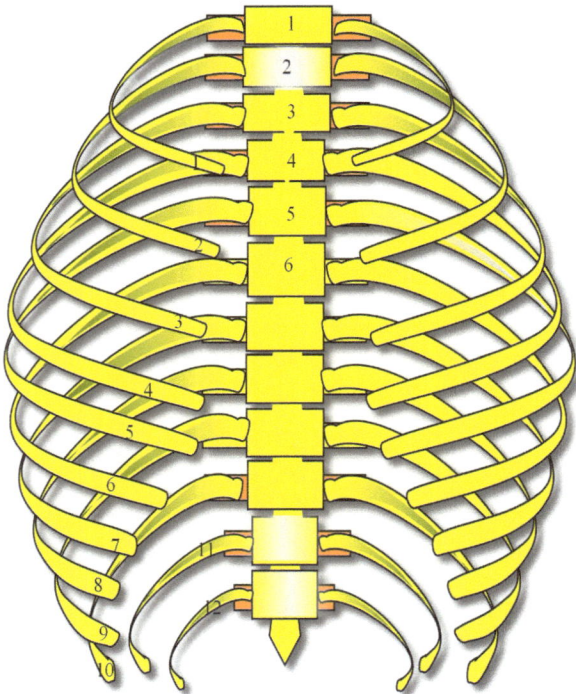

Figure TAN
Anterior view of the thoracic
spine and rib cage.

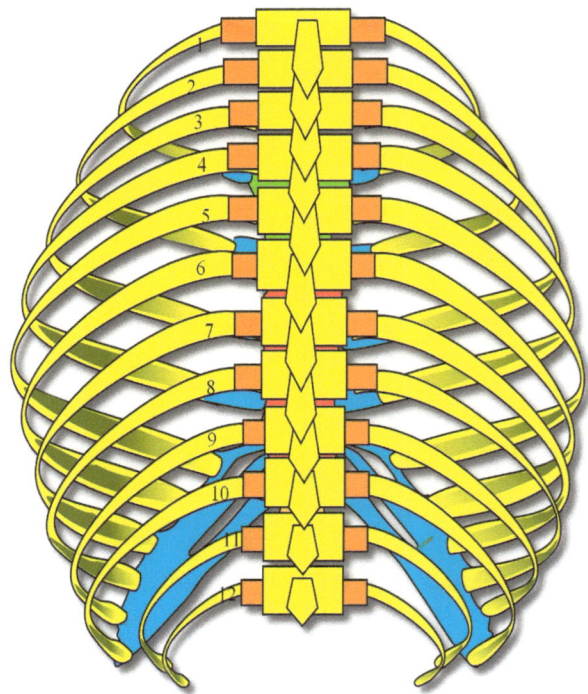

Figure TAP
Posterior view of the thoracic
spine and rib cage.

Generally the lower you go down the thoracic spine, the greater the rotation that takes place. The rib cage and thoracic vertebrae are illustrated in **figures TAN** and **TAP** to help you visualize and contrast the differences in the amount of rotation and side-shift possible. Also see page 15.

The upper five ribs allow for only small amounts of rotation. This is due to the flatter shape of the vertebral facets and the short length of cartilage at their anterior attachment to the sternum. Their main role is side-shift, with a degree of rotation.

The middle five ribs allow for more side-shift and a greater amount of rotation. This is due to the increased flexibility of the suspended cartilage. Their flexibility allows for equal amounts of side-bending and rotation, though the lower ribs in this area should produce a greater rotation and side-shift.

The lower two ribs are not joined to the sternum and this allows them much greater freedom of movement. The more rounded facet shapes of their corresponding vertebrae and their freedom of movement dictate that their primary role is rotation with adequate flexibility to take up the side-shift overspill. See page 198.

Chapter Seven
Physiology of the
Cervical Joints

The cervical vertebrae are different from the thoracic and lumbar vertebrae. This is because side-shift does not initiate their rotational or side-bending movements. Their movements are entirely dependant upon muscles, which provides them with an independence of movement from the spine below.

For example, a person leaning forward or backward can turn their head to the opposite side their body is facing.

The cervical spine is concave posteriorly with a similar curve to that of the lumbar spine.

C7 to C2 have the ability to side-bend and rotate in extension. In flexion these same vertebrae are limited to singular flexion movements only.

C2 and C1 are rotators and have no obvious allowance for extension or flexion movements. They have the ability to also arc laterally.

The occiput can flex and extend to a small degree. In neutral it has the ability to rotate.

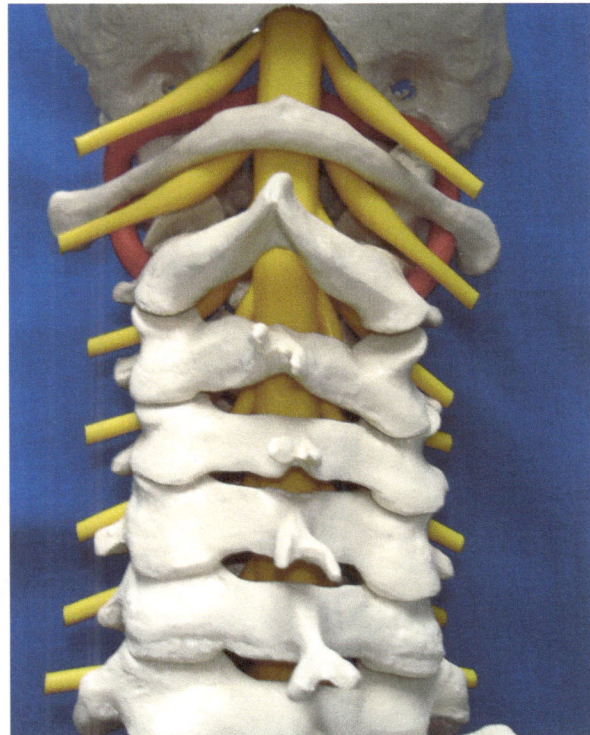

Cervical Reference

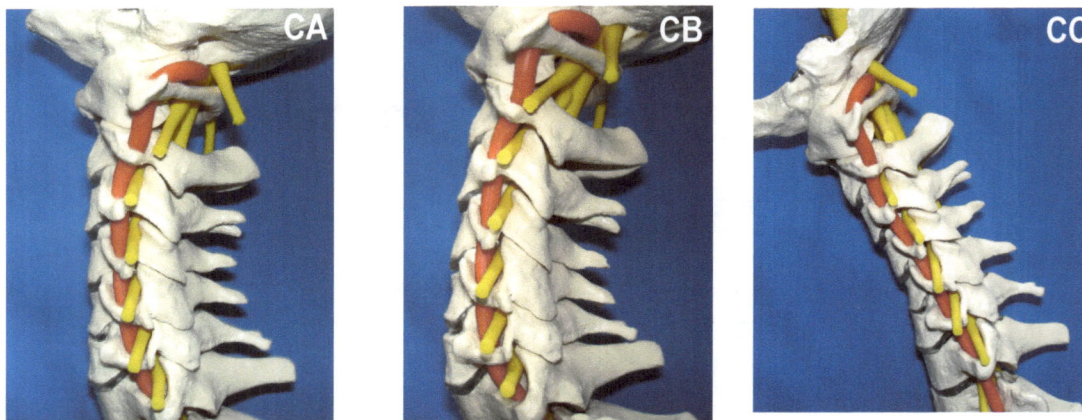

Figure CA is a side-view of the cervical spine in neutral. **Figure CB** is a side-view of the cervical spine in flexion. Cervical flexion is backward bending. **Figure CC** is a side-view of the cervical spine in extension. Cervical extension is forward bending.

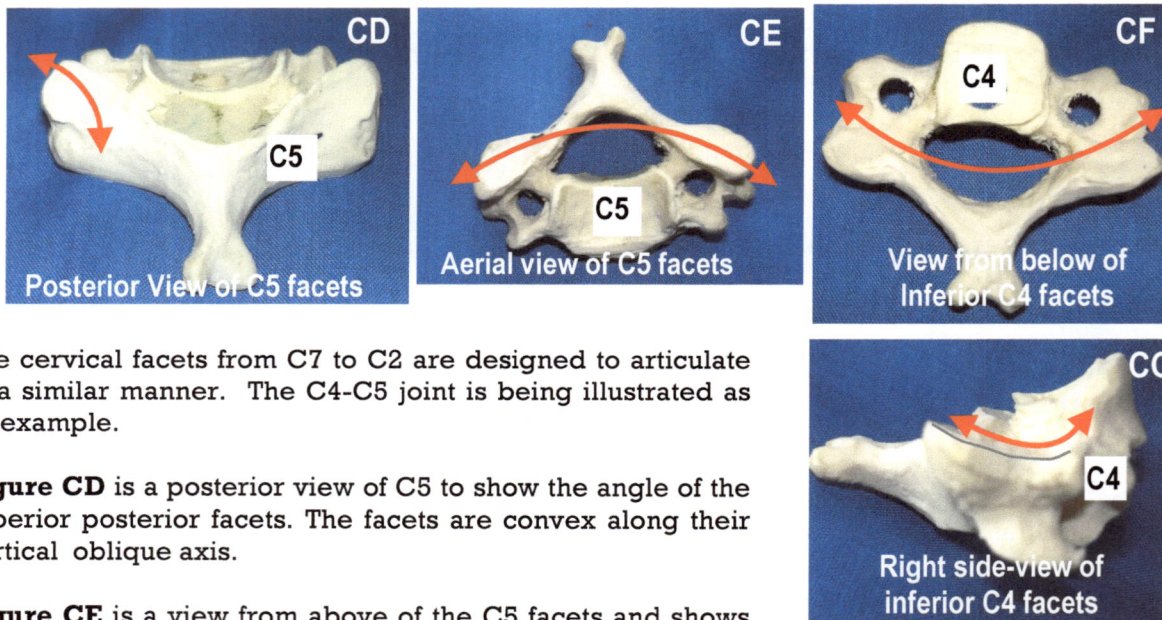

The cervical facets from C7 to C2 are designed to articulate in a similar manner. The C4-C5 joint is being illustrated as an example.

Figure CD is a posterior view of C5 to show the angle of the superior posterior facets. The facets are convex along their vertical oblique axis.

Figure CE is a view from above of the C5 facets and shows the convex shape of the facets along their horizontal axis.

Figure CF is a view of the inferior C4 facets across their horizontal axis and illiterates their concave shape.

Figure CG is a side-view of the inferior C4 facets, and shows the concave shape of the anterior facets along their vertical axis.

Cervical Flexion and Extension

Figure CH is a posterior view of C5. Note that the body of C5 is concave which means the physiology allows for limited side-shift. The capsule is placed in the centre of the body. There is little room between the nucleus and the spinal cord, which presumably explains why disc-related problems have the potential to occur in the cervical spine.

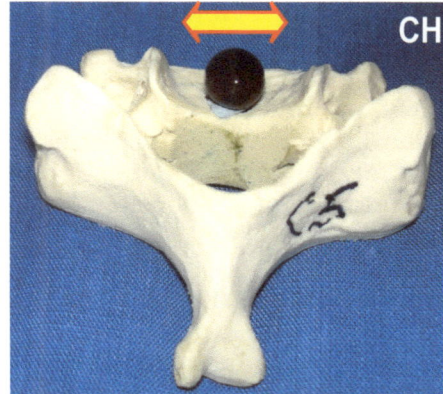

View of C5 nucleus placement

Figure CJ shows C4 in flexion. The facets and spinous process of C4 are approximated to those of C5.

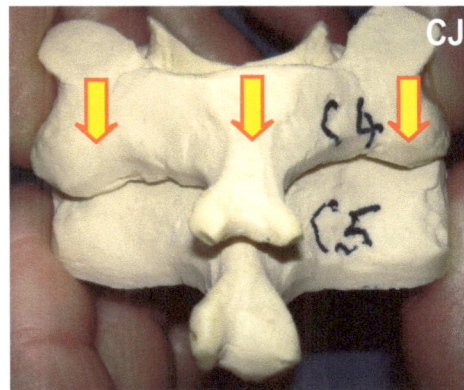

View of C4 in flexion

Figure CK shows C4 in extension. The facets and spinous process of C4 are separated from those of C5.

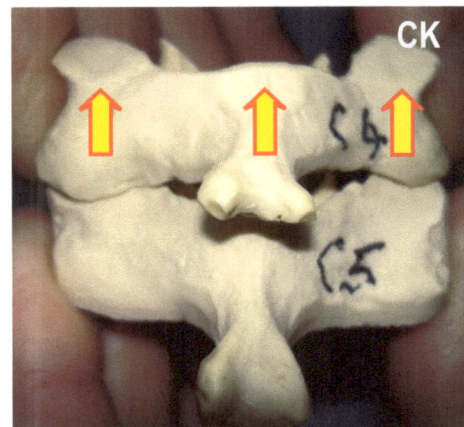

View of C4 in extension

81

Cervical Rotation:
Flexion and Extension

Overview

The cervical facet shapes between C7 and C2 do not allow for rotation in flexion. This is because the horizontal axes of the facets are designed purely for rotation and side-bending to the same side; which is extension.

Rotation right in flexion

If flexion rotation was attempted, initially the inferior facets of C4 would approximate with the lamina of C5, as shown in **figure CJ.**

If rotation to the right was then attempted, the right inferior facets of C4 would grate against the lamina of C5 and prohibit movement. This is shown in **figure CL.**

Rotation right in extension

Initially the facets of C4-C5 separate as shown in **figure CK.**

The neck muscles lever the right hand facet of C4 inferiorly, medially and posteriorly over the right C5 facet. On the left, the left C4 facet moves superiorly, laterally and anteriorly. This action causes C4 to rotate and side-bend to the right in extension, as shown in **figure CM.**

At the maximum point of this movement the C4 spinous process is separated and to the left of the C5 spinous process. The border of C4 on the left is superior, anterior and lateral. The right C4 facet is posterior. The convexity is on the right side.

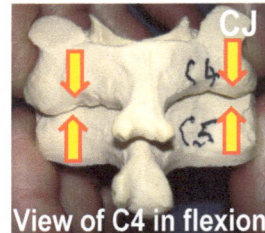

View of C4 in flexion

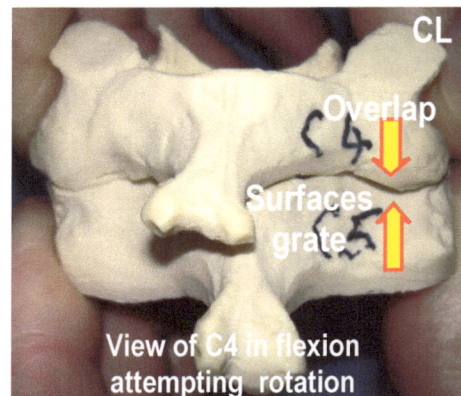

View of C4 in flexion attempting rotation

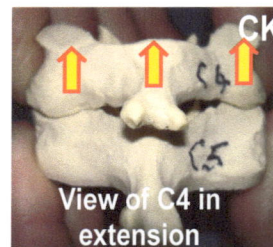

View of C4 in extension

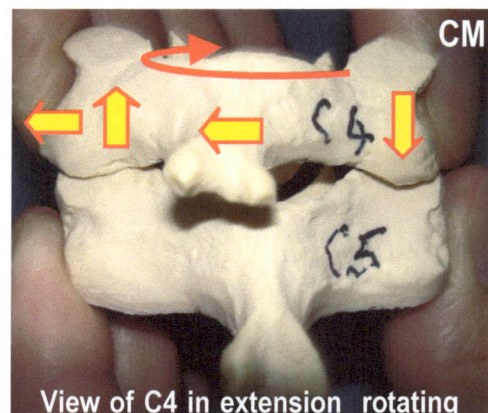

View of C4 in extension rotating

82

Cervical:
C2-1 Facet Anatomy

There is no disc or nucleus pulposus between the junction of C2 and C1. The odontoid peg of C2 replaces the nucleus pulposus as the point of pivot.

The facets of C1-C2 and the occiput, are designed specifically to rotate and side-shift in one movement, and allow for lateral arcing.

Figure CN is a posterior view of C2. The superior facets are convex across their horizontal medio-lateral axis.

Figure CO is a side view of C2. The facets are convex across their antero-posterior horizontal axis. The anterior surface banks in a gentle superior slope that drops away inferiorly.

Figures CP and CQ show the rounded shape of the inferior facets of C1. The anterior surface of the facets bank in a gentle inferior slope so that they can fit snugly against the superior facets of C2. Together they act as a form of ball and socket joint. Notice that the width of the facet of dens is designed to allow the odontoid peg to slide along as it rotates.

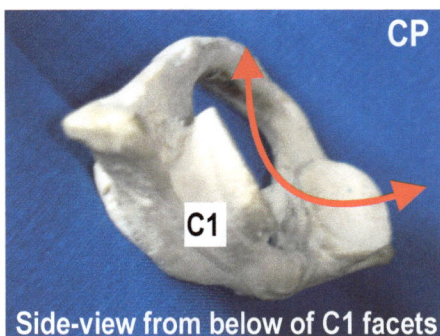
View from above of C2 facets — CN

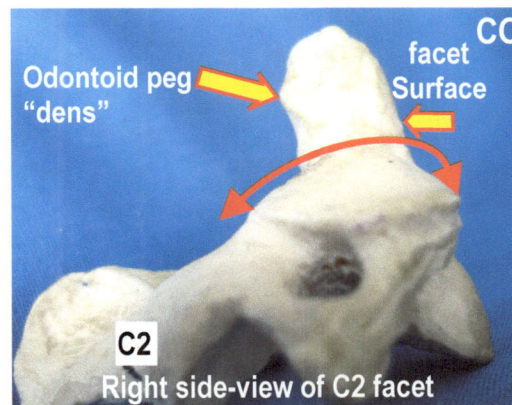
Odontoid peg "dens" — facet Surface — C2 — Right side-view of C2 facet — CO

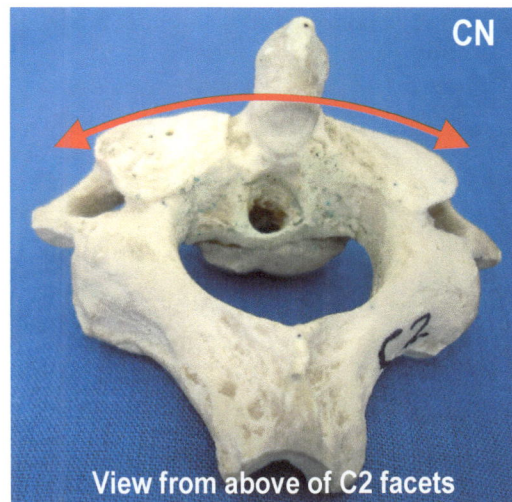
C1 — Side-view from below of C1 facets — CP

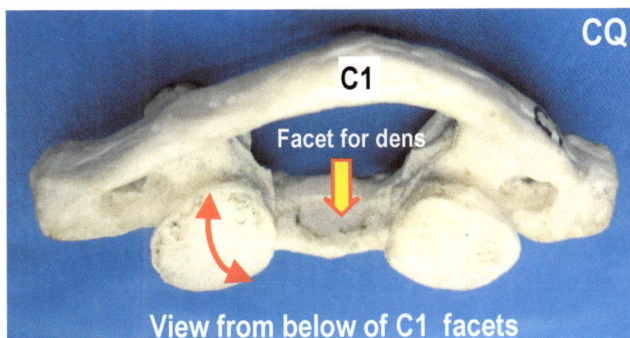
C1 — Facet for dens — View from below of C1 facets — CQ

Cervical:
Odontoid Peg

Figure CR is a posterior view of the C2-C1 joint. It shows the alignment of the facets which are angled inferiorly and laterally.

The odontoid peg at its articulation with C1 prohibits C1 from sliding posteriorly and injuring the spinal cord. This is an important safeguard to limit the effects of whiplash.

Figure CS is an aerial view of the C2-C1 joint. It identifies the position of the odontoid peg at its articulation with the anterior arch of C2. The joint is held firmly in place by the cruciform ligament. The joint is designed for the odontoid peg to simultaneously rotate and side-shift.

Figure CT is a side-view, taken from below, of the inferior anterior slope of the C2 body.

Figure CU is a side-view above C3 and shows the inferior anterior slope of the body.

Below is a side-view drawing of the C3-C2 vertebrae showing the way the C2 body is designed to resist posterior shift.

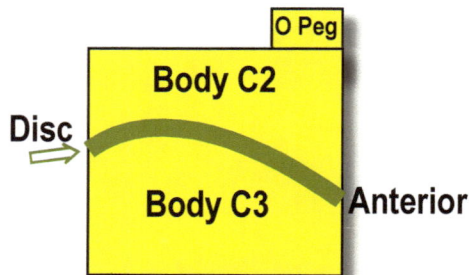

O Peg

Body C2

Disc

Body C3 Anterior

Figure CV is a supero-anterior view of the vertebral bodies of C3 and C2. It is the combination of the rounded shape of the bodies and the cruciform ligament that gives the odontoid peg its rigid stability.

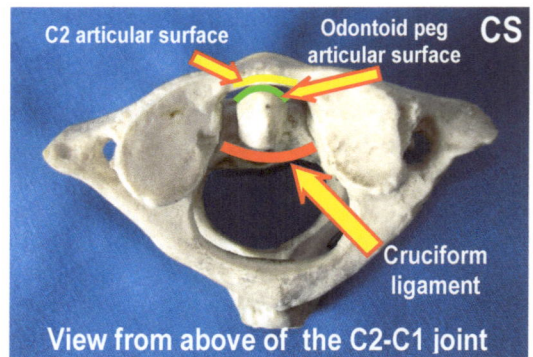
Posterior view of the C2-1 joint

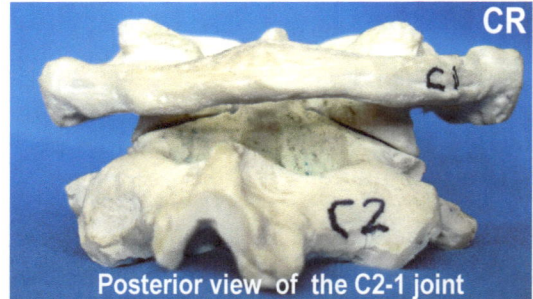
C2 articular surface
Odontoid peg articular surface
Cruciform ligament
View from above of the C2-C1 joint

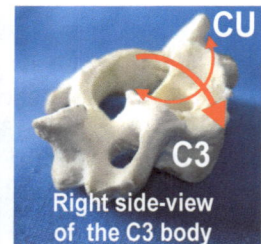
C2
View from below of the C2 body

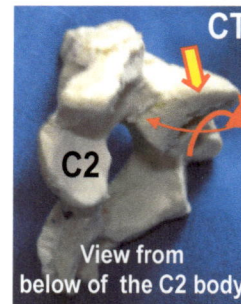
C3
Right side-view of the C3 body

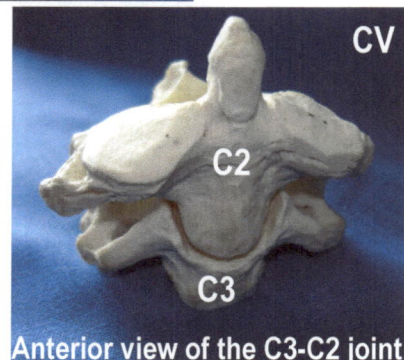
C2
C3
Anterior view of the C3-C2 joint

Cervical Extension:
Rotation Right at C1

Figure CR is a posterior view of the C2-C1 joint. Note that the spinous processes are in very close proximity when aligned correctly.

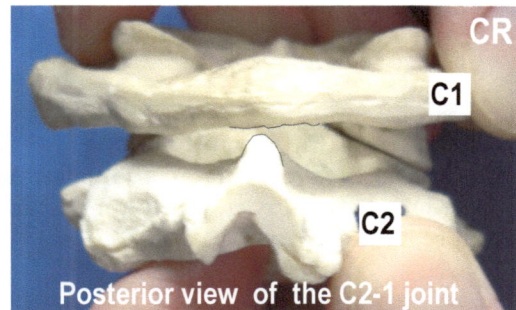

Posterior view of the C2-1 joint

Figure CW is a view from above of the C2-C1 joint in neutral. Note that the spinous process of C1 is anterior to that of C2. This is to avoid collision when C1 rotates and side-shifts.

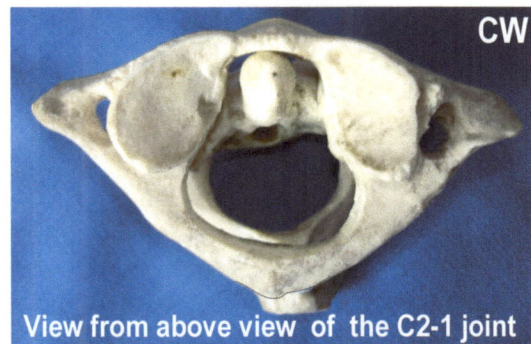

View from above view of the C2-1 joint

Figure CX is a posterior view of C1 rotating to the right. The facet shapes of C2 dictate that C1 has to side-shift laterally to the left for rotation to take place.

Position-wise, the left transverse process of C1 is anterior, inferior and side-shifted to the left. The C1 spinous process is to the left of the C2 spinous process.

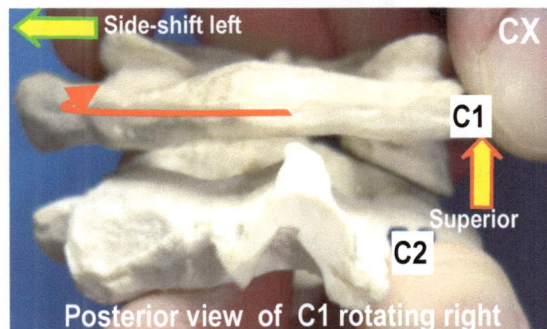

Side-shift left

Superior

Posterior view of C1 rotating right

In order for the C1 facets to follow the line of sideways arcing, the odontoid peg has to side-shift left along the articular facet of C2. This is shown more clearly in **figure CY.**

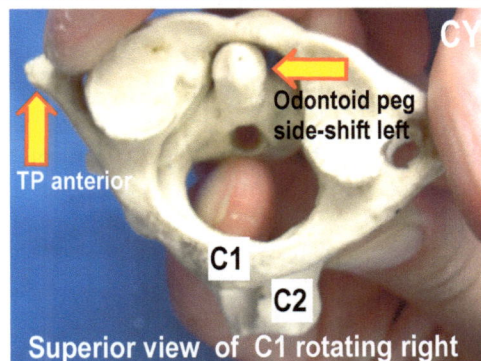

Odontoid peg side-shift left

TP anterior

Superior view of C1 rotating right

85

Cervical:
C1 Facet Anatomy

Figure CY shows the superior facets of C1. Occipital rotation takes place against these facets in neutral, as illustrated by the circular movement of the arrows .

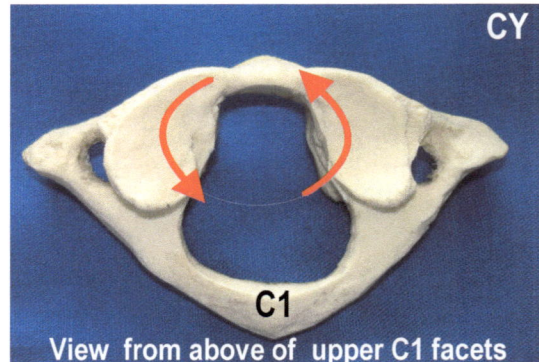

View from above of upper C1 facets

Figure CAA shows the varying concave shapes of the superior articular surfaces of C1. The arrow in green illustrates the more scooped shape at the anterior part of the facet. The red arrow shows the less scooped general concave shape.

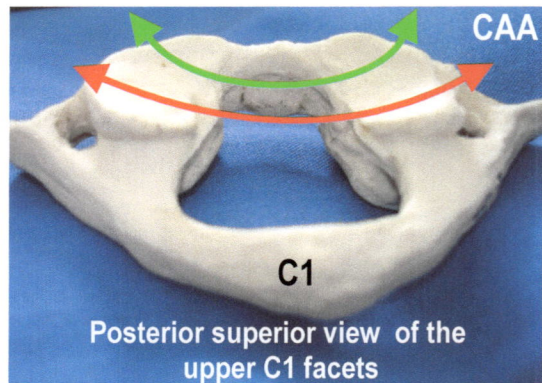

Posterior superior view of the upper C1 facets

Figure CAB is a side-view of the superior articular surface of C1. The facets are concave along their antero-posteriorly axis. The anterior surface of the facet is angled more acutely than at the medial and posterior surface. The anterior shape allows for chin nodding to take place.

The socket shape of the upper C1 facets allow for extension and flexion movements, along with rotation in neutral.   Rotation cannot take place when the occiput is positioned in either extension or flexion. Although it may be possible, movements laterally are very unlikely.

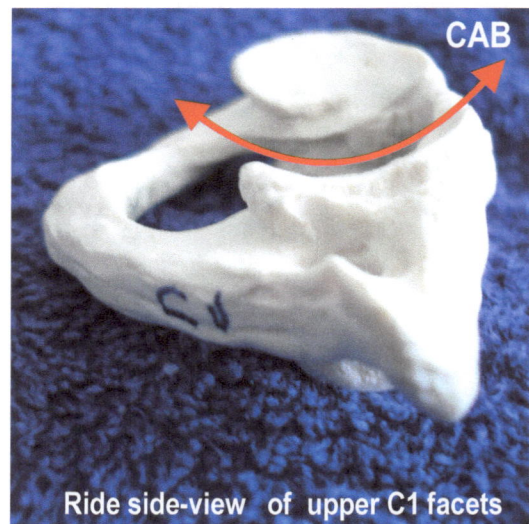

Ride side-view of upper C1 facets

Occiput:
Facet Anatomy

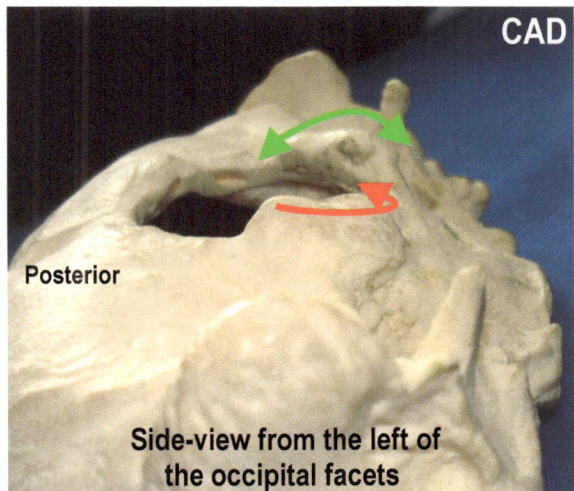

CAC

Styloid process

Posterior view of the occipital facets

Figure CAC is a posterior view of the occiput and shows the inferior convex shape of the facets. The styloid process is indicated for reference purposes only.

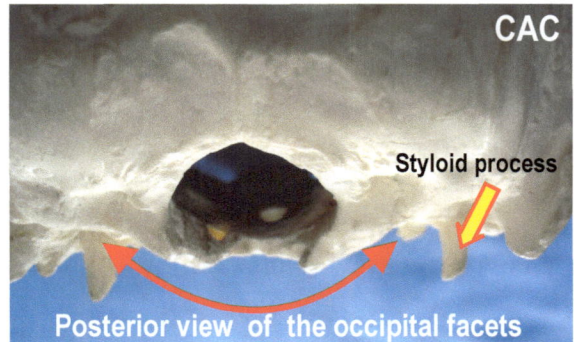

CAD

Posterior

Side-view from the left of the occipital facets

Figure CAD is a side-view taken from underneath, of the occipital facets. The green arrow follows the antero-posterior axis and highlights the change in articular curves. The red arrow shows the area where rotation takes place.

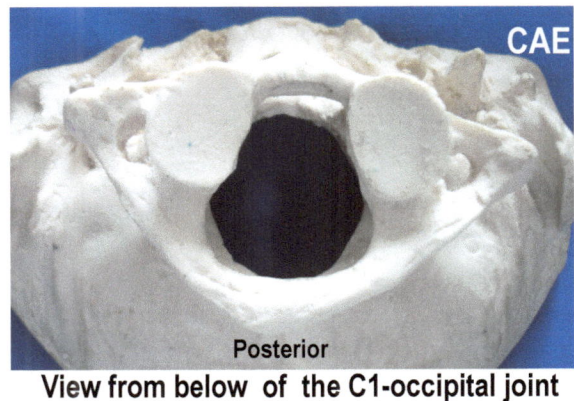

CAE

Posterior

View from below of the C1-occipital joint

Figure CAE is a posterior view taken from underneath of the facets of C1 engaged against the occipital facets, in neutral. There is no disc between C1 and the Occiput.

87

C1-Occipital:
Articulation

Overview

The C1-Occipital joint allows for the following movements:

1) Forward bending of the head
2) Backward bending of the head
3) Rotation of the head in neutral only

Figure CAF is a view from below of the C1 occipital joint in neutral.

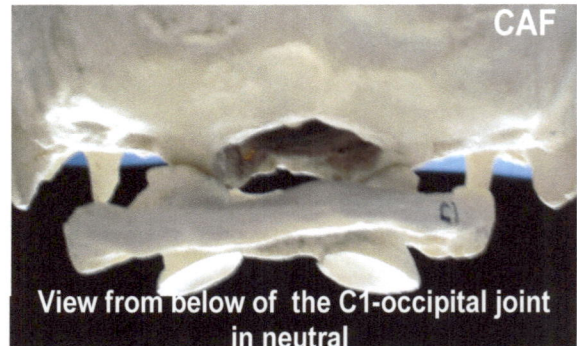

View from below of the C1-occipital joint in neutral

Figure CAG is a posterior view of the occipital bone in flexion (backward bending). The posterior surface of the C1-occipital articulation allows for a gentle decline of the head when backward leaning.

In flexion no rotation can take place.

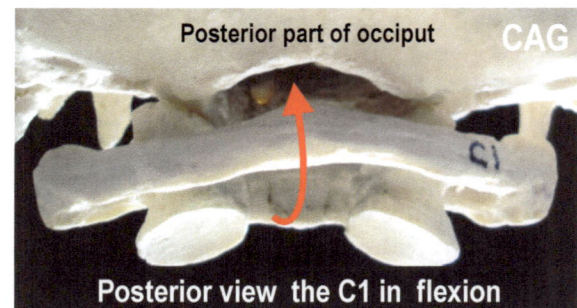

Posterior part of occiput

Posterior view the C1 in flexion

Figure CAH is a posterior view of the occiput in extension (forward bending). The anterior surface of the C1-occipital articulation dips down sharply, to accommodate the action of chin nodding.

In extension no rotation can take place.

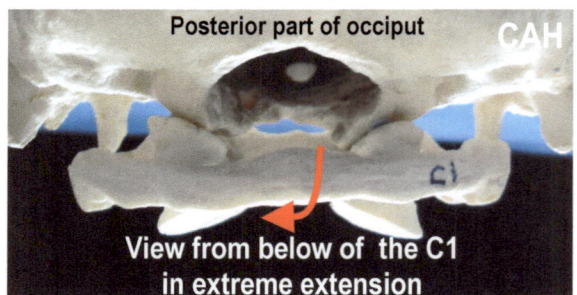

Posterior part of occiput

View from below of the C1 in extreme extension

Figure CAJ is a view from below of the occiput rotated to the left. For rotation to take place the C1 and occipital facets must be in neutral.

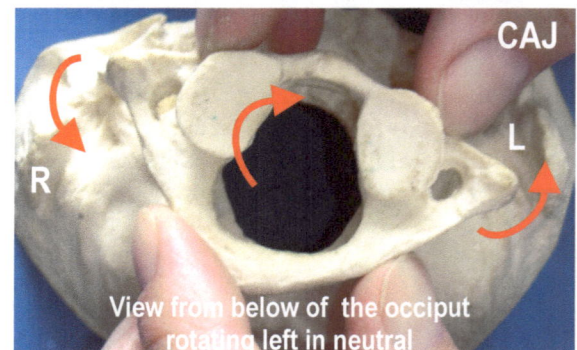

View from below of the occiput rotating left in neutral

88

Chapter Eight
L3-Left-Right
Flexion Subluxations
of the
Lower Back

Flexion subluxations in the lumbar vertebrae are caused when extension is forced on the joints, when weight bearing and side-shift dictate that flexion should take place.

Figure 1 is an illustration of the lower back in flexion with rotation to the right.

It can be seen that L4-L3 takes the maximum side-bending and stress. The secondary areas of stress are taken above at L2-L1 and below in the left sacroiliac joint. L4-L3 is therefore the area of prime torsion.

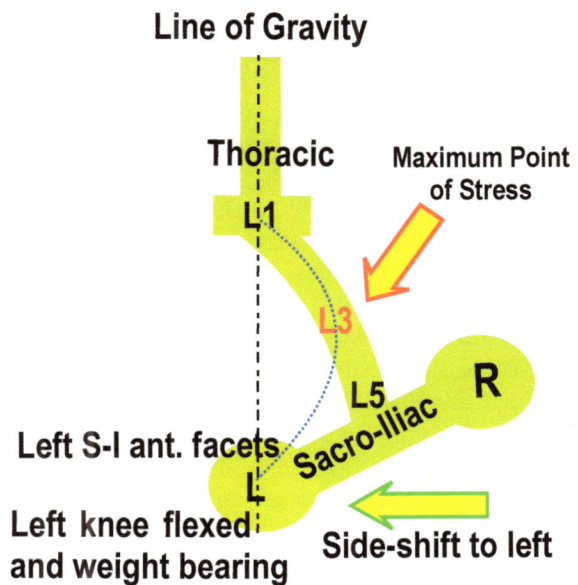

Line of Gravity

Thoracic

L1

Maximum Point
of Stress

L3

L5

R

Left S-I ant. facets

Sacro-Iliac

L

Left knee flexed
and weight bearing

Side-shift to left

Figure 1

89

Experiments to Illustrate
the Principles of Locking

1) *Flexion Recap* . Sit in front of a desk and place a book about 2 inches (5 cm) thick in front of you and to your immediate right. Now rest your elbows as follows; the left elbow on the desk and the right one on the book and then clasp your hands together tightly by interleaving your fingers. You should find that your hands at this point naturally side-bent to the left.

2) *Flexion Recap.* Place your weight on the left elbow whilst keeping your hands in this mid-air position and then side-shift your right elbow towards the left. You should find that your hands naturally veer towards your body as they rotate comfortably to the right.

3) This time remove the book to prohibit the initial side-bending then repeat the experiment. The weight should be on the left elbow and your elbows level. Now bring your hands towards your body slightly and side-shift your right elbow towards the left. *You should notice immediately that the rotation of your hands is restricted and to the right to the point of making your fingers begin to tighten. The further to the left you side-shift your right elbow the more your fingers tighten and veer towards your body. This illustration presents the backward curve of the lumbar.

* If you push your hands away from your body slightly your rotation will be to the left. The further to the left you side-shift your right elbow the more your fingers tighten and veer towards your body. This illustration represents the forward curve of the thoracic.

4) You can compound of this tightening still further if you keep your hands in the tightened position described in 3) and then push your hands away from your body to simulate forward bending. Notice that the further away from your body your hands go the tighter your fingers become. Note that you can side-shift your hands left but not right.

What can be deduced from this experiment?

Whilst the shapes of the hands do not represent any of the sacroiliac or spinal joint facets, this simple flexion experiment highlights the locking affect singular side-shift accompanied by forward bending can have in compounding the locking. It is this locking principle that I used to explain how individual joints initially lock on each other.

The 'consequence' shown in the next chapter describes the influence a forced reversal of side-shift together with backward bending can inflict on the already subluxated joint. To understand the affect of these changes, we can do one last experiment.

5) With your hands away from your body as described in 4) side-shift your left elbow towards the right. Notice how your hands veer to the right and away from your body as your hands locally rotate further right. This action really tightens to the point of discomfort. Now draw your hands towards your body to simulate extension and feel the bite. Your hands should now be closer to your body and to the right of their original starting position. If you side-shift your fingers to the left the joint moves in that direction but tightens and blocks to the right.

This last experiment provides a likely explanation for how bony locking can become so severe that it creates changes to the local tissue chemistry.

The extension version of this experiment has the weight on the right elbow, which causes side-bending right and the rest is in essence a mirror image of the above. See page 164.

Lower Back:
Flexion Rotation Rules

Before getting further into subluxations, set out below is a brief recap of how normal rotation to the right is performed in flexion (backward leaning).

When a person is standing upright and reaches behind them and rotates to the right, these movements take place.

The left knee flexes and the pelvis side-bends left.

The body weight is taken on the left side of the pelvis.

The left side 'A' anterior sacroiliac facets engage and angle the acetabulum and head of the femur anteriorly, medially and superiorly.

The lumbar vertebrae side-bend to the left and align the lumbar facets for flexion rotation to follow.

The pelvis then side-shifts to the left.

The lumbar vertebrae facets rotate right.

It was shown that the L4-L3 joint is the primary area of torsion. To fully recap on the normal physiological movement of the lumbar vertebrae refer to chapter four.

Briefly, the pelvis, with the left knee flexed, causes the facets of L4-L3 to side-bend left as shown in **figure LK.** Then, when body weight is directed through the left side of the pelvis, the lumbar facets align in preparation for rotation. The pelvis then side-shifts to the left and drags L4 in the same direction. The counter force of balance, to the right from above, causes the right facets of L3 to bank and rotate up the right L4 facets. This causes L3 to rotate to the right, as shown in **figure LL.**

When side-bending and rotation are taken to their physiological extreme limits, as shown in **Figure LL,** the L4-L3 joint is still mobile. Therefore, taking the joint to its physiological limit is not the answer to why the L3 joint becomes subluxated.

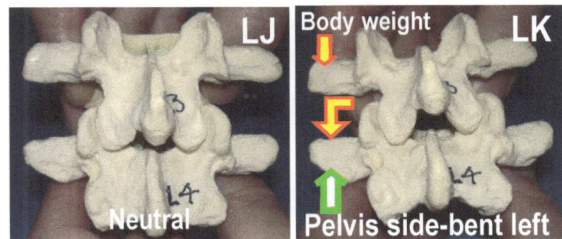

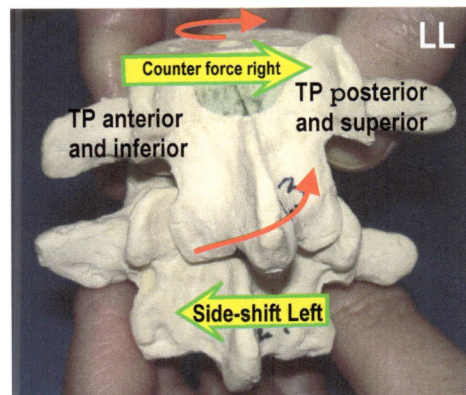

LJ — Neutral

LK — Body weight / Pelvis side-bent left

LL — Counter force right / TP anterior and inferior / TP posterior and superior / Side-shift Left

L4-L3:
Flexion Subluxation to the Right

If the left knee is not flexed for reasons of lack of space or bad practice, and body weight is directed to the left side of the pelvis, the lumbar facets cannot align into the correct position for flexion rotation to follow.

Backward leaning takes place and the L3 facets flex inferiorly. The flexing of the left knee should have caused the lumbar vertebrae to side-bend left. But without this, the body weight and ground resistance on the left can only approximate the left facets of L3 and L4 to a small degree. Therefore the facets are not in the correct starting position for normal flexion rotation to follow. This is shown in **figure FSA.**

When the pelvis side-shifts to the left as shown in **figure FSB,** L4 follows. The counter force to the right from above causes the L3 facets to move across the facets of L4, where they collide and impact into the side of the right L4 facet and left L4 lamina. This causes the joint to buckle.

Compare the difference in rotation between the normal physiological movement shown at its limit in **figure FSC** with the subluxated version, shown in **figure FSB.**

It can be seen from the illustrations in the top left hand corners of each photograph that the possible rotation to the right of the subluxated vertebra is much less than the normal rotation.

The illustrations in the bottom right hand corners of each photograph are of the right L3 facet trajectory. In the subluxated vertebra side-bending is virtually eliminated.

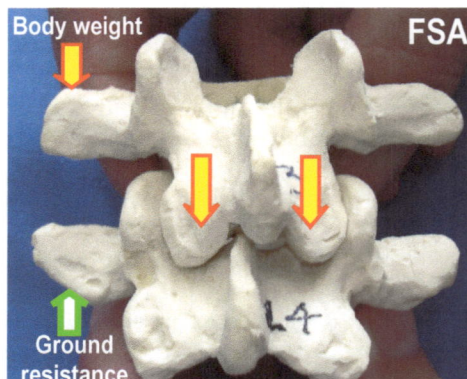

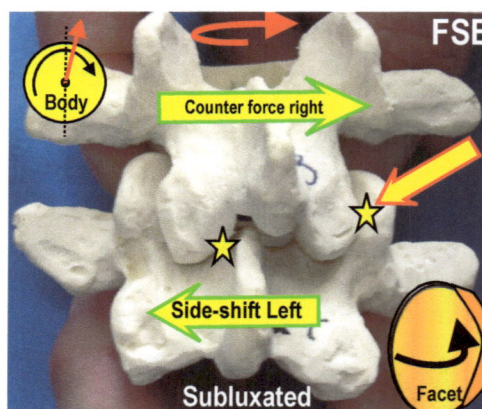

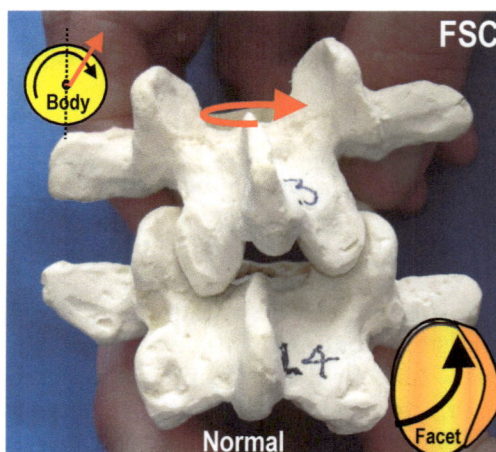

Line of Gravity Changes due to Flexion Right Subluxation

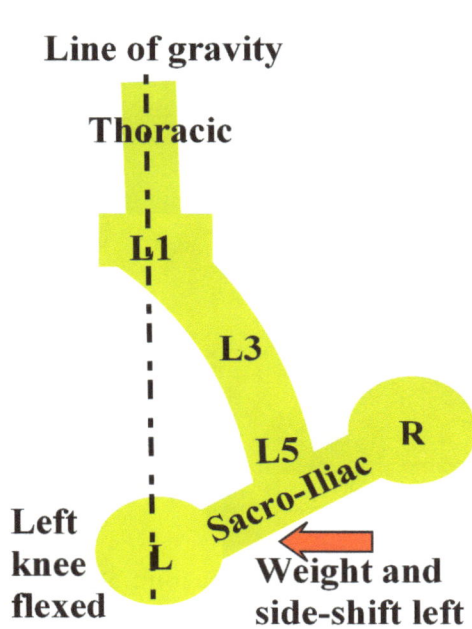

Line of gravity

Thoracic

L1

L3

L5

R

Sacro-Iliac

Left knee flexed

L

Weight and side-shift left

Figure 3a
Normal

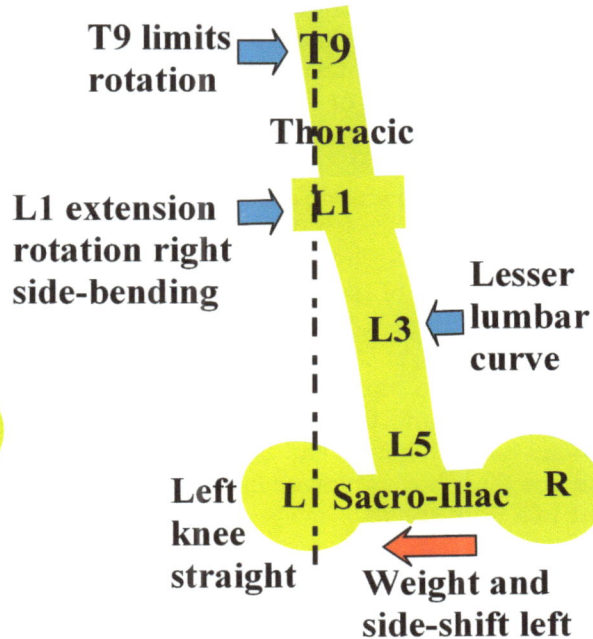

T9 limits rotation → T9

Thoracic

L1 extension rotation right side-bending → L1

Lesser lumbar curve

L3

L5

R

Left knee straight

L | Sacro-Iliac

Weight and side-shift left

Figure 3b
Group subluxation

Figures 3a and 3b above contrast the differences in the lumbar curve when the L3-L4 vertebrae becomes subluxated in flexion and a normal curve. The implication of the lesser side-bending curve of the subluxated vertebrae, is that the weight bearing line of gravity is not dissipated at L1 and is allowed to continue up the thoracic spine to approximately T9.

Illegal thoracic rotation left

If a persons intension is to rotate right in backward bending, using T10 as our example, when both pelvic weight bearing and side-shift are to the left, T11 side-shifts to the left. Counter resistance from above, side-shifts T10 to the right across the facets of T11. This contravenes the thoracic extension laws of movement and causes T10 to rotate and side-bend to the left, which is the opposite direction the person wanted to rotate. Understandably, this creates an area of extreme torsion and is shown in **figure FSD.**

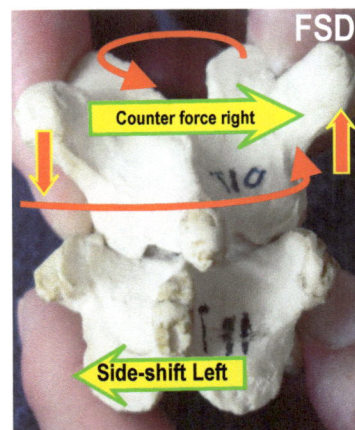

FSD
Counter force right
Side-shift Left

T10 Rotation and Side-bending to the left

Typical L3:
Flexion Subluxation to the Right

Returning to L4-L3, in the subluxated joint the physiological flexion law is broken if side-shift to the left is maintained and the person bends forward. The right facets of L3 attempt to move superiorly, as shown in **figure FSE**. This forces the right L3 facets into the right L4 facets where they compact and subluxate.

A nice practical example for the layman and pro alike of this type of subluxation occurs when a person stands in a backward leaning position with their weight distributed on their left leg and rotates to the far right without flexing their left knee and then bends forward. Commonly this type of action can be traced to people who use their hover mower incorrectly. or load vans in a tight space.

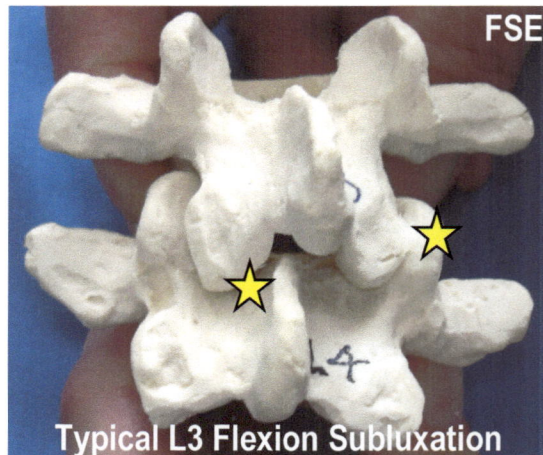

Typical L3 Flexion Subluxation

The forces that are placed on L4-L3 are also placed on L2-L1 and the sacroiliac joint. So let's look at the L2-L1 joint next.

To briefly recap on the normal physiological movement of the L2-L1 joint, L1 acts as a counter lever in the vertical position during lumbar rotation and side-bending movements. When the left knee flexes, L2 follows the side-bending of the weight-bearing left pelvis. This aligns the right L2 facets to the middle of the right L1 facet, as shown in **figure LY.** When the pelvis side-shifts left, L2 is dragged in the same direction and the two aligned facets engage to block the side-shift. This is shown in **figure LZ**. If these movements are taken to their physiological limit, they do not lock; therefore, this is not how the L2-L1 joint becomes subluxated.

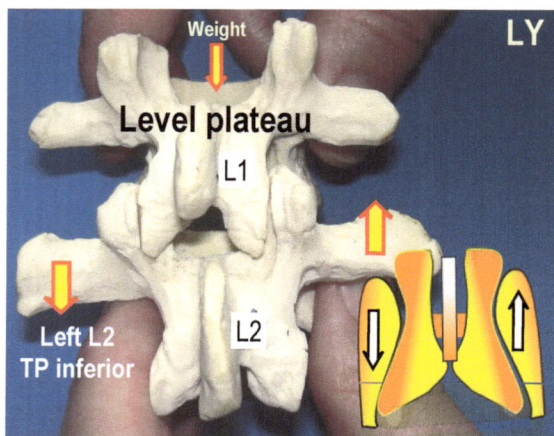

L2 side-bends left

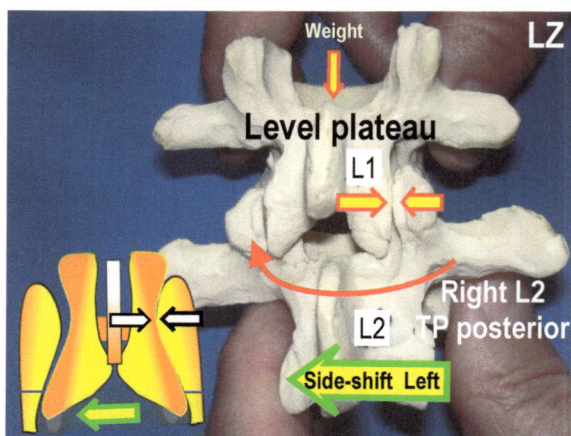

L2 rotates right whilst L1 blocks this movement to protect the thoracic vertebrae from rotating left.

L2-L1:
Flexion Subluxation to the Right

If the weight bearing left knee is not flexed and the lumbar is flexed in readiness to rotate right, the facets of L2 and L1 approximate in parallel. The inferior border of the L1 facets are brought into close proximity with the L2 lamina. Due to weight bearing on the left, the left facet of L2 is marginally side-bent left. This is an incorrect starting point and is shown in **figure FSF** and **FSFa**.

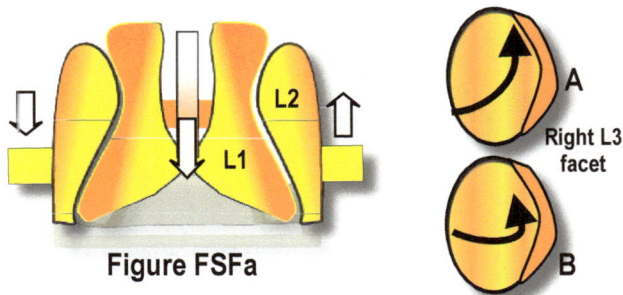

FSF

Weight

Lamina

Ground resistance

Posterior view of L2-L1 joint

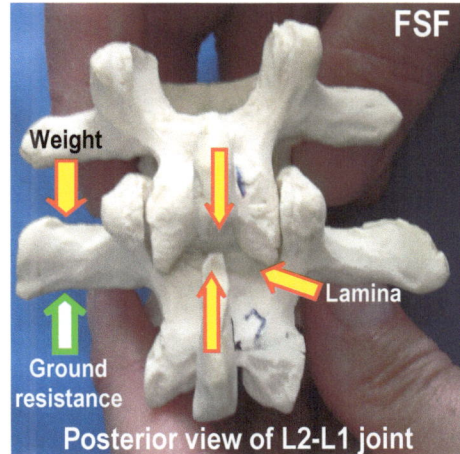

Figure FSFa

A

B

Right L3 facet

Figures FSG and **FSGa** show L2 following the pelvic side-shift left. *A quick reminder of what happened at L3 below. The facet of L3 should have rotated in an arc, as shown in 'A' above but instead subluxated and only marginally rotated and side-bent, as shown in 'B' without arcing.* This has the knock-on effect of stopping the right facets of L1 from following the rotation arc of L3 and smoothly sliding up the right L2 facet. As L2 rotates right, the right facet of L1 becomes wedged against the L2 facet, as shown in **figure FSGb**. Because the right facet of L2 cannot move up the right facet of L1, L1 is forced to side-bend right.

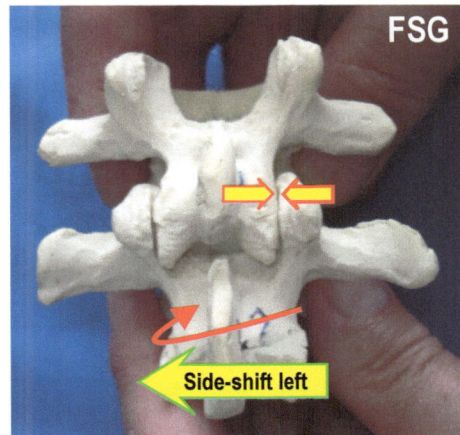

FSG

Side-shift left

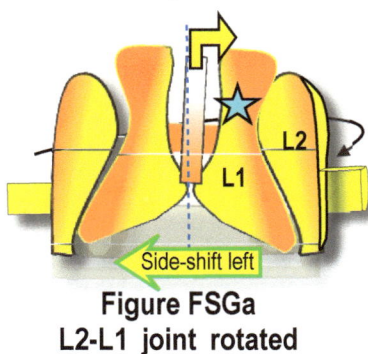

Side-shift left

Figure FSGa
L2-L1 joint rotated

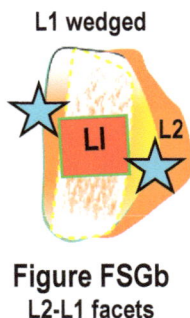

L1 wedged

Figure FSGb
L2-L1 facets

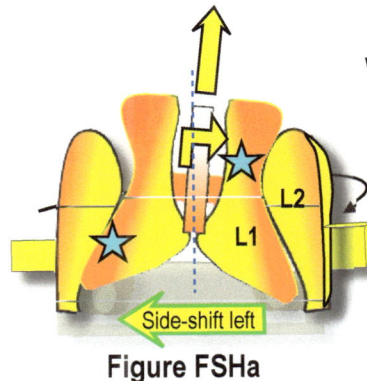

Side-shift left

Figure FSHa

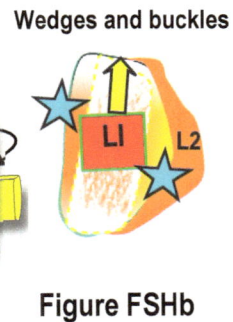

Wedges and buckles

Figure FSHb

L1-T12:
Flexion Subluxation to the Right

Continuing on from the previous page, **figure FSGb** showed how the L1 facet got wedged just over halfway up the L2 facet and caused a minor subluxation. This subluxation is further compounded when the person leans forward without changing their direction of side-shift. The thoracic column levers the facets of L1 superiorly as shown on the previous page in **figures FSHa** and **FSHb.** As the misaligned right facet of L1 gets dragged superiorly, the joint buckles. The force of the side-shift to the left rotates and side-bends the destabilized L1 vertebra to the right. A photograph of this final stage is shown in **figure FSH**.

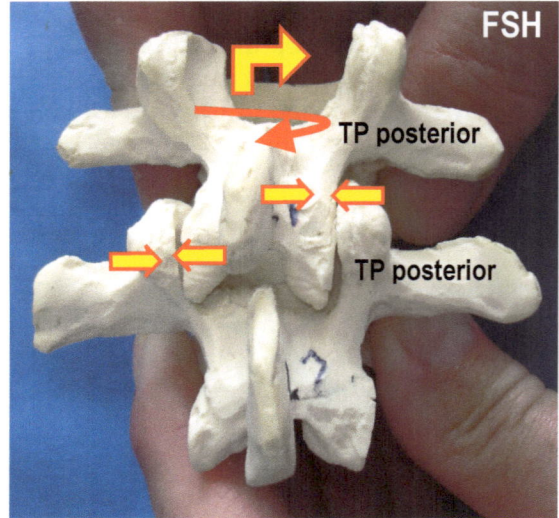

The L1-T12 joint

As was explained in chapter four, because normal physiological pelvic side-shift is blocked at L1, T12 has no way of rotating. However, **figure 3b** showed how the misaligned subluxated lumbar spine allowed the pelvic side-shift to pass to the left of L1.

The pelvic side-shift to the left does not come back into the mid-line until approximately T9 to T7 and therefore creates huge stability problems.

For reference, **figures LCH** and **LCHa** show the L1-T12 joint in neutral.

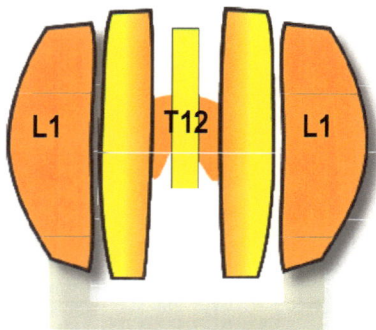

Figure LCHa
L1-T12 in neutral

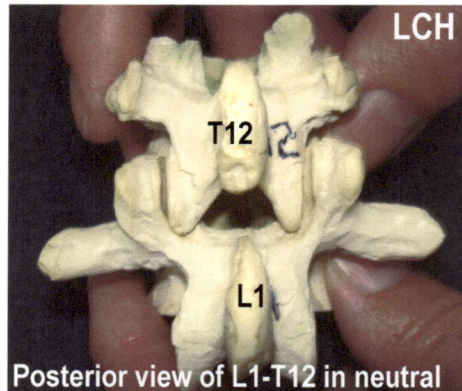

Posterior view of L1-T12 in neutral

96

L1-T12:
Flexion Subluxation to the Right

Stage one

In thoracic extension (backward bending) T12 approximates with L1. **Figure FSR** illustrates the facet angles of L1. It can be seen that the rotation and side-bending to the right of the L1 facets is followed by the superior facets. The superior facets of L1 do not touch the T12 facets, as shown in **figure FSS**. However, this is an incorrect starting point for T12 to rotate right.

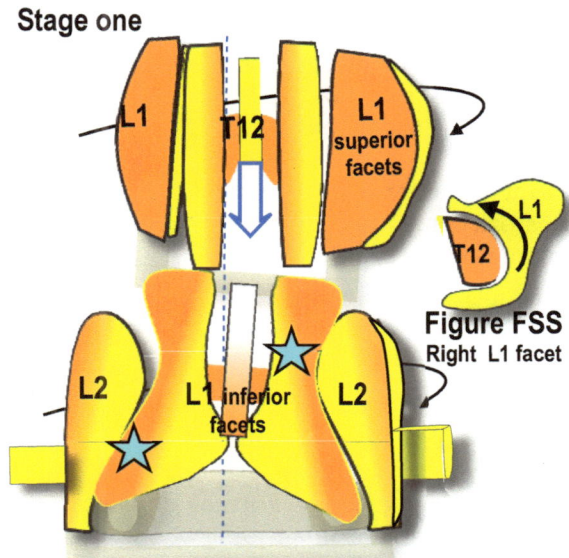

Stage two

Figure FST illustrates the next stage when pelvic side-shift forces L1 to the left. As L1 side-shifts to the left the inferior part of the right L1 facet engages against the inferior part of the right T12 facet. As side-shift continues, T12 buckles and rotates up the L1 facet, as shown in **figure FSU** and **FSV**.

Figure FSR
Posterior view of L2-L1-T12 facets

Figure FSS
Right L1 facet

Stage three

Figure FSW illustrates the upward pull on the right side of the T12 facet when the person leans forward without change in side shift. The distorted T12 facet is dragged up the L1 right facet where it becomes firmly wedged. This is the final stage of the subluxation. **Figure FSX** illustrates T12 being forced to rotate right as the side-shift to the left buckles and side-bends T12 left. **Figure FSY** illustrates T12 subluxated approximately one third of the way up the L1 facet.

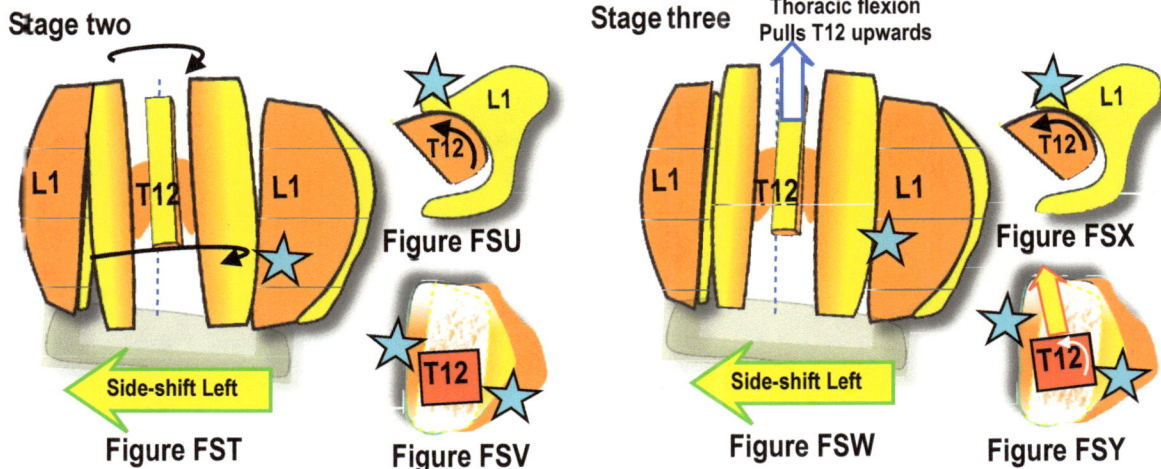

Stage two

Figure FSU

Figure FST

Figure FSV

Side-shift Left

Stage three

Thoracic flexion
Pulls T12 upwards

Figure FSX

Figure FSW

Figure FSY

Side-shift Left

Sacroiliac:
Flexion Subluxation to the Right

Figure FSZ is a photograph of the final stage of the T12 subluxation. T12 is rotated and side-bent to the right in thoracic extension.

The right transverse processes of L1 and T12 are posterior and the spinous processes are approximated.

The sacroiliac joint

Figure FSK illustrates the normal physiological movement of the sacroiliac joint when a person rotates to the right in flexion.

To briefly recap, when the left knee is flexed and body weight is taken on the left, the left anterior 'A' sacroiliac facets engage and the pelvis as a whole side-bends to the left.

Then, when pelvic side-shift to the left takes place the 'A' anterior facets compress and cause the pelvis to side-bend still further to the left, whilst causing the acetabulum and head of the femur to move anteriorly, medially and superiorly. Plus, the lumbar vertebrae are provided with the necessary side-shift they need to rotate to the right.

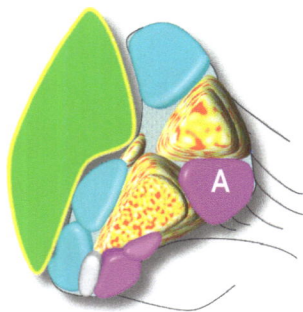

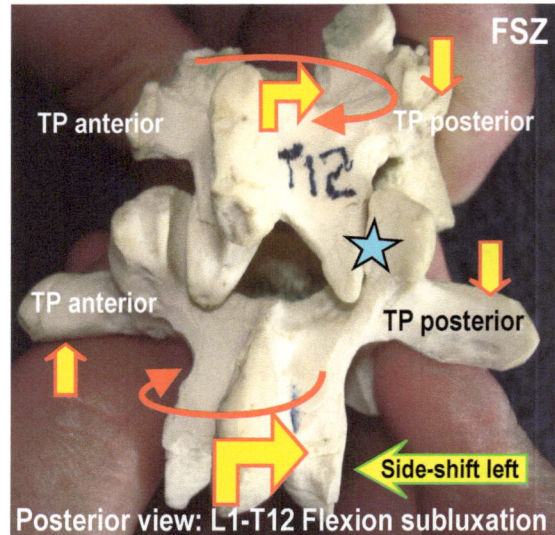

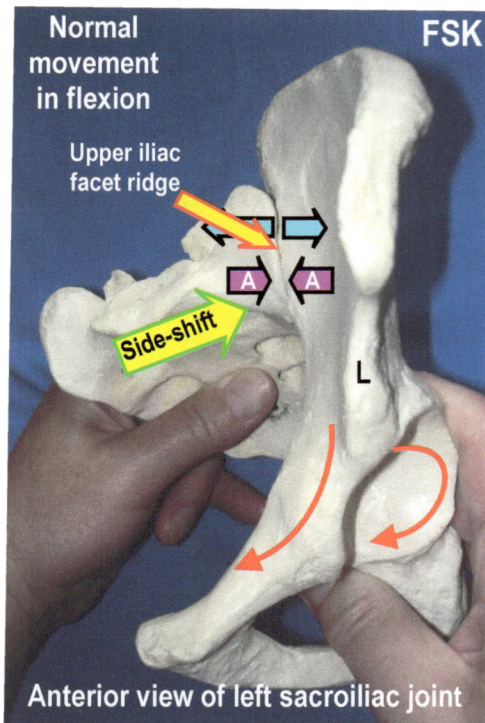

Sacroiliac:
Flexion Subluxation

The sacroiliac subluxation takes place if the left knee is kept straight. This prohibits the ilium and acetabulum from moving anteriorly, medially and superiorly. Therefore, when body weight is brought to bear on the left side of the pelvis against the left anterior 'A' sacroiliac facets, the sacral base continues to remain level.

When the hips sway to the left as shown in **figure FSL,** the left anterior 'A' sacroiliac facets become over compressed. Whilst conversely, the left posterior 'F' facets become over-separated. The left sacroiliac joint is thus destabilized.

Figure FSM shows the consequences when the person leans forward without changing the direction of side shift. Because L4-L3 and L2-L1 are subluxated, the lumbar vertebrae become locked and act like a forward bending lever that forces the base of the sacrum anteriorly. With the sacroiliac joint destabilized, the 'A' anterior sacroiliac facets act as a pivot that rotates the sacrum anteriorly over the upper facet ridge, and posteriorly over the iliac protuberance. Thus the sacrum is forced to ride up the anterior inferior edge of the iliac bony mass, as illustrated in **figure FSMa,** where it impacts fractionally above the iliac anterior protuberance and the anterior part of the posterior 'F' facet.

The subluxation is wedged firmly in place by bone against bone and reinforced by the ultra strong anterior and posterior sacroiliac ligaments. As a result the subluxations in the lumbar vertebrae above are permanently locked in. This subluxation is caused by the sacrum moving against the ilium therefore, the subluxation is classified as **sacroiliac**.

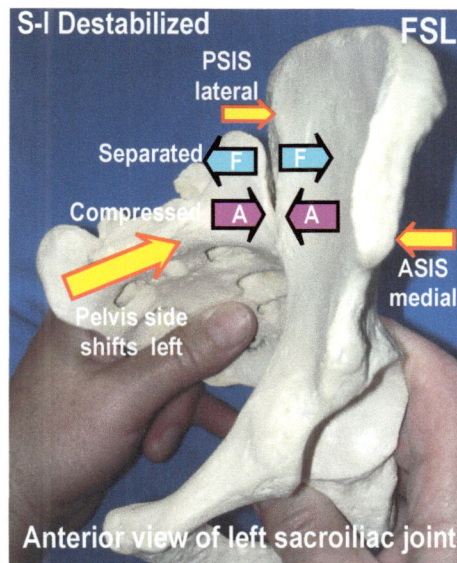

S-I Destabilized — FSL
PSIS lateral
Separated — F — F
Compressed — A — A
ASIS medial
Pelvis side shifts left
Anterior view of left sacroiliac joint

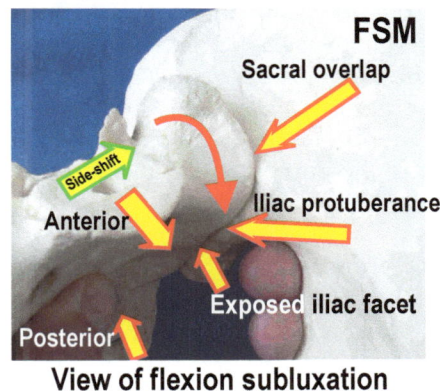

FSM
Sacral overlap
Side-shift
Anterior
Iliac protuberance
Exposed iliac facet
Posterior
View of flexion subluxation

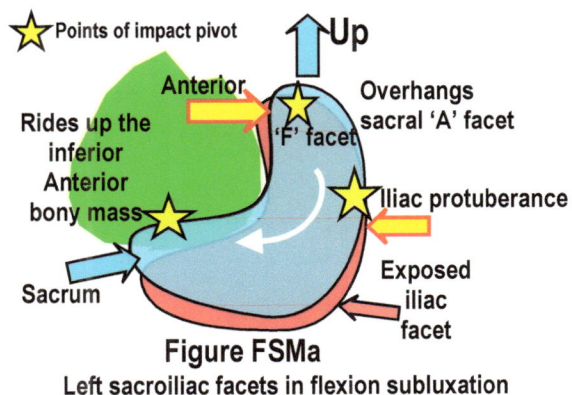

Points of impact pivot
Up
Anterior
Overhangs sacral 'A' facet
Rides up the inferior Anterior bony mass
'F' facet
Iliac protuberance
Sacrum
Exposed iliac facet

Figure FSMa
Left sacroiliac facets in flexion subluxation

Sacroiliac:
Flexion Subluxation

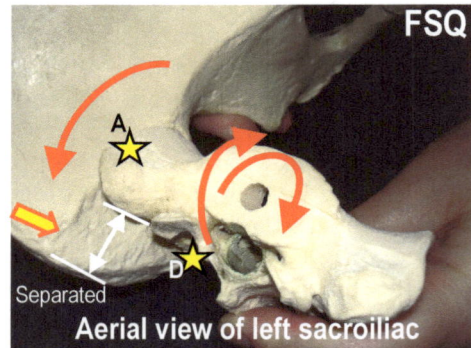

FSN Anterior view

Normal physiological movement

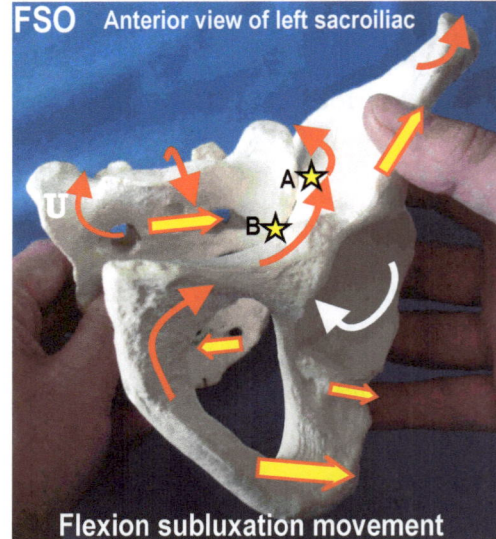

FSO Anterior view of left sacroiliac

Flexion subluxation movement

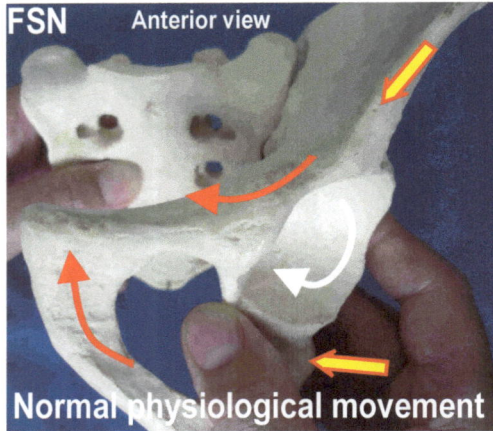

FSQ

Separated

Aerial view of left sacroiliac

For comparison purposes, **figure FSN** shows the direction of forces during normal physiological flexion. **Figure FSO** shows the buckled position of the left ilium and its affect on the angle of the acetabulum, pubic ramous and iliac crest in the flexion subluxation. The yellow stars show the points of impact. The upward arrow (U) shown in white on the right side of the sacral base denotes the minor upward tilt that takes place.

Figure FSQ shows the subluxated sacrum in relation to the ilium from above. Note that the base of the sacrum on the left side is anterior in relation to the left ilium and that the posterior superior iliac crest is medial.

Two stages take place simultaneously to create the flexion subluxation. To make it easier to understand, **figure FSQa** illustrates the two stages in blocks:

Stage one, the inferior part of the innominate is pushed outward to create side-bending to the left;

Stage two, the left innominate is forced posteriorly. It is important to remember that it is the sacrum that moves on the weight bearing ilium.

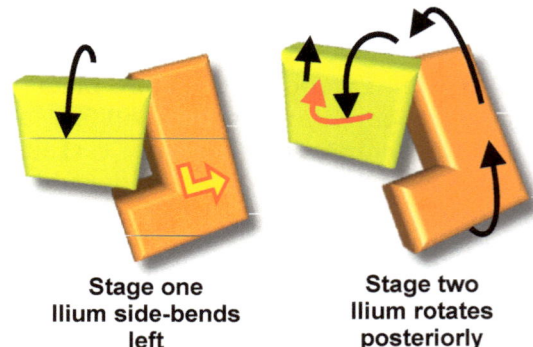

Stage one
Ilium side-bends left

Stage two
Ilium rotates posteriorly

**Figure FSQa
Anterior view of the left
sacroiliac subluxation**

Chapter Nine
Consequences of the
L3-Left-Right
Flexion Subluxation Pattern

In the last chapter it was shown how the left flexion subluxation caused the sacral 'A' facet to dislocate and impact over the anterior iliac ridge of the anterior 'A' facet, whilst simultaneously the sacral apex became forcibly levered posteriorly. This exposed the left anterior 'B' iliac facets and impacted the posterior sacral D' facets against the inferior iliac bony mass. This was shown in **figures FSO** and **FSQ** on page 100, and at facet level to the right in **figure FSMa**.

In relation to the subluxated displacement of the sacrum, the ilium is side-bent right and rotated posteriorly, as shown in **figure 9c**. As this is a sacroiliac subluxation, it is the sacrum that is incorrectly placed, as shown in **figure 9b**.

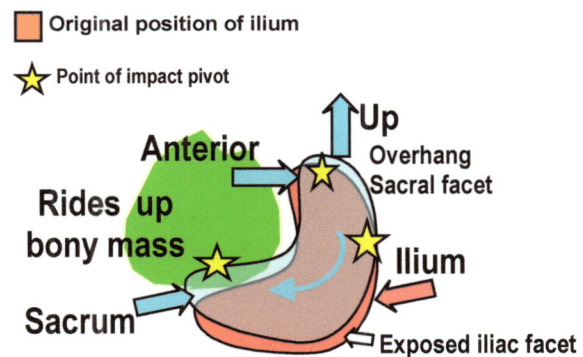

□ Original position of ilium

⭐ Point of impact pivot

Figure FSMa
Subluxated left sacroiliac facets

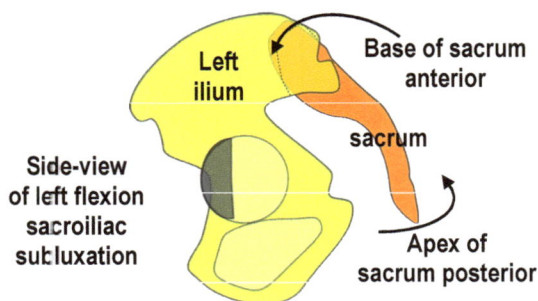

Figure 9b

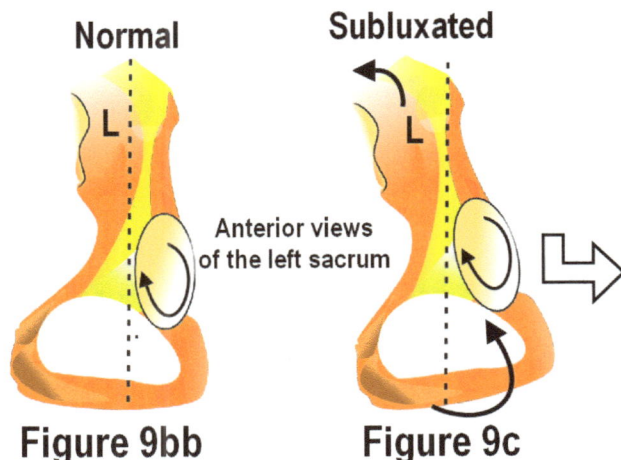

Figure 9bb   **Figure 9c**

101

Left Flexion Further Explanation

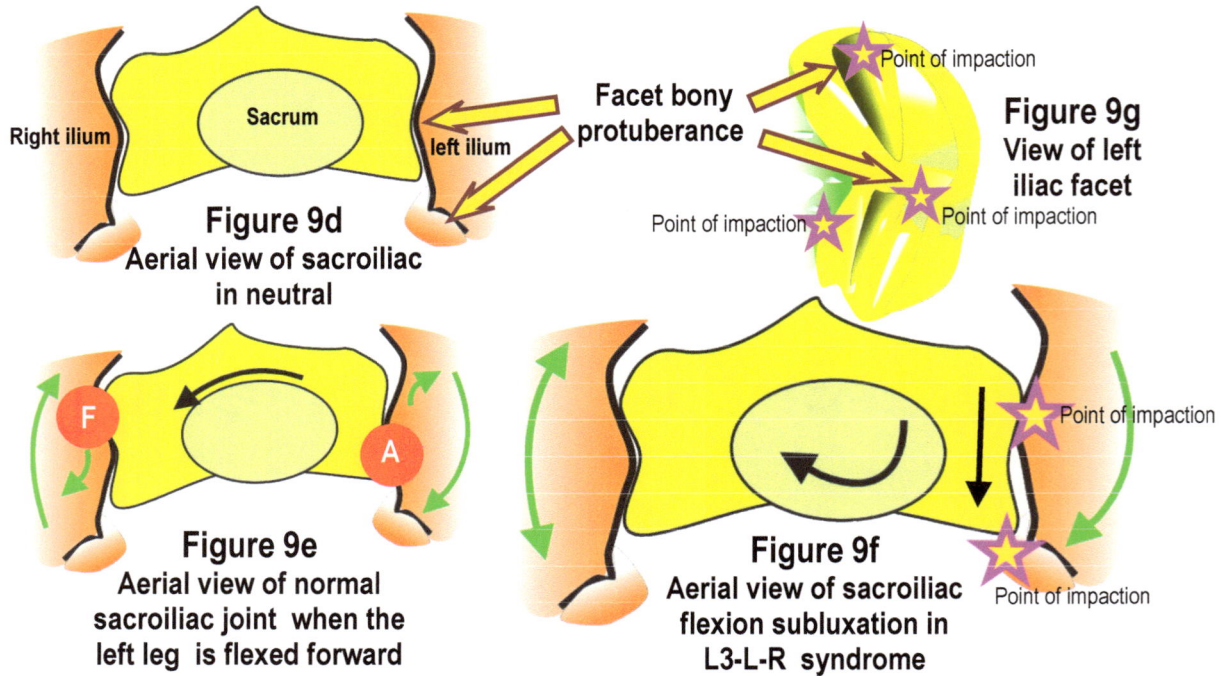

Figure 9d
Aerial view of sacroiliac
in neutral

Right ilium   Sacrum   left ilium

Facet bony
protuberance   Point of impaction

Figure 9g
View of left
iliac facet

Point of impaction   Point of impaction

Figure 9e
Aerial view of normal
sacroiliac joint when the
left leg is flexed forward

Figure 9f
Aerial view of sacroiliac
flexion subluxation in
L3-L-R syndrome

Point of impaction

Point of impaction

Above are aerial views of the sacroiliac joint for comparison. **Figure 9d** shows the joint in neutral, which is the normal standing position. **Figure 9e** shows the normal physiological facet contact when the left knee is flexed.

Figure 9f shows the impacted position of the sacrum when the left knee is kept straight in the flexion subluxation pattern described in the last chapter. The force levering the sacrum anteriorly, together with the weight bearing and side-shift on the left drag the left side of the sacrum over the left iliac facet. This causes it to impact against the bony protuberance, between the iliac facets 'F' and 'A' and half way down the anterior facet ridge. This is further illustrated in **figure 9g**. The compressed angle of the sacroiliac joint on the right side is in apparent alignment.

Figure 9h continues on from **figure 9b** on page 101 page and shows the consequences of the anteriorly rotated left sacrum. When the person straightens into an upright position the sacrum pulls the ilium back with it in a scooping action. It is this that causes the person to have an upright posture together with a loss in height.

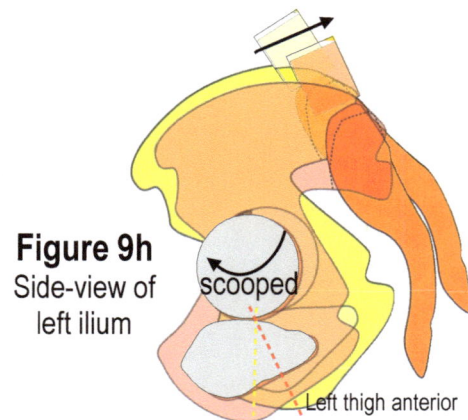

Figure 9h
Side-view of
left ilium

scooped

Left thigh anterior

Consequences:
Flexion Subluxation to the Right Ilium

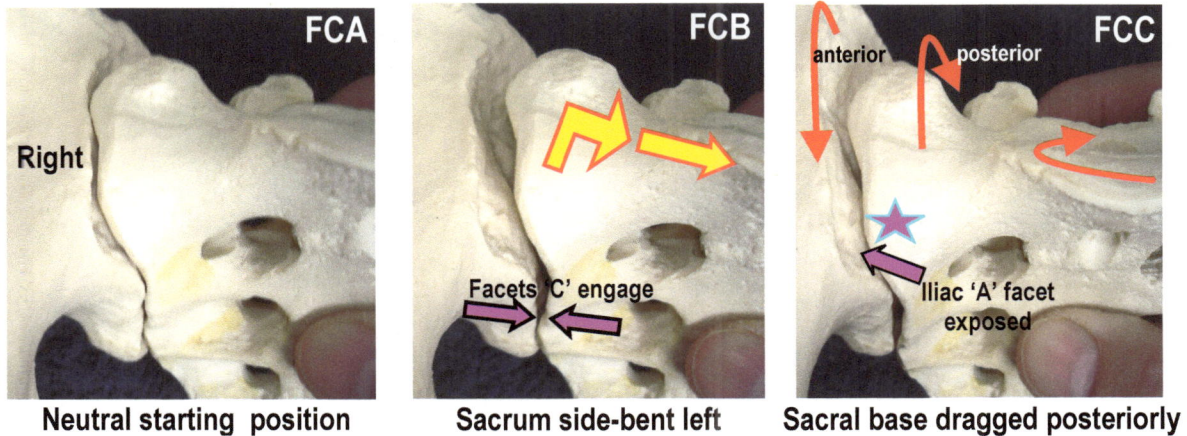

Neutral starting position

Sacrum side-bent left

Sacral base dragged posteriorly

Figure FCA is the neutral position for reference purposes. As the pelvic side-shift and weight-bearing begin to transfer to the right leg, the locked and defectively angled sacrum is prized away from the upper half of the iliac facets on the right, as shown in **figure FCB**. This creates a point of impacted pivot in the area of the anterior 'C' facets.

As side-shift continues to transfer to the right, the weight bearing ground resistance returning up the right leg rotates the acetabulum posteriorly, inferiorly and medially. Whilst at the same time, as the person straightens, the base of the sacrum

is drawn back as shown in **figure 9h** on the previous page. These two opposite forces tip the upper half of the ilium anteriorly and medially, as shown in **figure FCD**. It is this movement that forces the right superior anterior border of the right bony mass of the ilium to impact against the right posterior sacral 'F' facets, as shown in **figure FCC**.

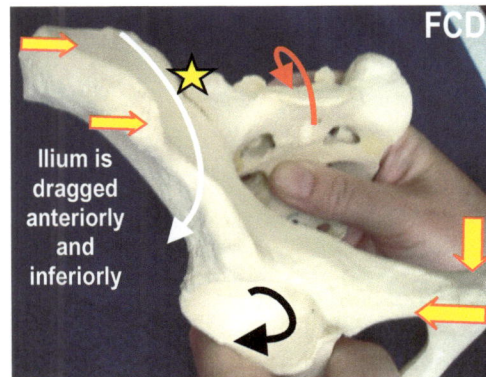

This is a **sacroiliac** subluxation.

Figure FCD shows the position of the right acetabulum and ilium. The acetabulum is inferior, medial and posterior and brings the right leg backwards. The anterior superior iliac spine is medial, anterior and inferior and the pubic tubercle is posterior, inferior and medial.

Illustrations:
Right Iliac Flexion Subluxation

Figure 9J shows the position of the right sacral facet as it rides up and impacts against the right superior bony mass of the ilium. Note that there are three points of impact pivot:

1) The anterior superior iliac bony mass

2) The mound between the 'A' anterior iliac facet and the 'F' posterior iliac facet.

3) The 'B' anterior iliac facet.

For clarity **figure 9K** illustrates how the edge of the sacrum becomes wedged behind the iliac bony protuberance. It is this that locks the subluxation in.

Figure 9L illustrates the position of the right innominate immediately after the flexion subluxation has taken place on the left.

Figure 9M illustrates the position of the ilium when the person leans backward in order to stand upright. The 'F' posterior facet of the sacrum is levered posteriorly over the 'F' posterior facet of the ilium into the bony mass.

The innominate is side-bent right and tipped anteriorly. This rotates the acetabulum posteriorly, medially and inferiorly and places the weight of the person standing on their right leg, on their toes.

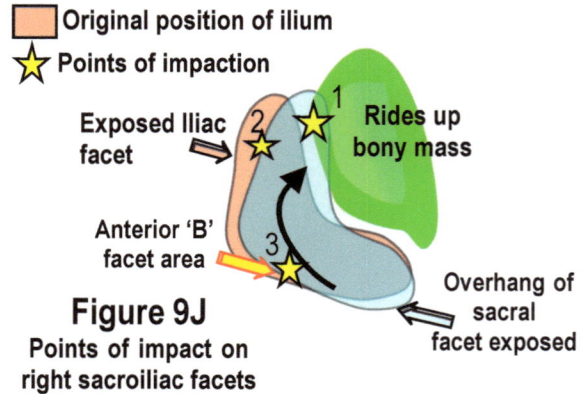

Original position of ilium
Points of impaction

Exposed Iliac facet

Rides up bony mass

Anterior 'B' facet area

Overhang of sacral facet exposed

Figure 9J
Points of impact on right sacroiliac facets

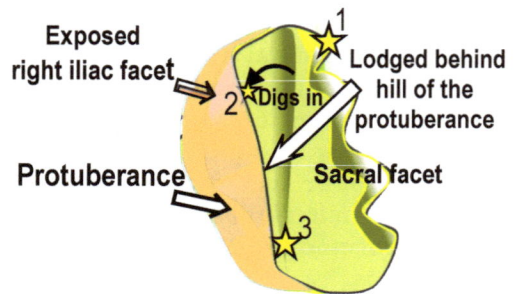

Exposed right iliac facet

Lodged behind hill of the protuberance

Digs in

Protuberance

Sacral facet

Figure 9K
Side-view showing the subluxated anterior right sacral facet wedged against the contours of the right iliac facet

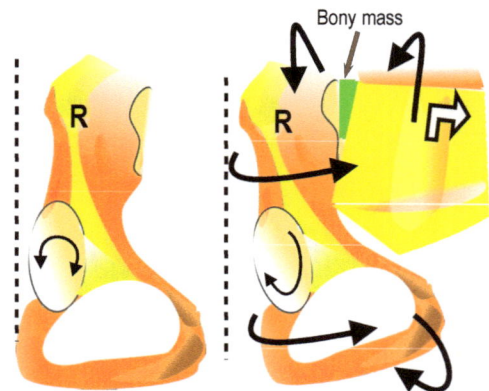

Bony mass

R

R

Figure 9L   **Figure 9M**

Anterior views, showing the effect the left flexion subluxated pattern has on the right

The Pelvis and Legs:
Right Flexion Subluxation

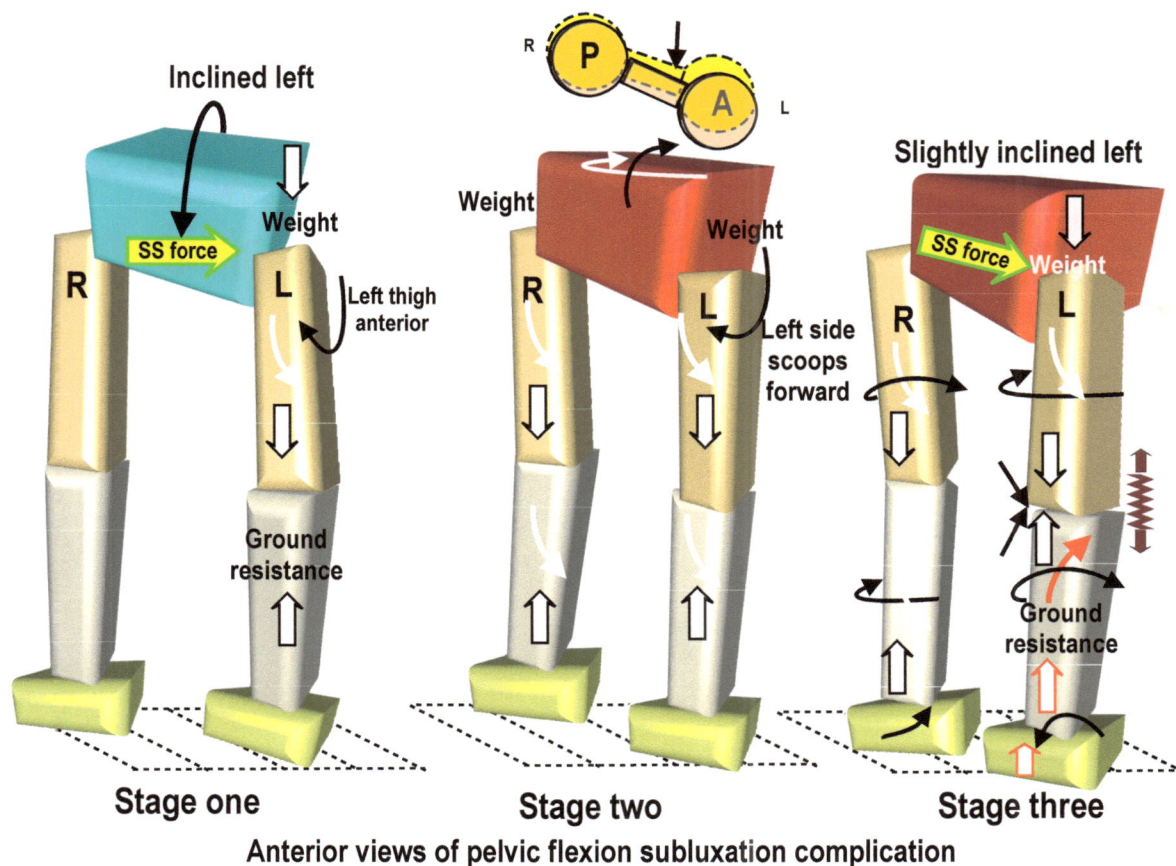

Anterior views of pelvic flexion subluxation complication

Stage one: is an illustration of the pelvis and legs just after a person has side-shifted left and lent forwards without bending their knees. It shows the left leg forward in accordance with flexion subluxations illustrated in **figures 9f and 9h** on page 102. This locks the person in forward leaning.

Stage two: As the person straightens, the left side of the pelvis is scooped forward to draw the sacrum backwards in order that the spine can remain upright. This causes the base of sacrum to move backwards and subluxate on the weight bearing right sacroiliac joint, as illustrated in **figures 9L** and **9M** on the previous page. The right knee becomes angled medially and posteriorly.

Stage three: Is an illustration of how the pelvis deals with the opposing forces. The left side of the pelvis is pushed further anteriorly and rotated to the right in an attempt to level the side-bending of the sacral base. In doing this the left knee is forced to flex anteriorly and laterally. As ground resistance travels back up the inside of the left leg the tibia is rotated externally and compressed medially.

Flexion Feet

Figure 9N shows the backward leaning posture the upper body takes in order to accommodate the angle of the pelvis. Notice how the upper thighs are angled anteriorly.

Figure 5 illustrates the effect the flexion subluxation pattern has on the feet. The position of the left foot is forward and pronated. Weight bearing is taken from the middle towards the front of the foot.

Figure 9p and **FCG** illustrate the mechanism whereby the pelvis side-shifts to the left and causes an upward force to drive up the left side of the torso. See also **figure IADa** on page 108.

In the left flexion subluxation pattern the sacral base side-bending is fairly minimal and therefore the amount of side-shift to the left to correct it means that the force applied upwards goes straight into the persons left shoulder/cervico-dorsal junction.

A person with the L3-left-right pattern will generally have relatively level shoulders though the area to the left side of T1 will be higher than the right.

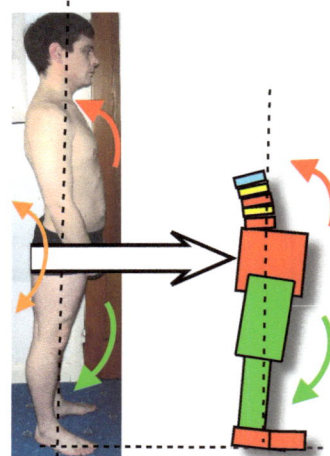

Figure 9N

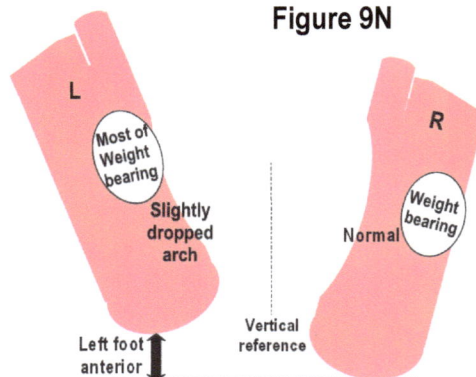

Figure 5
Typical flexion feet

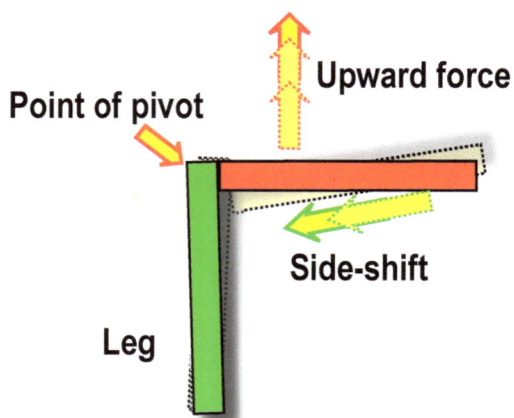

Figure 9p
Upward force

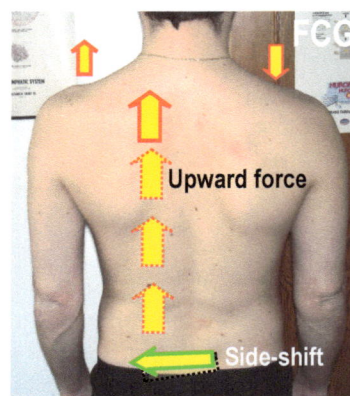

Lumbar Flexion Subluxation Pattern

All of the transverse processes are posterior on the right

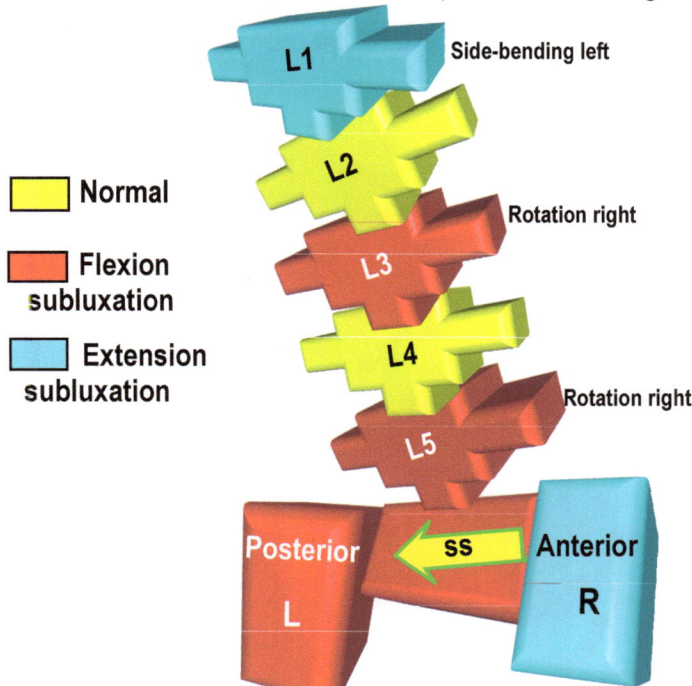

L1 — Side-bending left

L2

Rotation right

L3

L4

Rotation right

L5

Normal

Flexion subluxation

Extension subluxation

Posterior — L — ss — Anterior — R

Figure 6
Posterior view of lumbar
and sacroiliac joints

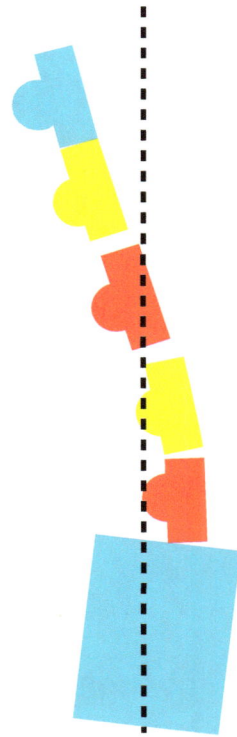

Figure 6a
Right side-view of lumbar
and sacroiliac joints

Putting all the subluxation elements of the lumbar and sacroiliac joints together, **figure 6** shows the theoretical lumbar vertebrae flexion subluxation pattern.   The flexion subluxations are in red.

Although L1 is backward bent, because the subluxation locked with side-bending and rotation to the right, (the same side) it is technically an extension subluxation.

Figure 6a provides a right side-view of the sacroiliac and lumbar joints. L1 is shown in backward bending, which is the angle it is seen and felt.

Finally, the side-bending left and the rotation right of the pelvis rotates L4 to the right against L3. In doing this the right superior facet of L4 becomes further compacted against the subluxated inferior right L3 facet. This double locks in the L3 subluxation.   For the same reason the L5 subluxation also becomes double locked. The further the base of the sacrum moves anteriorly the greater the torsion on L4.   This can make visual and palpable differentiation of L4-L3 very confusing, as it feels and looks as if L4-3 has side-bent right.

Lines of Upward Ground Force
Created by Side-Shift

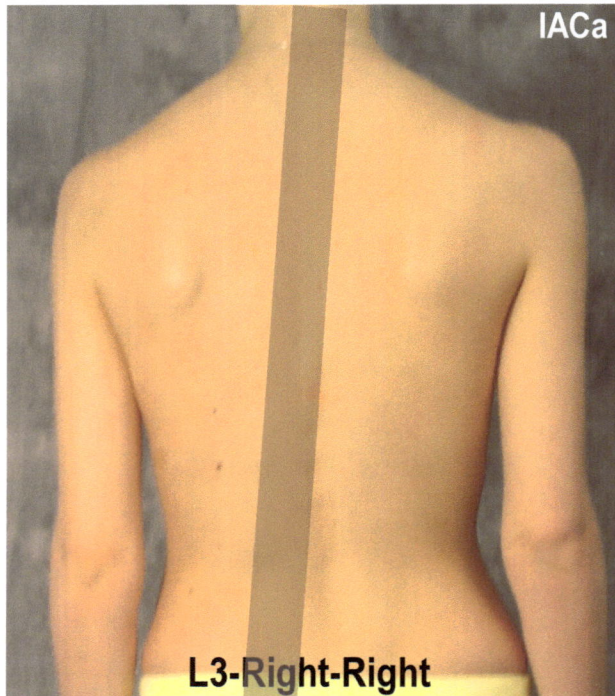

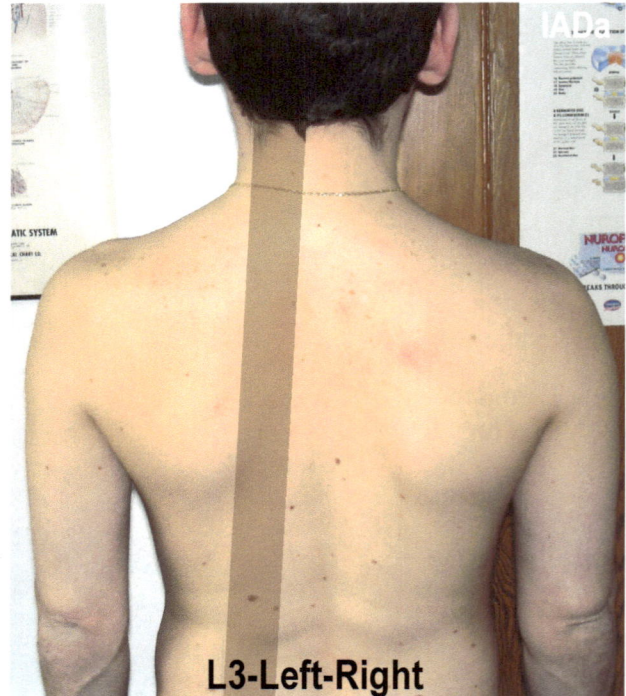

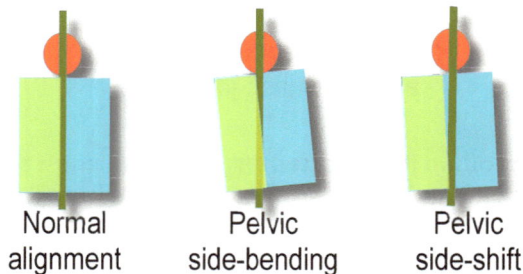

IACa

L3-Right-Right

IADa

L3-Left-Right

Normal alignment	Pelvic side-bending	Pelvic side-shift

Figure IACb
L3-right-right

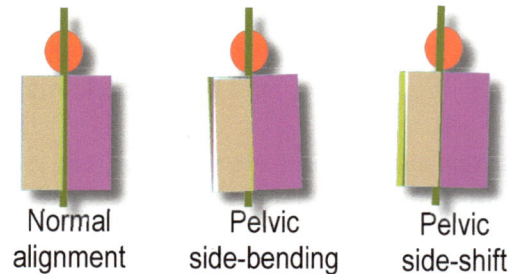

Normal alignment	Pelvic side-bending	Pelvic side-shift

Figure IADb
L3-left-right

Figures IACa and **IADa** show the two subluxation pattern models for comparison with the lines of returning ground force drawn in over their spines. See pages 106 and 124.

In the L3-right-right pattern the pelvic side-bending and therefore side-shift is more exaggerated than that seen in the L3-left-right pattern. With such excessive side-shift to compensate for, the line of returning ground force has to cross over to the right side of the cervico-dorsal junction at approximately T3.

The illustrations in **figures IACb** and **IADb** show how the mechanism of how these lines of returning ground force established themselves.

Chapter Ten
L3-Right-Right
Extension Subluxations
of the Lower Back

Subluxation patterns are created when backward leaning is forced on a forward leaning spine, without change in rotation, weight bearing and side-shift.

Figure 2 is an illustration of the hypothetical forces placed on the lumbar and sacroiliac joints in extension (forward leaning), with rotation to the right.

It can be seen that L3 takes the maximum bending and stress and that the secondary areas of stress are taken at L2-L1 and the right sacroiliac joint. L3-L4 is therefore the area of prime torsion.

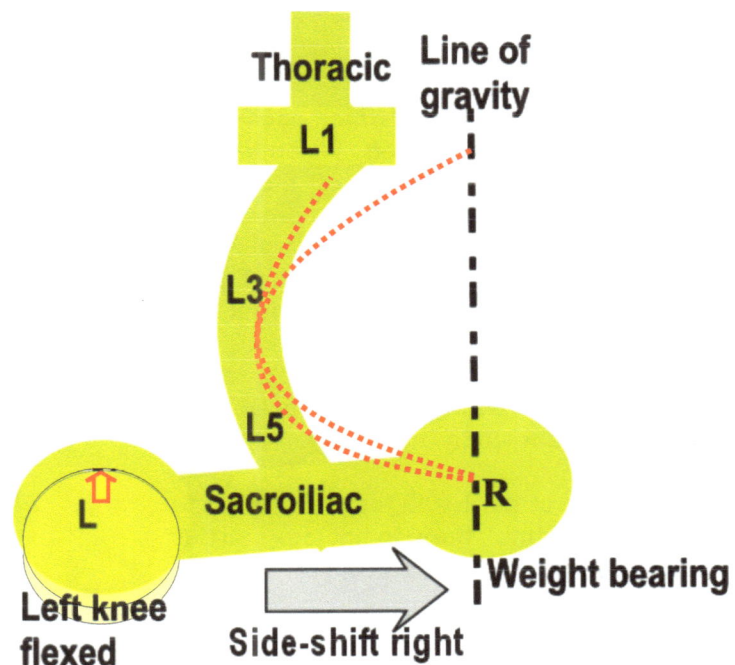

Figure 2

Extension Lower Back Rules

Below is a recap on how normal rotation to the right is performed in forward bending. When a person is standing or leaning forward and rotates to the right, these movements take place:

The left knee flexes and the pelvis side-bends left.

The body weight is taken on the right side of the pelvis.

The right posterior 'F' sacroiliac facets engage, which angles the right acetabulum and head of the femur posteriorly, laterally and inferiorly.

Ground resistance travels up the right leg and pushes the head of the femur superiorly.

The pelvis becomes elevated, which partially levels and rotates to the pelvis right.

The lumbar vertebrae follow the movement of the pelvis and rotate to the right.

The pelvic side-shift to the right aligns the lumbar facets for extension side-bending to follow.

It was shown that the L4-L3 joint is the primary area of torsion. To fully recap on the normal physiological movement of the lumbar vertebrae, refer to chapter four.

Briefly, the left knee is flexed, which causes the facets of L4-L3 to side-bend left. When weight is directed through the right side of the pelvis the pelvis becomes level and automatically rotates to the right and takes the lumbar vertebrae in the same direction, as shown in **figure LN**. The pelvis then side-shifts to the right and this forces L4 to move in the same direction. The counter force from above levers the left facets of L3 to bank up the left L4 facets and causes L3 to side-bend left, as shown in **figure LO**.

If the movements of the L4-L3 joint are taken to their physiological limit, they do not lock, so this is not how the joint subluxates.

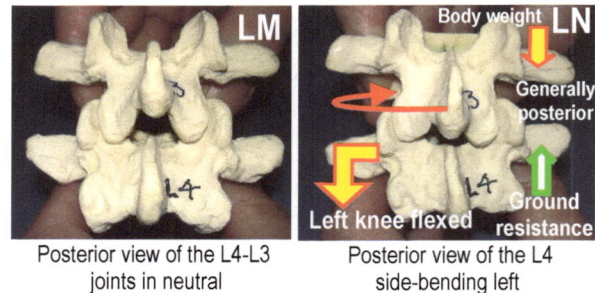

Posterior view of the L4-L3 joints in neutral

Posterior view of the L4 side-bending left

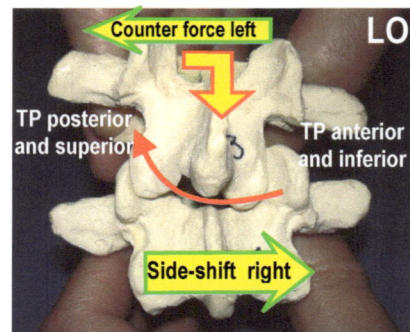

Posterior view of the L4 side-side-shifting right

110

L4-L3:
Extension Subluxation to the Right

If the left knee is not flexed for reasons of lack of space or bad practice and weight is placed on the right side, the pelvis cannot rotate to the right. Thus the left facets of L4-L3 are not rotated to the right and aligned in readiness for extension side-bending to follow. This incorrect starting point is shown in **figure ESA** along with the forward leaning that takes place.

Figure ESB shows when the pelvis side-shifts to the right and L4 is dragged in the same direction. The L3 facets are forced across the facets of L4 where they impact into the side of the left L4 facet. With weight still on the right side, the joint tends to side-bend slightly and buckle to the right.

If the pelvic side-shift to the right is maintained and the person straightens as shown in **figure ESC**, the thoracic vertebrae act as a long lever and force the left hand facet of L3 inferiorly on the left L4 facet and impact further. The more the person straightens the tighter the subluxation.

The illustrations in the bottom left side corners of the photographs are of the left L3 facet trajectory. The 'body' in the top left hand corners shows the degree of rotation. Whilst there is some degree of side-bending right there is no rotation in the extension subluxation. However, there could be a minimal amount of rotation left.

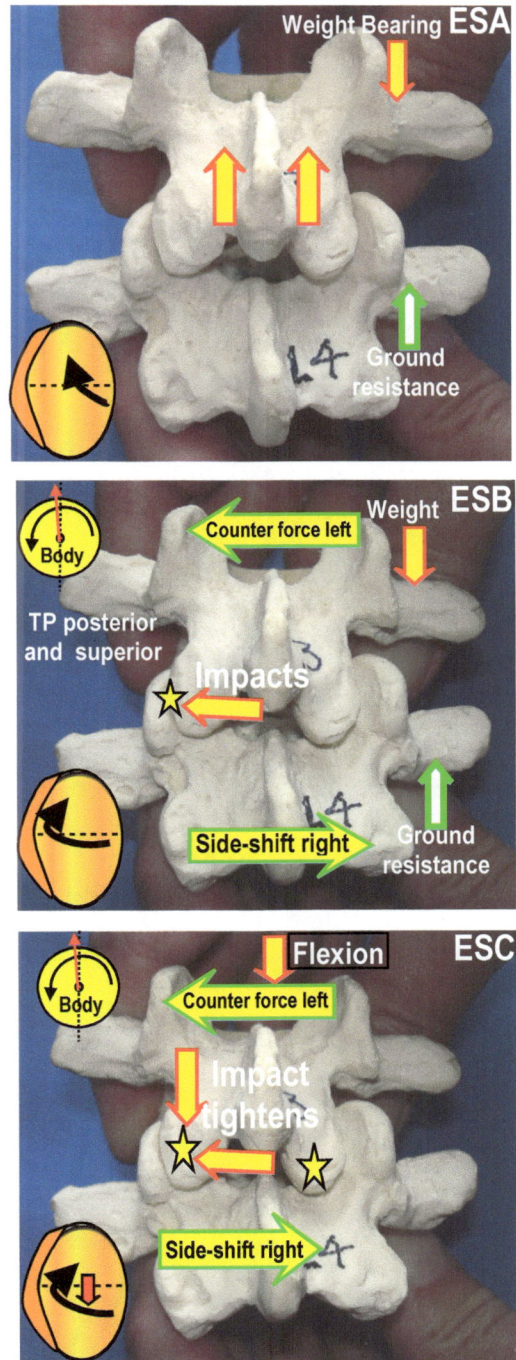

111

L4-L3 Subluxation Vs Normal Rotation

A practical example of this type of subluxation occurs when a standing person keeps their legs straight and bends forward as they side-shift their pelvis right and rotate their torso to the right. If the person then straightens, whist continuing to keep their pelvic side-shift and torso rotation to the right the sacroiliac and spinal joints lock on each other and subluxate.

Commonly this type of action can be traced to people who dig or shovel incorrectly or lift when rotated in a tight space.

Figure ESD is an exaggeration of the normal extension rotation to the right movement and is shown for comparison against the subluxated version shown in **figure ESC.**

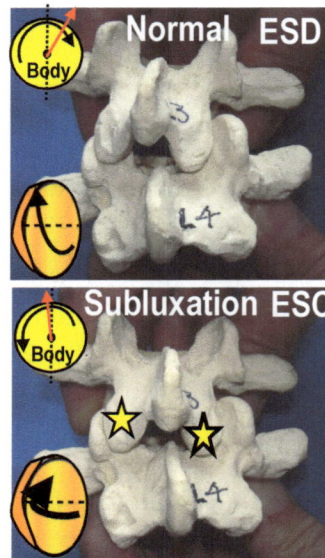

The forces that are placed on L4-L3 are also placed on L2-L1 and the sacroiliac joint. So let's look at the L2-L1 joint next. To briefly recap on the normal physiological movement of the L2-L1 joint, L1 acts as a counter lever in the vertical position during lumbar rotation movements. When the left knee flexes, L2 follows the pelvic side-bending. However, the weight bearing down the right side of the body meets the upward ground resistance at the pelvis and counters this side-bending to a point. L1-L2 rotate right along with the pelvis and the combination of this movement positions the left L2 facet just below the upper part of the left L1 facet, as shown in **figure ESD**.

When the pelvis side-shifts to the right, it fully levels the pelvis and side-shifts L2 in the same direction. This causes L2 to side-bend right and engage against the level left L1 facet. This is shown in **figure ESDa.** If these movements are taken to their physiological limit, they do not lock; therefore this is not how the L2-L1 joint becomes subluxated in extension to the right.

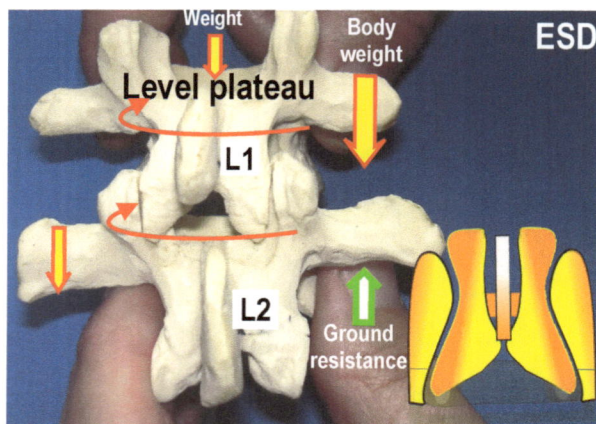

General rotation right

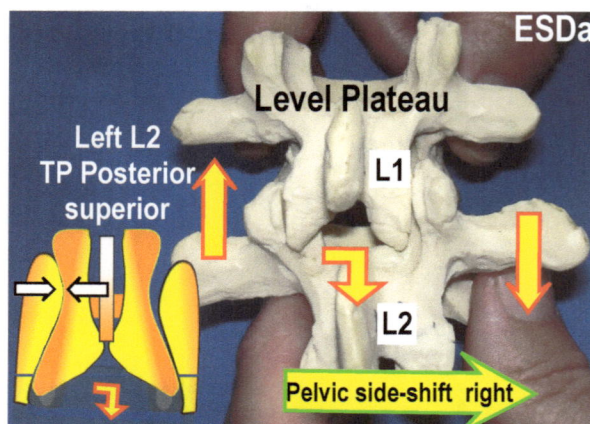

L2 side-bends right and L1 remains level

L2-L1:
Extension Subluxation to the Right

If the left knee is not flexed and the body weight is taken on the right leg, no lumbar side-bending to the left or pelvic rotation to the right can take place. Due to the weight bearing on the right, the left facets of L2 become marginally side-bent right. This is an incorrect starting point and is shown **figures ESE** and **ESEa**. See **figures LBB** and **LBBa** on page 51 for comparison.

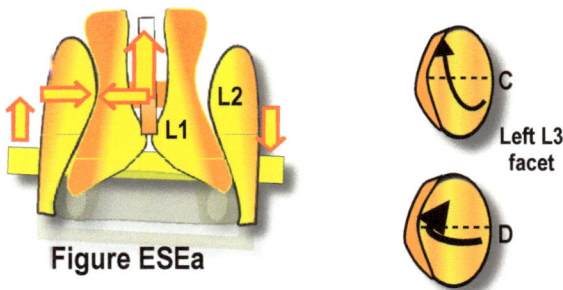

Figure ESEa

Left L3 facet

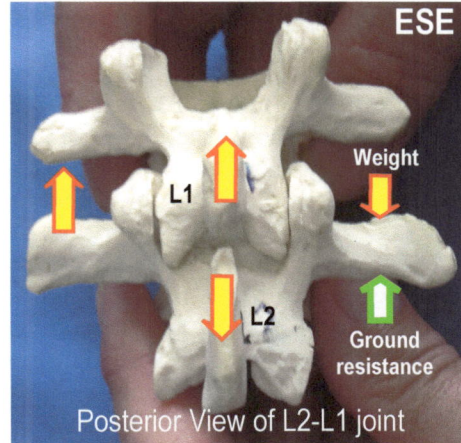

ESE

Weight

Ground resistance

Posterior View of L2-L1 joint

Figure ESG and **ESGa** show L2 following the pelvic side-shift right. *A reminder of what happened at L3 below. The left facet of L3 should have side-bent in an arc, as shown in 'C' above but it subluxated and side-bent as shown 'D' without arcing.* This has the knock-on effect of stopping the facets of L1 from following the side-bending arc of L3 and sliding smoothly up the L2 facet. As L2 side-bends right the left facet of L1 becomes wedged against the L2 facet as shown in **figure ESGb**. Because the left facet of L2 cannot move up the left facet of L1, L1 is forced to side-bend left as shown in **figure ESGa**.

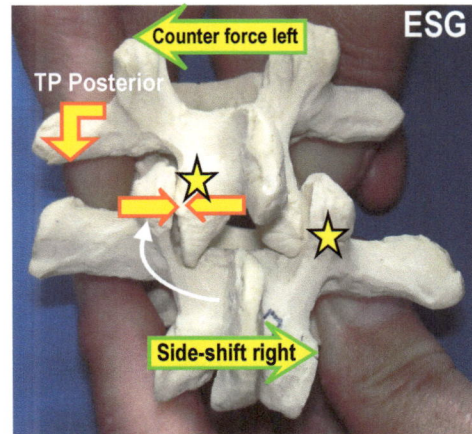

ESG

Counter force left

TP Posterior

Side-shift right

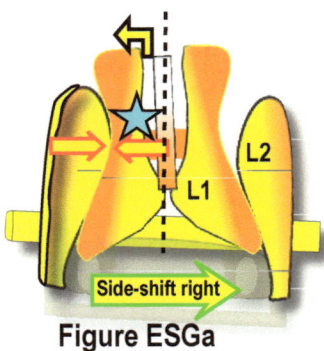

Side-shift right

Figure ESGa

L1 wedged

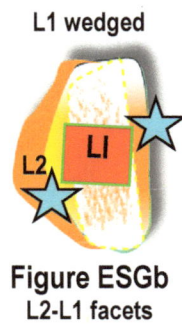

Figure ESGb
L2-L1 facets

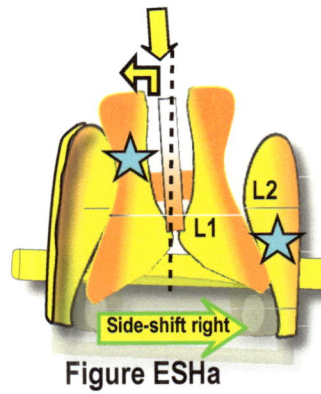

Side-shift right

Figure ESHa

L1 wedge and buckles

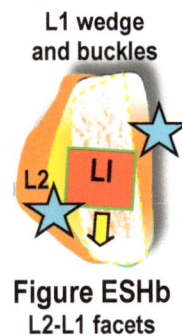

Figure ESHb
L2-L1 facets

L2-L1:
Extension Subluxation to the Right

Continuing on from the previous page **figure ESGb** showed how the L1 facet got wedged just over halfway up the left L2 facet and caused a minor subluxation. This subluxation is further compounded when the person leans backwards without changing the direction of side-shift. The thoracic column levers the facets of L1 inferiorly as shown on the previous page in **figures ESHa** and **ESHb**. As the misaligned left facet of L1 gets dragged inferiorly, the joint buckles. The force caused by the side-shift to the right, side-bends the destabilized L1 vertebra to the left. A photograph of the final stage of this subluxation is shown in **figure ESH**.

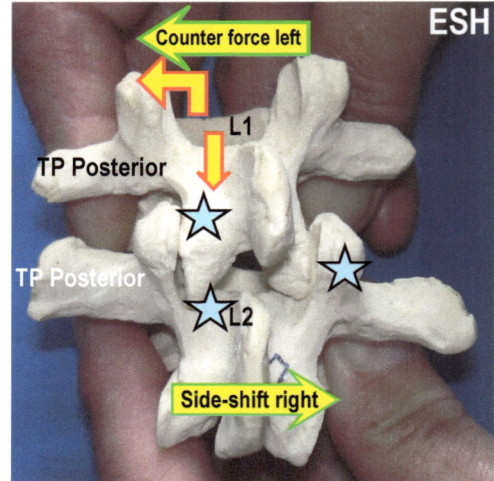

The L1-T12 joint

As was explained in chapter four, in normal physiological lumbar extension, side-shift passes to the right of L1. This provides T12 along with all the thoracic vertebrae above with the ability to rotate. This side-shift is not blocked in the subluxated lumbar vertebrae.

For reference, **figures LCH** and **LCHa** show the L1-T12 joint in neutral.

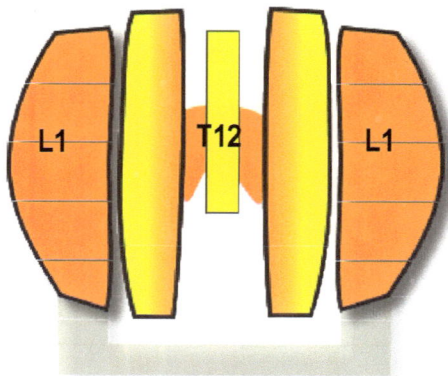

Figure LCHa
L1-T12 in neutral

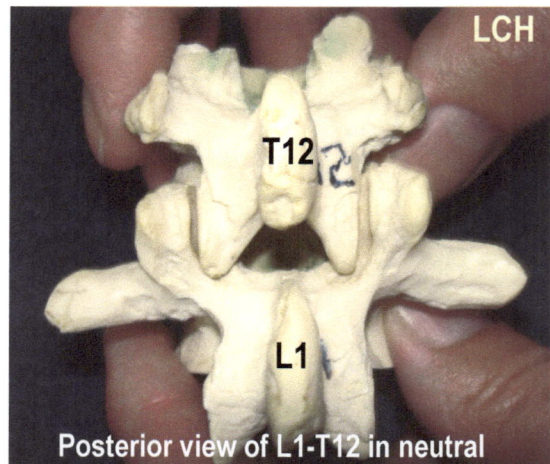

Posterior view of L1-T12 in neutral

L1-T12:
Extension Subluxation to the Right

Stage one

In thoracic flexion, (forward bending) T12 separates with L1. **Figure ESF** illustrates the subluxated angles of the L1 facets. It can be seen that the rotation and side-bending to the left by the inferior L1 facets is reflected in the superior L1 facets. The superior facets of L1 do not touch the T12 facets, as shown in **figure ESFa.** However, this is an incorrect starting point for T12 to rotate left.

Stage two

Figure EFSb illustrates the next stage when pelvic side-shift forces L1 to the right. As L1 side-shifts to the right the inferior part of the left L1 facet engages against the inferior part of the left T12 facet. As side-shift continues, T12 buckles and rotates up the L1 facet, as shown in **figures EFSc** and **EFSd**.

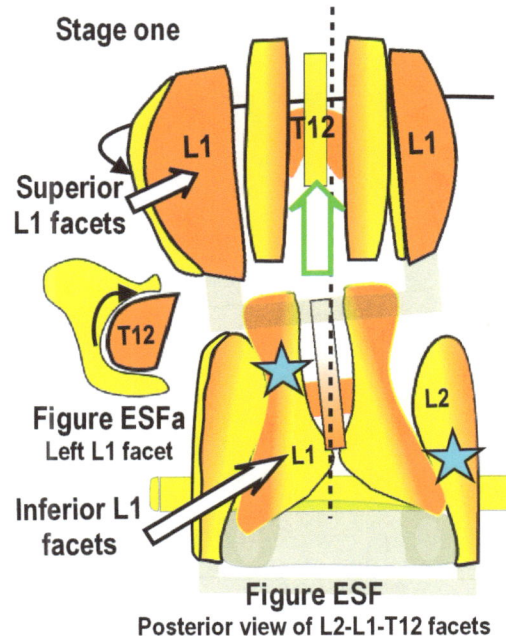

Figure ESF
Posterior view of L2-L1-T12 facets

Stage three

Figure ESFe illustrates the downward thrust on the left side of the T12 facet when the person leans backwards without change in side shift. The distorted T12 facet is dragged down the L1 right facet where it becomes more firmly wedged. This is the final stage of the subluxation. **Figure ESFf** illustrates T12 being forced to rotate left as the side-shift right buckles and side-bends T12 left. **Figure FSY** illustrates T12 subluxated one third of the way up the L1 facet.

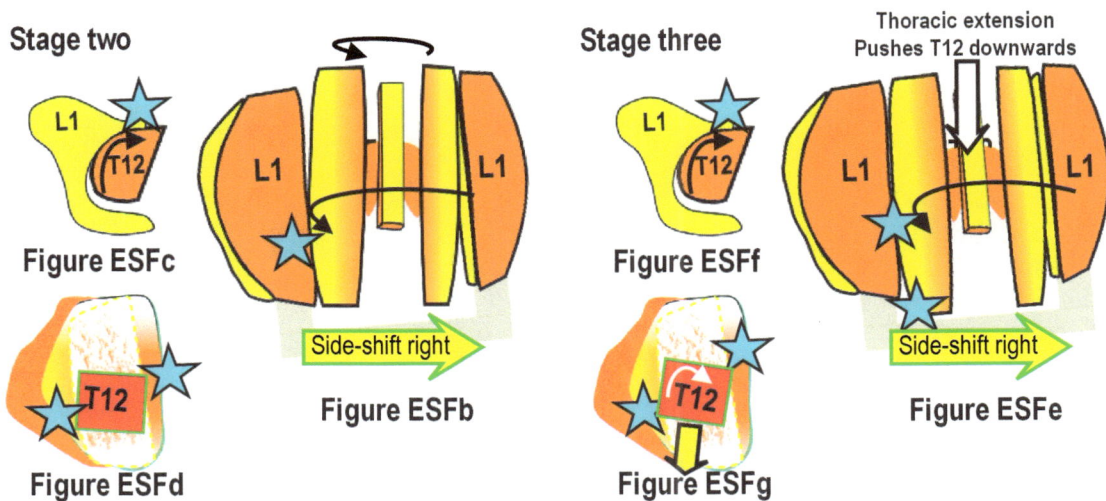

Sacroiliac:
Extension Subluxation to the Right

Figure ESJ is a photograph of the final stage of the T12 subluxation. T12 is rotated and side-bent to the left in thoracic flexion.

The left transverse processes of L1 and T12 are posterior and the spinous processes are separated.

Sacroiliac extension rotation right

Figure ESK illustrates the normal physiological movement of the sacroiliac joint when a person rotates to the right in extension.

To briefly recap, when the left knee is flexed and body weight is taken on the right, the right posterior 'F' sacroiliac facets engage and the whole pelvis rotates to the right.

Then, when pelvic side-shift to the right takes place the 'F' posterior facets compress and cause the pelvis to rotate still further to the right, whilst causing the acetabulum and head of the femur to move posteriorly, laterally and inferiorly. Plus, the lumbar vertebrae are provided with the necessary side-shift they need to side-bend to the right.

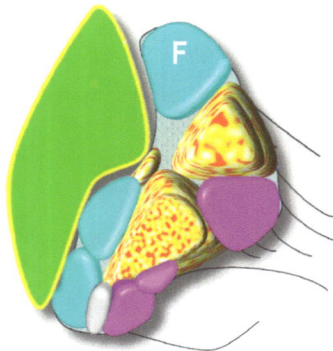

Posterior view:
Extension subluxation at L1-T12

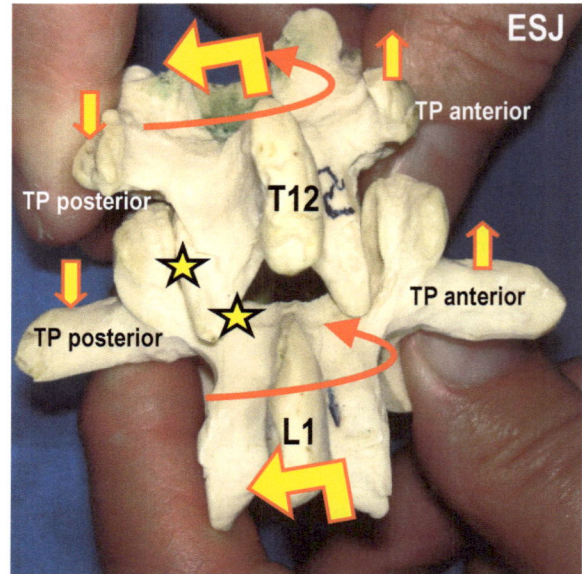

Anterior view of right sacroiliac joint

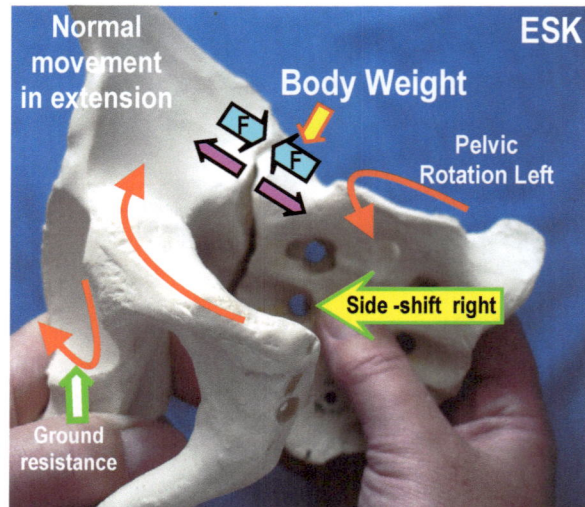

116

Sacroiliac:
Extension Subluxation to the Right

The sacroiliac subluxation takes place if the left knee is kept straight. This prohibits the ilium and acetabulum from moving superiorly, laterally and posteriorly. So when the body weight is brought to bear on the right side of the pelvis against the right posterior 'F' sacroiliac facets, the sacral base continues to remain level.

When the hips sway to the right as shown in figure **ESM,** the right posterior 'F' sacroiliac facets become over-compressed. Whilst, conversely, the right anterior 'A' sacroiliac facets become over-separated. The right sacroiliac joint is thus destabilized.

Figure ESN shows the consequences when the person leans backwards without changing the direction of side shift. Because L4-L3 and L2-L1 are subluxated, the lumbar vertebrae become locked and act like a backward bending lever that forces the base of the sacrum posteriorly. With the sacroiliac joint destabilized, the 'F' anterior sacroiliac facets act as a pivot that rotates the sacrum posteriorly under the upper facet ridge, and anteriorly over the medial iliac protuberance.

The sacrum is forced to ride up the anterior superior edge of the iliac bony mass, as per the illustration in **figure ESNa** where it impacts just under the iliac anterior protuberance and the anterior part of the posterior 'E' facet.

The subluxation is wedged firmly in place by bone against bone and reinforced by the ultra-strong anterior and posterior sacroiliac ligaments. As a result the subluxations in the lumbar vertebrae above are permanently locked in. This subluxation is caused by the sacrum moving against the ilium therefore, the subluxation is classified as **sacroiliac**.

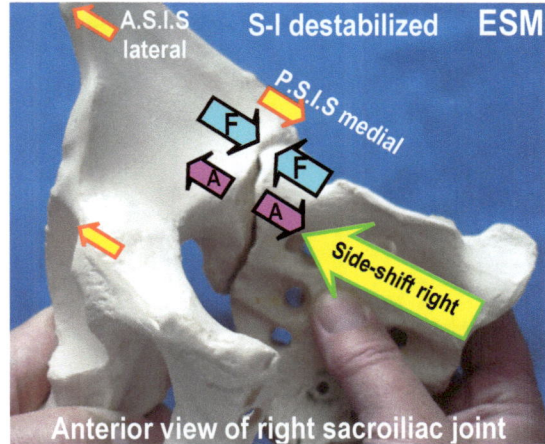

Anterior view of right sacroiliac joint

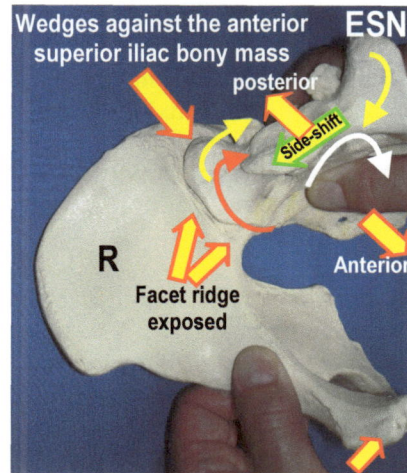

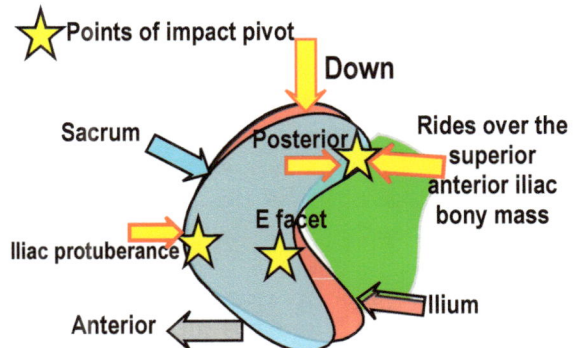

Figure ESNa
Right sacroiliac facets in extension subluxation

Sacroiliac:
Extension Subluxation to the Right

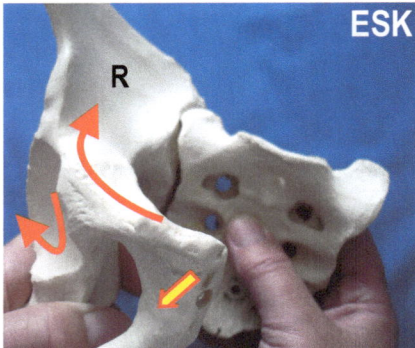

Normal physiological movement

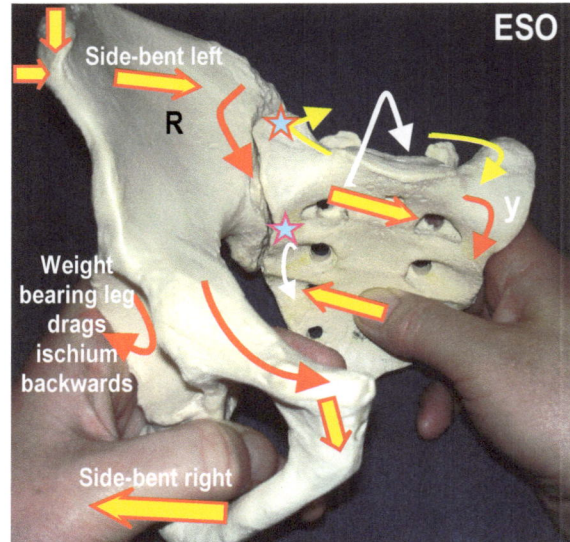

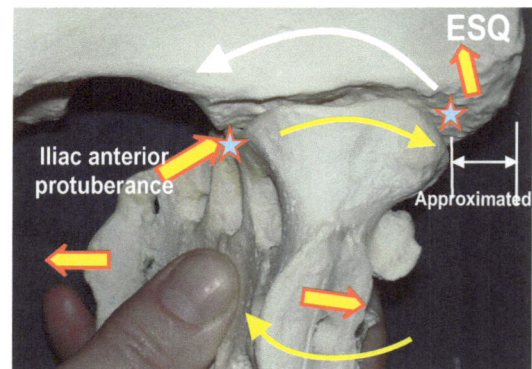

For comparison purposes, **figure ESK** shows the direction of forces during normal physiological extension. **Figure ESO** shows the buckled position of the right ilium and its affect on the angle of the acetabulum, pubic ramous and iliac crest in the extension subluxation. The blue stars show the points of impact. The downward arrow (y) shown in white on the left side of the sacral base denotes the minor downward tilt that takes place.

Figure ESQ shows the subluxated sacrum in relation to the ilium from above. The base of the sacrum on the right side is posterior in relation to the right ilium and the posterior superior iliac crest lateral.

Two stages take place simultaneously to create the extension subluxation. To make it easier to understand **figure ESQa** illustrates the two stages in blocks:

Stage one, the base of the sacrum subluxates posteriorly and causes the right innominate to rotate to the left, and;

Stage two, the sacrum rides up the right anterior iliac protuberance and side-bends the inferior part of the ilium, left. The sacrum subluxates against the weight bearing ilium.

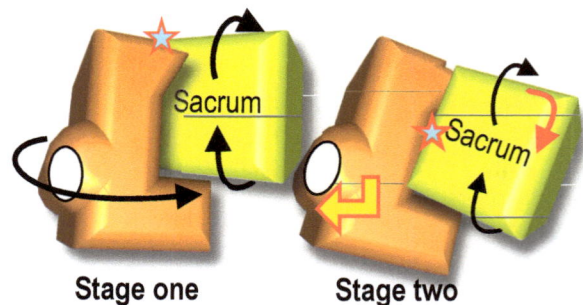

Stage one   Stage two

Figure ESQa
Anterior view of right sacroiliac extension subluxation

Chapter Eleven
Consequences of the Lower Back
L3-Right-Right
Extension Subluxation Pattern

In the last chapter it was shown how the right posterior sacroiliac subluxation caused the sacral base to rotate posteriorly and the apex anteriorly, as shown in **figure CSEA.**

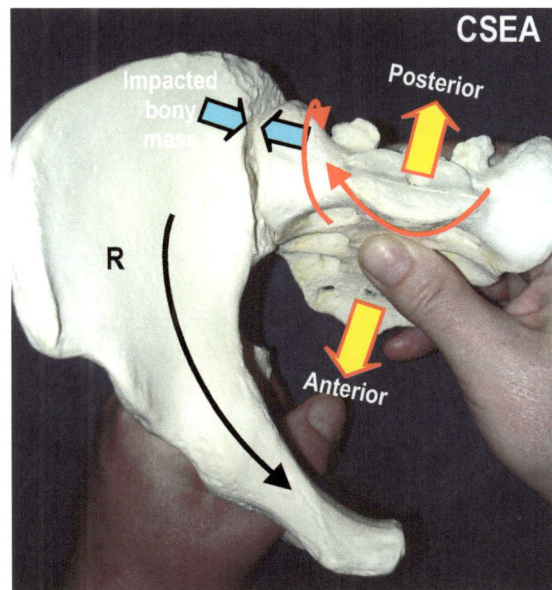

Because the base of the sacrum became locked posteriorly by the right sacroiliac joint, the left non subluxated ilium was forced to rotate posteriorly. This lifted the left leg anteriorly as shown in **figure 9b**.

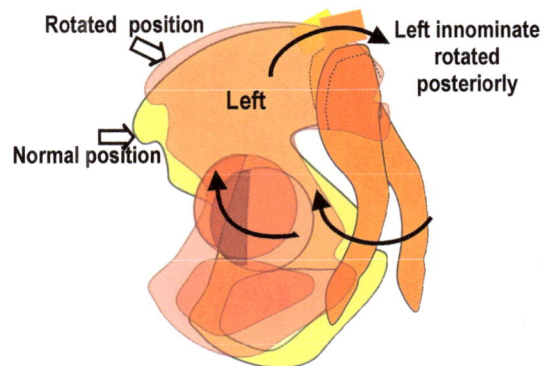

Figure 9b

Extension Subluxation Pattern
from Right to Left Ilium

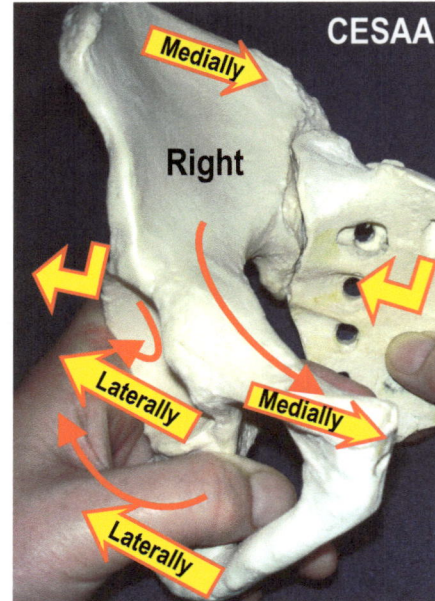

In the right extension subluxation, the posterior 'F' sacral facet impacted against the superior anterior bony mass of the ilium. This caused the superior half of the innominate to distort and rotate medially, whilst the inferior half moved laterally. This distortion is shown in **figures CESAA** and **9BA.**

A further consequence of the right sacroiliac extension subluxation is that the sacrum becomes side-bent left as shown in **figure 9BB** and **figure CESBB** on the next page. This has the effect of buckling the inferior part of the left ilium medially.

There is yet another consequence of the right sacroiliac subluxation. Because the sacrum is rotated right and not left as in the normal physiological movement, the left 'F' sacroiliac facets are levered into engagement. This is illustrated in **figures 9BA** and **CESB**.

In summary the distorted pelvis as a whole is side-bent right and rotated left.

Because at this point the left posterior 'F' sacroiliac facets are not weight bearing and side-shift to the left has not taken place, no subluxation is present yet.

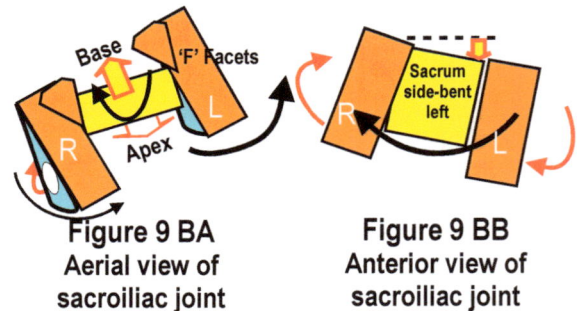

Figure 9 BA
Aerial view of sacroiliac joint

Figure 9 BB
Anterior view of sacroiliac joint

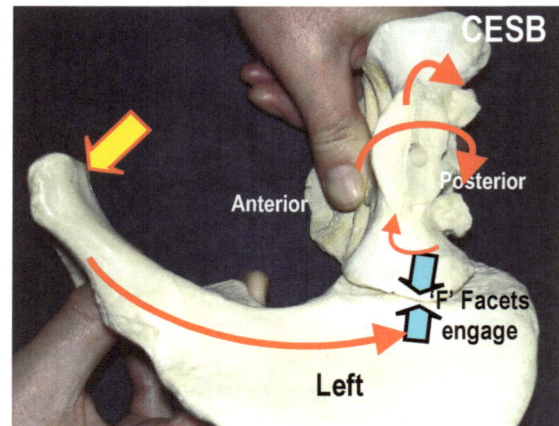

120

Forces on Left Ilium:
Extension Subluxation Pattern

Figure 9C recaps on the starting point where the left innominate and leg are generally tilted posteriorly by the base of the sacrum.

Figure CESBB is an aerial view of the left ilium at this same point. The acetabulum is rotated posteriorly, superiorly and laterally, as would occur in the normal physiology when the 'F' posterior sacroiliac facets engaged. However, because the sacrum is side-bent left, the innominate is also forced to side-bend left. This causes the acetabulum to buckle medially. At this point even though the sacrum and ilium are distorted, there is no subluxation on the left.

As the person straightens the sacral base is levered anteriorly and weight is brought to bear on the left sacroiliac joint and leg. This is illustrated in **figure 9Ca**.

As ground resistance returns up the left leg the acetabulum is lifted superiorly, which causes the innominate to rotate posteriorly. This is illustrated in **figure 9Cb**.

The forces shown in **figure CESSBC,** cause the left sacral 'F' posterior facet to be dragged anteriorly over the 'F' posterior iliac facet, where it impacts and subluxates against the superior iliac protuberance. This action prizes the anterior sacral facets away from the anterior iliac facets and causes the left innominate to buckle and side-bend to the right but not enough to counter the overall side-bending left. Simultaneously, the sacral 'D' posterior facet impacts against the inferior anterior bony mass.

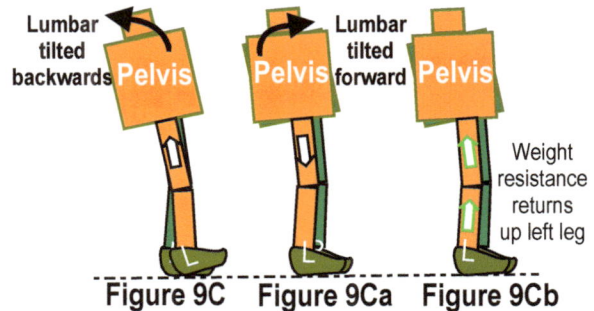

Lumbar tilted backwards | Pelvis — Lumbar tilted forward | Pelvis — Pelvis

Weight resistance returns up left leg

Figure 9C   **Figure 9Ca**   **Figure 9Cb**

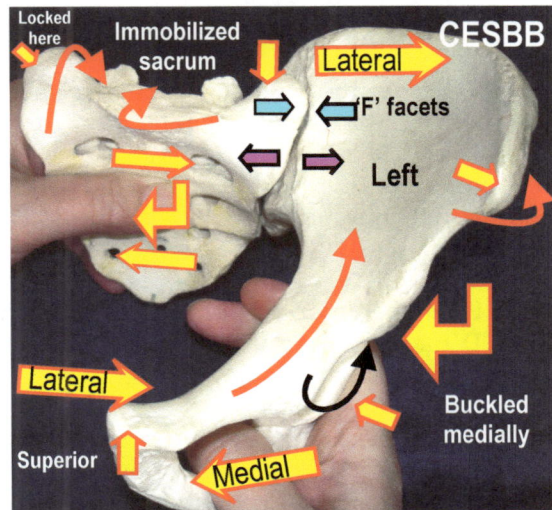

Locked here — Immobilized sacrum — **CESBB** — Lateral — 'F' facets — Left — Lateral — Superior — Medial — Buckled medially

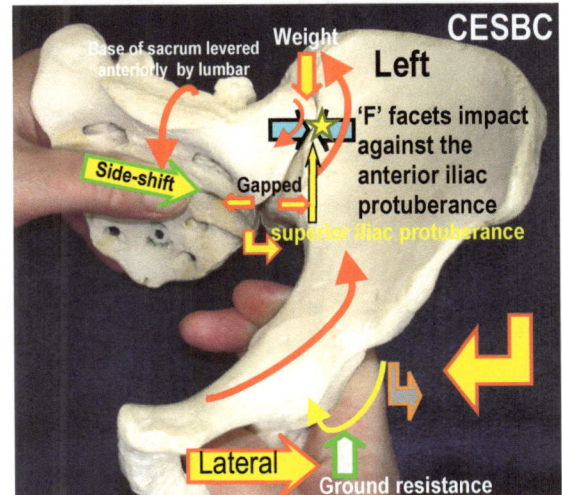

Base of sacrum levered anteriorly by lumbar — Weight — **CESBC** — **Left** — 'F' facets impact against the anterior iliac protuberance — Side-shift — Gapped — superior iliac protuberance — Lateral — Ground resistance

Points of Facet Impact:
Left Ilium

As weight continues to bear down on the left, because the left leg is lifted, as shown in **figure 9B** on page 119, the left innominate has further to travel inferiorly. This causes side-shift to automatically transfer to the left sacroiliac joint which forces the subluxations to become wedged in still further. This is illustrated in **figure 9D.** The extra distance the left leg has to travel to reach the ground also means that the upper pelvis ends up angled anteriorly and inferiorly, giving the person a forward bent posture.

Figure 9E shows the points where the sacral facets impact against the iliac facets.

Point 1) is at the anterior perimeter of the iliac 'F' facet at the meeting with the superior iliac protuberance.

Point 2) is at the inferior posterior border of the iliac 'D' facet, where it meets the foot hills of the inferior anterior iliac bony mass.

Points 3) form the anterior border of the iliac facets. These are pseudo points of subluxation. As the weight bearing innominate forces the anterior inferior bony mass of the ilium to rotate anteriorly, the sacral 'D' facets are forced to ride up the iliac bony mass. This clamps the lower anterior halves of the sacroiliac facets together at **point 3)** with the pivot subluxation at **point 1)**. This is illustrated in **figures 9G** and **9Ga.** When weight is taken off the left leg, the anterior sacroiliac facets at **point 3)** snap open. This is shown in **figures 9F** and **9Fa**. This phenomenon produces a judder within the left sacroiliac joint during the walking action. Care must be taken not to mis-diagnose this as an over-worn sacroiliac joint.

This subluxation is classified as **iliosacral.**

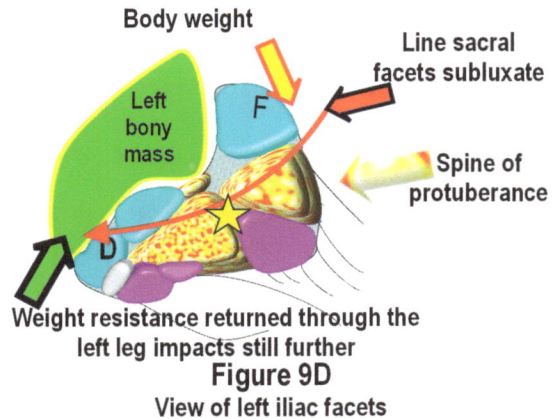

Figure 9D
View of left iliac facets

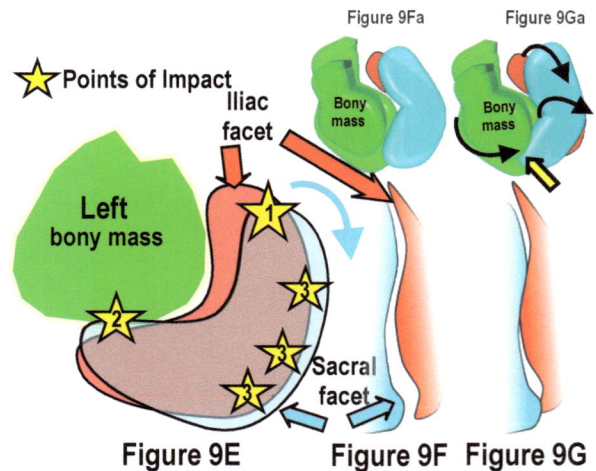

Figure 9E   Figure 9F   Figure 9G

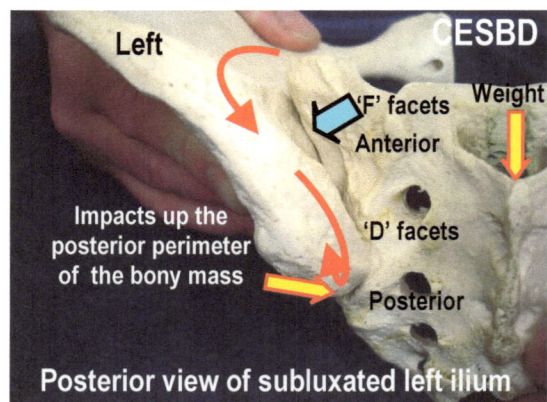

Posterior view of subluxated left ilium

122

Extension Subluxation
when Side-Shifted Left

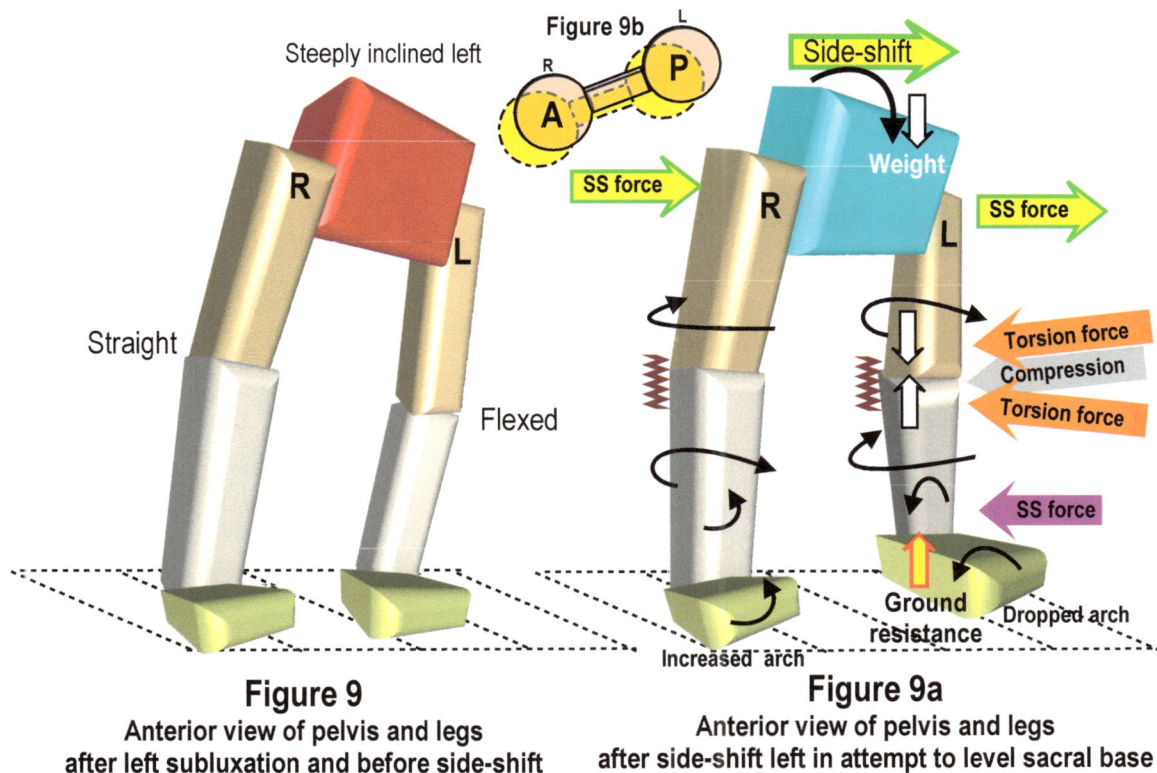

Figure 9
Anterior view of pelvis and legs
after left subluxation and before side-shift

Figure 9a
Anterior view of pelvis and legs
after side-shift left in attempt to level sacral base

Figure 9 illustrates in blocks the angles of the pelvis, legs and feet just as the left iliosacral subluxation has taken place. See **figures 9BA** and **9BB**. At this point weight bearing is changing from the right foot to the left. Note that the right foot is anterior to the left. The pelvis a whole is side-bent left and rotated left.

Figures 9a illustrates in blocks the conflicting angles of the pelvis, legs and feet after the body has tried to level the sacral base by side-shifting the weight distribution to the left, as shown in **figure CESBC**. In completing this manoeuvre the left side of the pelvis and feet are positioned further posteriorly which exaggerates the torsion placed on the pelvis. **Figure 9b** demonstrates how the side-shift to the left emphasises the posterior position of the left buttock.

Figure 9a also shows the adverse forces placed on the feet, knees and hips. The right foot is turned inward causing ground resistance to return up the posterior lateral side of the foot and leg, whilst the more weight bearing left foot has the ground force resistance travelling up the medial anterior foot. This resistance puts a myriad of strains and counter-strains on the instep of the left foot, ankle knee, and hip, sacroiliac and above.

Changes after Side-Shift Left

Figure 10 shows the pelvis and lumbar when the initial lower back subluxation pattern developed as weight bearing and ground resistance were applied. The overall lumbar concavity is on the right. The extension subluxations are shown in blue.

Figure 10a shows the complications that develop in the lower back when pelvic side-shift transfers to the left. Note that the shape of the lumbar curve is reduced as conflicting weight bearing and ground resistance meet. The flexion subluxation is shown in red.

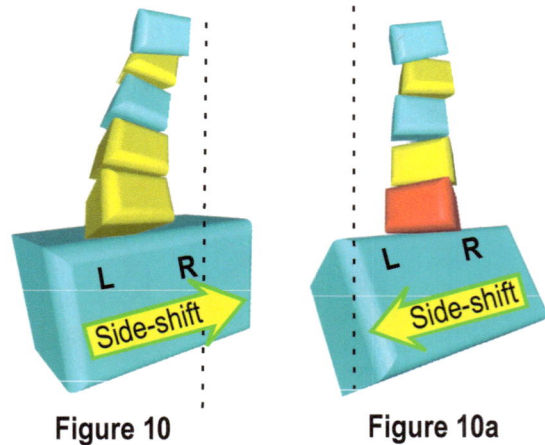

Figure 10

Figure 10a

Ground Force
Figure 10b, shows how the side-shift to the left attempts to level the sacral base. As the left leg becomes the dominant weight bearing leg, ground resistance returning up the left leg is referred up the left hand side of the spine where it crosses over to the right side at approximately T3, see page 108 for more information. The upward misalignment of the sacrum on the left together with the side-shift to the left as shown in **figure 3D**, creates a new set of movements and subluxations up the spine that are locked in by the subluxated left sacroiliac joint. This makes for very interesting subluxation permutations.

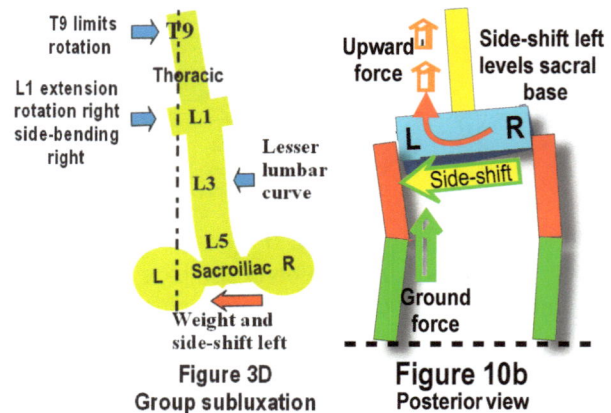

Figure 3D
Group subluxation

Figure 10b
Posterior view

Extension Feet
The positions of the feet shown in **figure 11** are of a person with an extension subluxation pattern. The right foot is anterior with an increased arch. Note that the weight bearing part of the right foot is towards the posterior lateral part of the foot. The left foot has a dropped arch due to the weight distribution on the medial anterior part of the foot. The toes of the left foot are angled laterally.

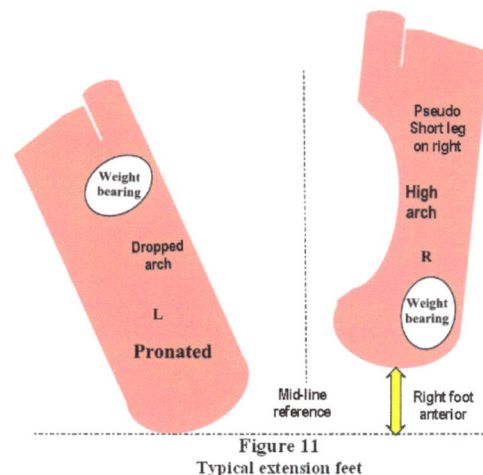

Figure 11
Typical extension feet

Left Leg Drag

Figure 11A illustrates the forward leaning posture of the L3-R-R person. If they stood or walked around like this they could have balance problems and fall forward.

Figure 11B shows the compensations the body makes to keep the body upright. In particular note how far the knees have to flex to keep the lumbar more vertical. Also note that the midline has moved further anteriorly. This is the posture Lisa has had to adopt to stand upright in **figure 11C.**

Figure 11C is a side-view of Lisa standing. Note how the line of gravity passes through the area of her cervico-dorsal junction and causes her shoulders to become rounded. Also note that her forward-bent posture causes the angle of her neck to be pushed forward.

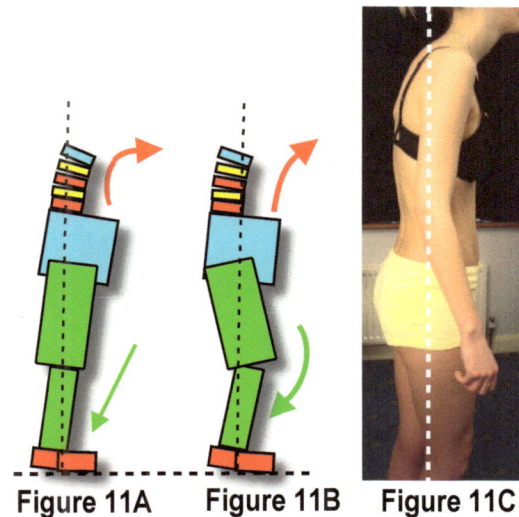

Figure 11A   Figure 11B   Figure 11C

Knee drop test

The standing feet are placed side by side and flat on the floor. Observe the sacrum and ask the person to keep their left leg straight and flex their right knee keeping their heel firmly on the floor. This directs all movement to the pelvis. The person should be able to do this with no detectable pain or restriction on the sacroiliac joint as the knee is being flexed in the direction of the left subluxation.

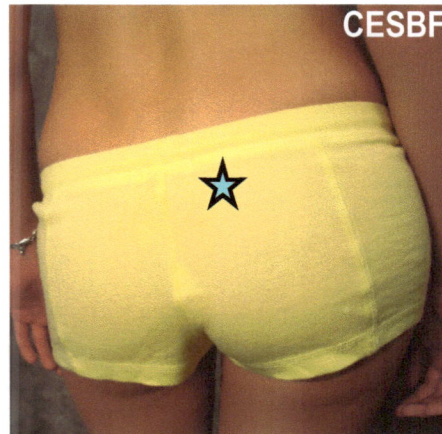

CESBF

When the person is asked to flex their left knee as shown in **figure CESBF** under the same circumstances the person will most often experience difficulty flexing the knee fully and feel pain at the posterior base of their right sacrum. This is because the sacrum on the right side cannot rotate posteriorly as it is blocked by the bony mass, as shown in **figure ESQa.**

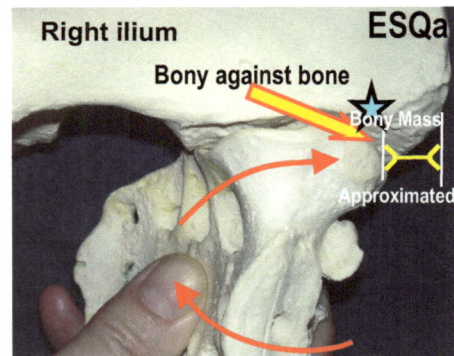

Right ilium   ESQa
Bony against bone
Bony Mass
Approximated

Theoretical Lumbar: Extension Subluxations

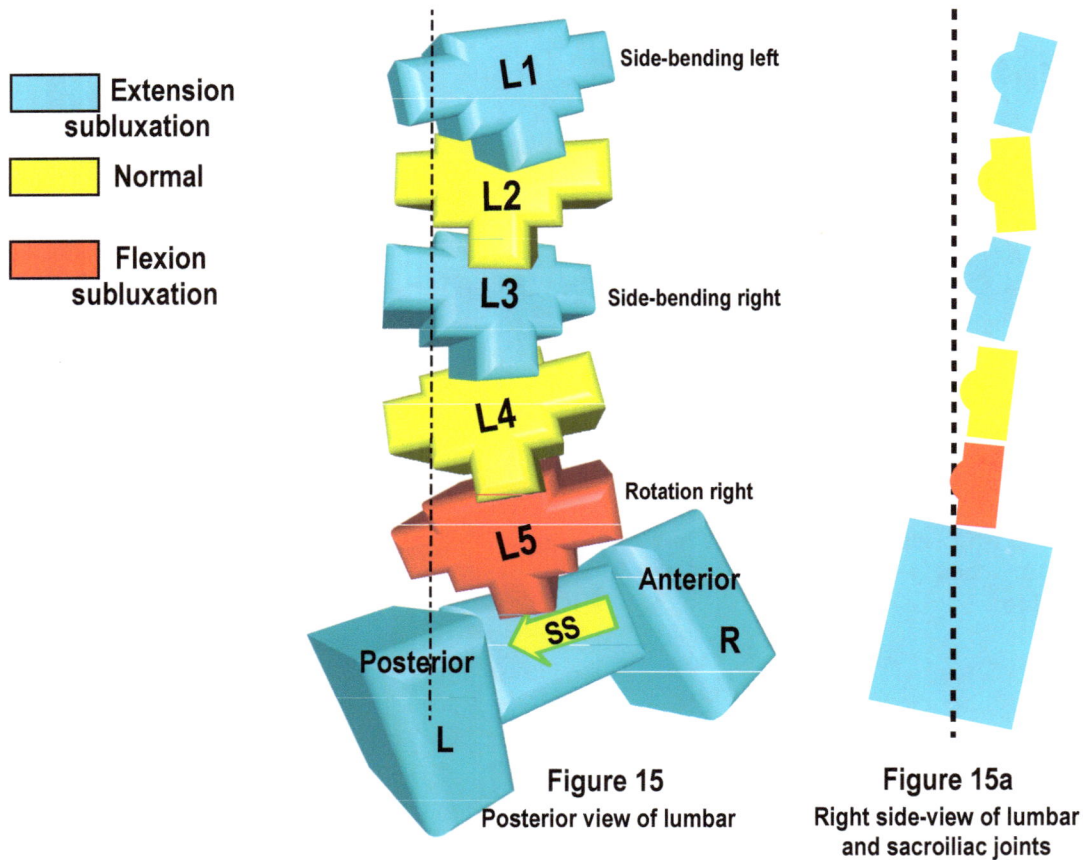

Legend:
- Blue: Extension subluxation
- Yellow: Normal
- Orange/Red: Flexion subluxation

L1 — Side-bending left
L2
L3 — Side-bending right
L4
L5 — Rotation right
SS
Posterior / Anterior
L / R

Figure 15
Posterior view of lumbar

Figure 15a
Right side-view of lumbar
and sacroiliac joints

Figure 15 shows the theoretical lumbar vertebrae extension subluxation pattern when all elements of the lumbar and sacroiliac joints are put together. The extension subluxations are in blue. L5 is not always subluxated but it is shown above in a state of subluxation and is therefore in red because it would be caused in flexion. If L5 subluxates, it can become compacted and unbalanced.

Figure 15a is a side-view taken from the right side. As can be seen, there is a loss of lumbar flexion and that the pelvis and lumbar are both leaning forward. L1 is forward bent and rotated and side-bent left.

Finally, because the pelvis has become rotated and side-bent left, L4 is forced to rotate left against L3. In doing this the left superior L4 facet is forced to compact still further against the subluxated left L3 facet. This double locks in the L3 subluxation. Conversely, for the same reason the L5 subluxation is prized open, which makes the joint unstable.

126

Chapter Twelve
Subluxations of the
Thoracic Joints

When looking at the almost flat surfaces of the anterior facets of T7 it is difficult to see how T6 can become subluxated. But it does.

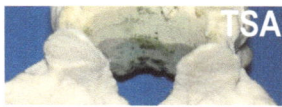

Figure 2 shows why weight-bearing and side-bending pass to the right of the thoracic column.

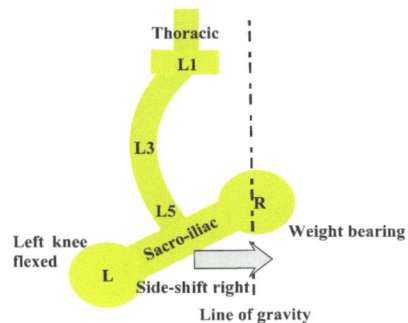

To fully recap on the normal physiology when rotation is to the right refer to chapter six. Briefly, **figure TSB** shows the facets of T6 positioned when the person is in neutral or leans forward. The ground resistance from below and the body weight from above marginally approximate the left facets, as shown in **figure TSC**. When pelvic side-shift takes place to the right, T7 follows and side-shifts left. T6 resists due to the balance mechanism and side-shifts to the left. This causes the left T6 facet to rotate right around the left T7 facet, as shown in **figure TSD**. The parallel ribs attached at either side of each vertebra, prohibit what would have otherwise been a pendulum arc, shown by the dotted red arrow.

When all these factors are taken to their physiological limit they do not lock. Therefore, this is not the answer to how the joints become subluxated.

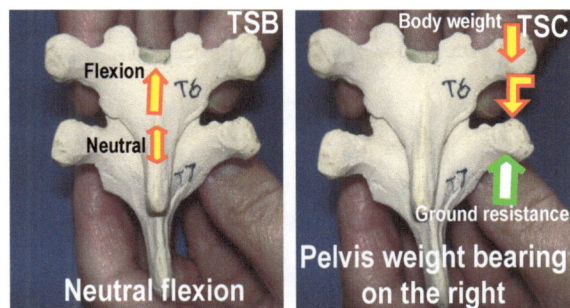

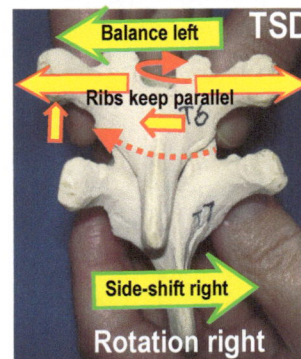

Figure 2
Lumbar Extension-Rotation Right

Theory:
Rotation Right in Thoracic Flexion

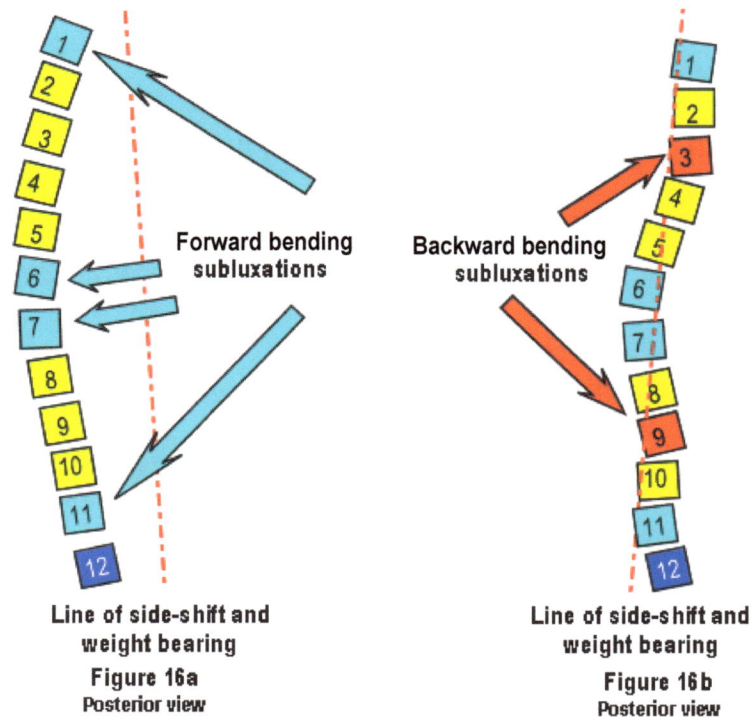

Forward bending subluxations

Backward bending subluxations

Line of side-shift and weight bearing
Figure 16a
Posterior view

Line of side-shift and weight bearing
Figure 16b
Posterior view

Figure 16a is an illustration of the points of maximum stress when a person bends forward and rotates right. *Pelvic side-shift is to the right.* Because T12 becomes locked as part of the lumbar vertebrae subluxations below, it is not considered as part of the thoracic flexion pattern. Therefore the lowest mobile thoracic vertebra is T11.

By simple division, the maximum bending and stress is taken at the mid point between T11 and T1, which is T6/T7, and the secondary areas of maximum stress are taken at the two ends, T1 and T11. These vertebrae will therefore be the most likely sites for flexion subluxations when the person straightens with no change in side-shift. This is because the side-shift would be locked in by the subluxated sacroiliac joints on the right.

These subluxations will cause the person to forward bend and are locked in by the right sacroiliac joint. When the person straightens as shown in **figure 16b,** the maximum bending and stress in the thoracic vertebrae focuses at T3 and T9. Again it is a simple division, the mid point between T1 and T6 is T3 and the mid point between T7 and T11 is T9.

When the person transfers their side-shift to the left, the free flexed vertebrae are forced to rotate left. If the side-shift becomes locked in by the sacroiliac subluxation on the left and the person straightens, they are in effect taking their back into extension. It is this action that causes T3 and T9 to rotate left and subluxate in extension.

T6:
Flexion Subluxation to the Right

The thoracic flexion subluxation begins when the person leans forward taking their weight on their right leg and keeping their left knee straight. To rotate right, they side-shift their pelvis to the right; this side-shift then passes up the right side of the spine and causes T7 to side-shift right. At the same time counter balance from above causes T6 to side-shift left across the T7 facets. Due to the mildly rounded shape of the T7 facets, T6 rotates right.

When the person straightens and maintains weight and pelvic side-shift to the right, the inferior edge of the left T6 facet collides with the left pedicle of the T7 transverse process. The more the person straightens, the tighter the compaction. This is shown in **figure TSE.**

In attempting to remain parallel, the ribs on both sides lock in the compaction still further. The subluxation is locked in place by the subluxations below. In relation to the spinous process of T7, T6 is separated and to the left. And in relation to the left transverse process of T7, T6 is anterior and separated. The left T7 rib is separated form the left rib of T6 and the right is approximated. Whilst the left T6 facet is compacted, the right facet is destabilized and loose.

Figure TSEa illustrates the effect the subluxated vertebra has on the ribs. The left rib is pushed laterally and inferiorly on the costo-transverse facet of T6 and causes the rib to subluxate in inspiration. Whilst on the right, the rib is pulled medially and superiorly which causes it to subluxate in an unstable expiration. **Figures TSEb** and **TSEc** are side views of the costo-transverse facets and illustrate how the ribs become subluxated in the angles of inspiration on the right and expiration on the left. T11, T7 and T1 will subluxate in exactly the same way as T6. More more detailed information about rib subluxations can be found in chapter 19.

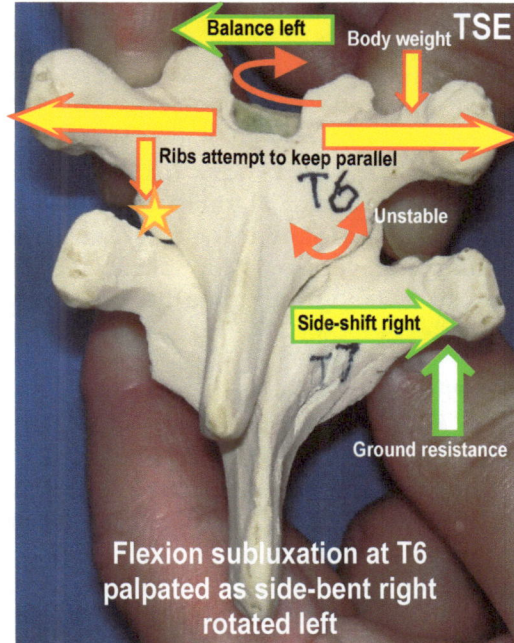

Flexion subluxation at T6 palpated as side-bent right rotated left

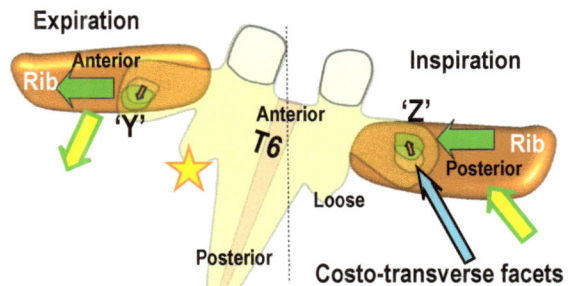

Figure TSEa
Posterior view of rib flexion subluxation

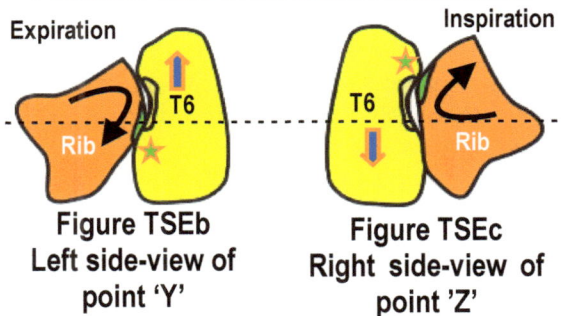

Figure TSEb
Left side-view of point 'Y'

Figure TSEc
Right side-view of point 'Z'

T3:
Extension Subluxation to the Left

Due to the flexion subluxations below that became locked in by the weight bearing and pelvic side-shift to the right, T4 is rotated right and side-bent right, as shown in **figure TSF**. **Figure TSG** shows what happens when the person straightens from forward bending and pelvic weight bearing is transferred to the left leg. The resistant ground force travels up the left side of the spine, where the opposing force from above on the left, approximates the left side facets of T3 with the T4 facets.

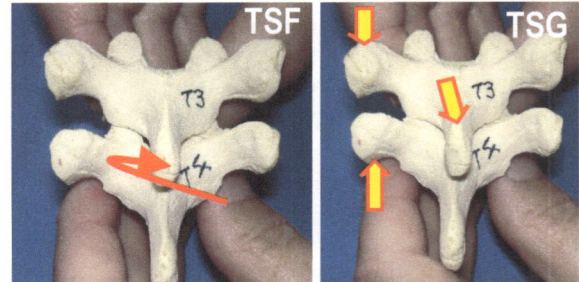

Figure TSH illustrates what happens when the pelvic side-shift sways to the left. T4 follows the side-shift of the pelvis and side-shifts to the left, whilst counter resistance from above causes the T3 facets to side-shift to the right across the convex facets of T4. This rotates and side-bends the body of T3 to the left and the right T3 facets impact against the lamina of T4. Because of the forward-bending arc caused by the already established flexion subluxations the ability of the thoracic spine to straighten is hindered. As the person forces their back to straighten, the facets of T3 are forced further inferiorly where they compact and ride up the T4 lamina. The ribs on either side fight to remain parallel and lock-in the subluxation further, particularly on the right. The T3 spinous processes are approximated and to the right of the T4 spinous process. The right transverse process of T3 is anterior and separated in relation to the right transverse process of T4. The right T4 rib is separated from the right rib of T3 and the left side is approximated.

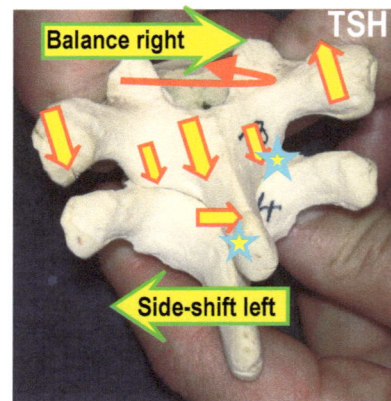

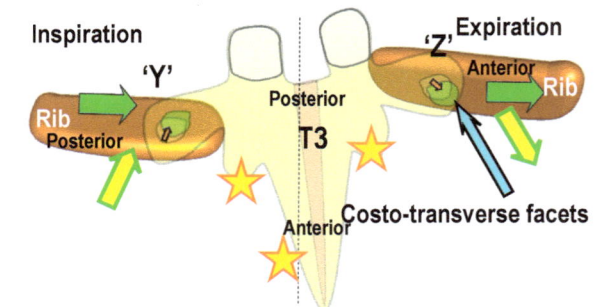

In this subluxation the ribs, as illustrated in **figures TSHa, TSHb** and **TSHc**, have no spare movement and become locked in expiration on the right and inspiration on the left.

T9 will subluxate in exactly the same way as T3.

Figure TSF, TSG, TSH

Figure TSHa
Posterior view of rib extension subluxation

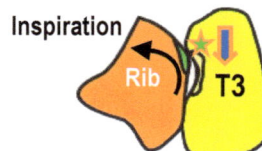

Figure TSHb
Left side-view of point 'Y'

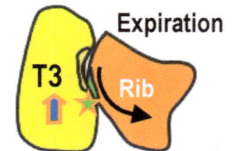

Figure TSHc
Right side-view of point 'Z'

Thoracic L3-Right-Right Overview

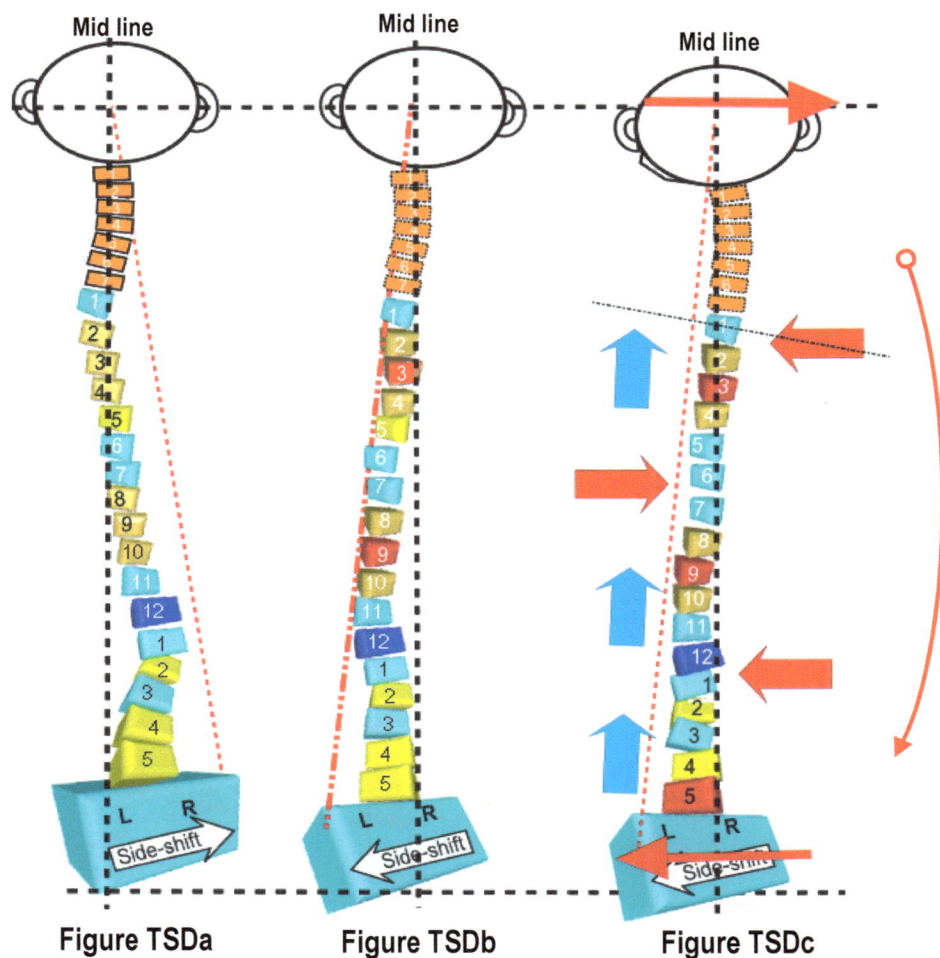

Figure TSDa   **Figure TSDb**   **Figure TSDc**

The above illustrations are an overview of how the thoracic vertebrae are affected by the forces that caused the L3-right-right subluxation pattern:

*(**Figure TSDa** corresponds to **figure 16a** and **figure TSDb** corresponds to **figure 16b** on page 128.)*

Figure TSDa illustrates in three dimensions the thoracic vertebrae when side-shift is to the right.

Figure TSDb illustrates in three dimensions the changes in the thoracic vertebrae when side-shift transfers to the left.

Figure TSDc illustrates in three dimensions the compensations that take place when the pelvis side-shifts further to the left in an attempt to level. This causes a bowing torsion to be exerted on the length of the spine. A consequence of this force could be that T5 additionally becomes subluxated.

Figure TSDc is typical of how a patient with the L3-right-right subluxation pattern presents.

L3-Right-Right Thoracic Spine in 3D and Scapulae Displacement

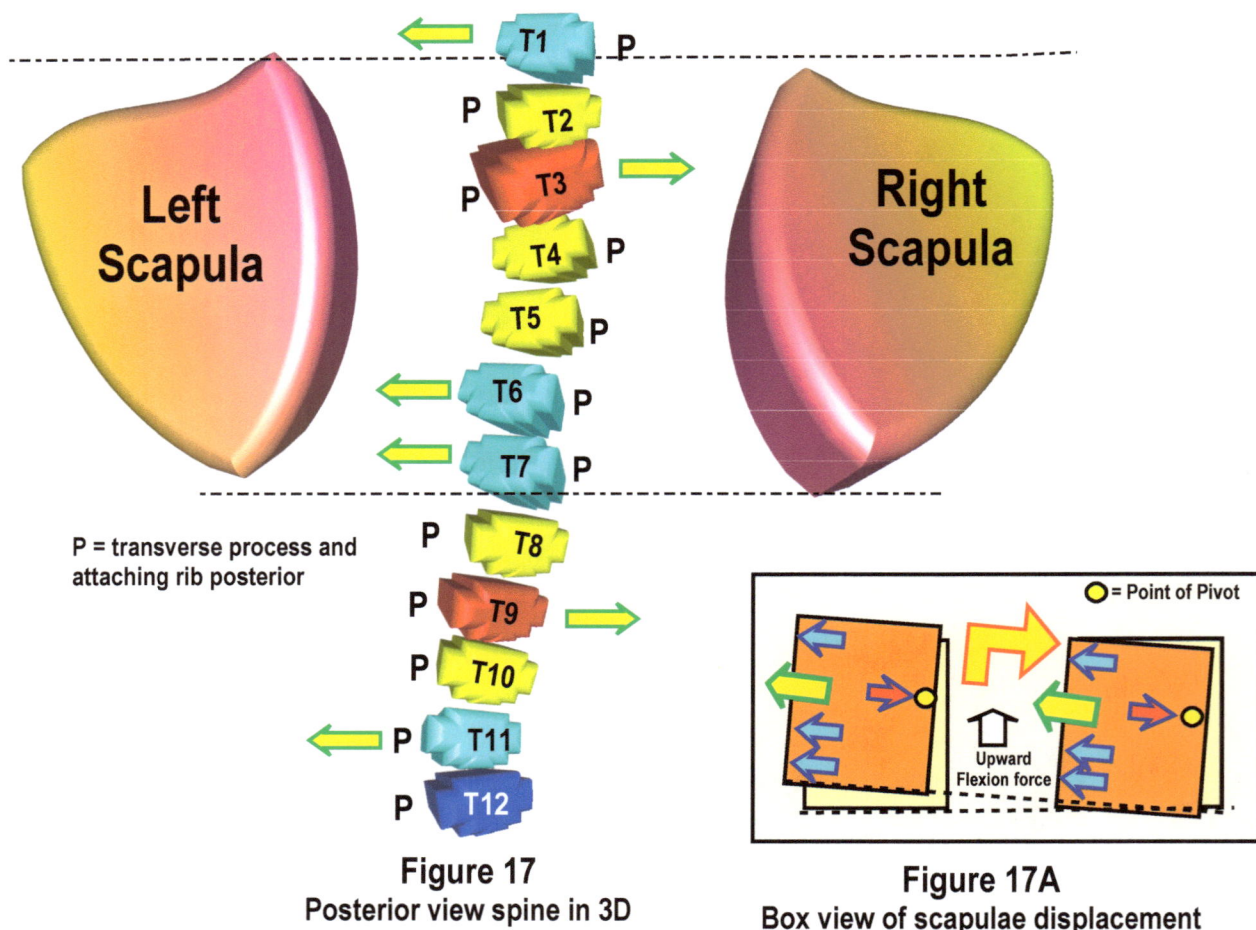

Left Scapula

Right Scapula

T1 — P
P — T2
P — T3
T4 — P
T5 — P
T6 — P
T7 — P

P = transverse process and attaching rib posterior

P — T8
P — T9
P — T10
P — T11
P — T12

Figure 17
Posterior view spine in 3D

○ = Point of Pivot

Upward Flexion force

Figure 17A
Box view of scapulae displacement

Figure 17 is a continuation of **figure TSDc** on the previous page and shows the rotation and side-bending in more detail along with the effect this pattern has on the scapula bones.

The scapulae follow the angles and side-shift of the spine, as simplified and demonstrated in **figure 17A**. The points of pivot although not shown in the illustration (for the sake of simplicity), attempt to de-side-bend the scapulae. Note that the subluxation pattern draws both shoulders superiorly, particularly on the left.

Note also that T11 follows the exaggerated rotation left of T12 even though it is rotated right.

The free vertebrae between the subluxated vertebrae are pulled in all directions and locked in a state of torsion.

L3-Right-Right Thoracic Theory Outcome

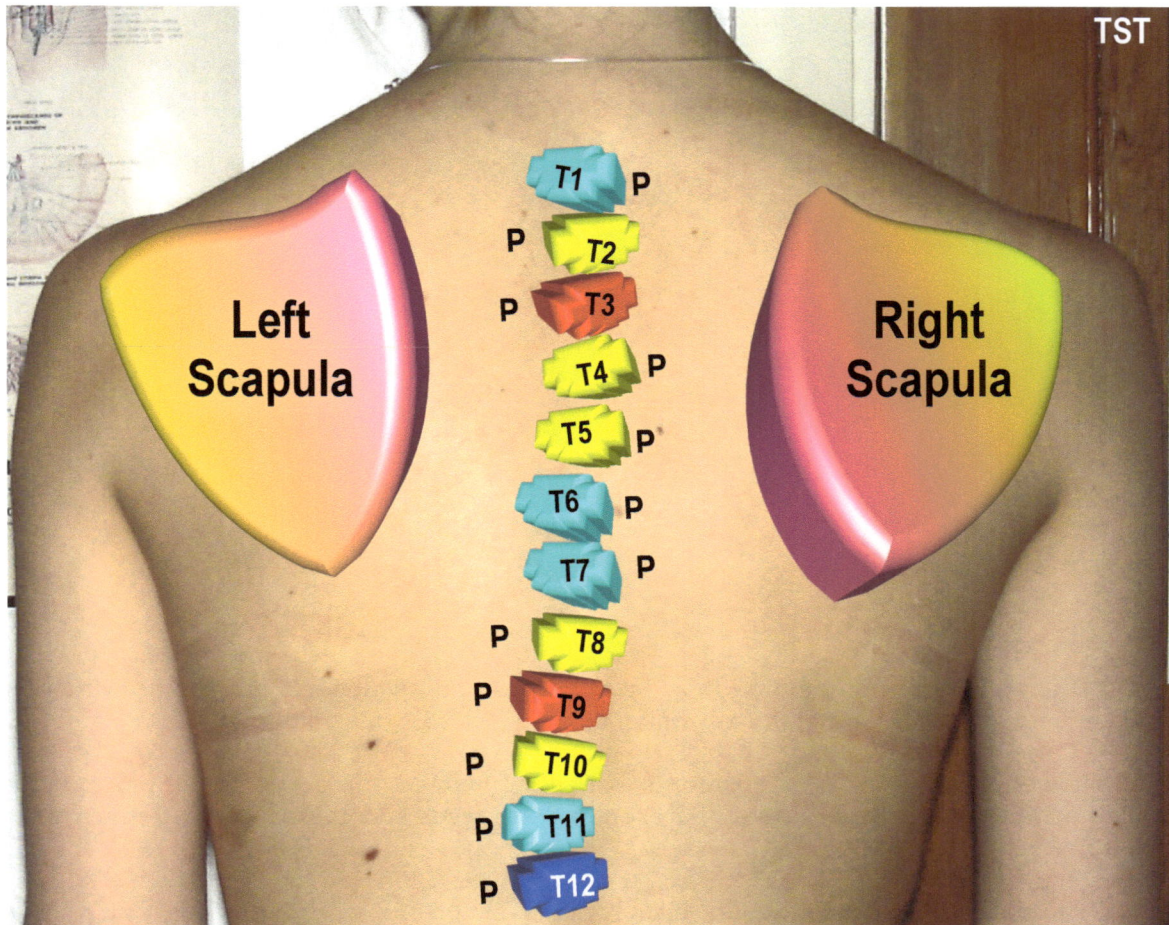

The above picture **figure TST** shows **figure 17**, transposed onto a picture of Lisa's back. It is not to scale.

The medial sides the scapulae follow the curves and shapes of the vertebrae and ribs. For example if you look at the right side of T6/7. The right transverse process is posterior which forces the attached rib posterior, therefore the medial inferior tip of the right scapula has no option other than to follow.

The angle of the right scapula has ramifications for the efficiency and integrity of the right gleno-humeral joint and bursa. The angle of the left scapula creates a torsion of opposite forces between the anterior transverse process of T1 and the posterior angle of the superior angle of the scapula.

Thoracic Posture:
L3-Right-Right Subluxation Pattern

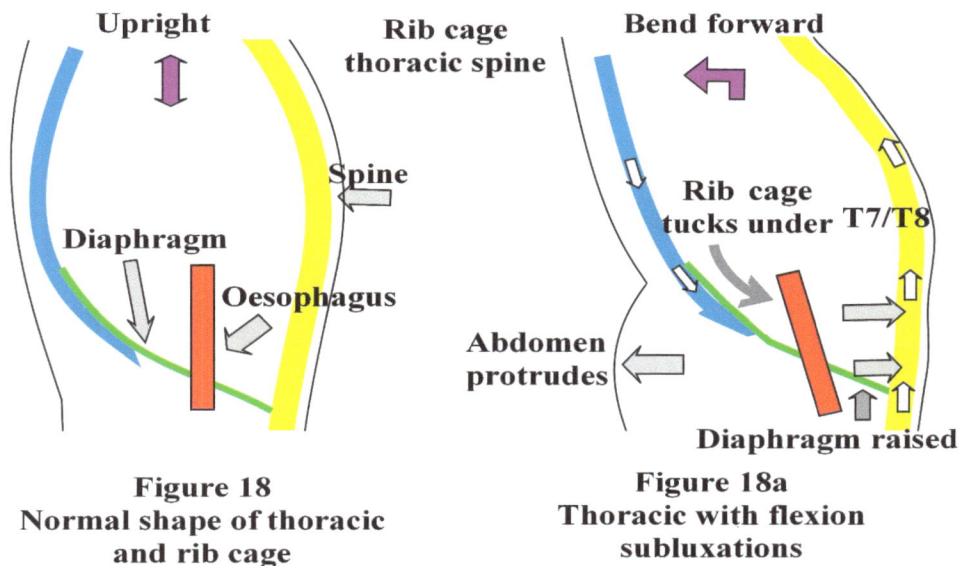

Figure 18
Normal shape of thoracic and rib cage

Figure 18a
Thoracic with flexion subluxations

Figure TSAD is a picture of Lisa sitting in a slouched position, which is a common position for people sitting and eating in front of the television or sitting in front of a computer VDU.

Figure 18 shows a side-view of the position of a non subluxated spine. Note the oesophagus is naturally positioned. It is illustrated to represent the soft tissue and vessels passing through the diaphragm.

The person who slouches forward extenuates the rounded shape of their shoulders and jutting jaw. The position also bulges their abdomen. Unlike the person free from the thoracic flexion subluxation pattern who can straighten, the person with the subluxation flexion pattern is constantly locked in a forward bent position. Therefore, the person feels more comfortable to slouch than sit up straight, which reinforces and adds to the problem.

If the person attempts to sit up straight it comes at the expense of exaggerating their thoracic extension subluxations, which can be very uncomfortable and therefore in a short time they will resume slouching forward again. No amount of pulling your shoulders back is going to correct this.

The diaphragm is dragged superiorly by the misaligned vertebrae and is therefore likely to affect the oesophagus in some way as it passes through.

Theory:
Rotation Right in Thoracic Extension

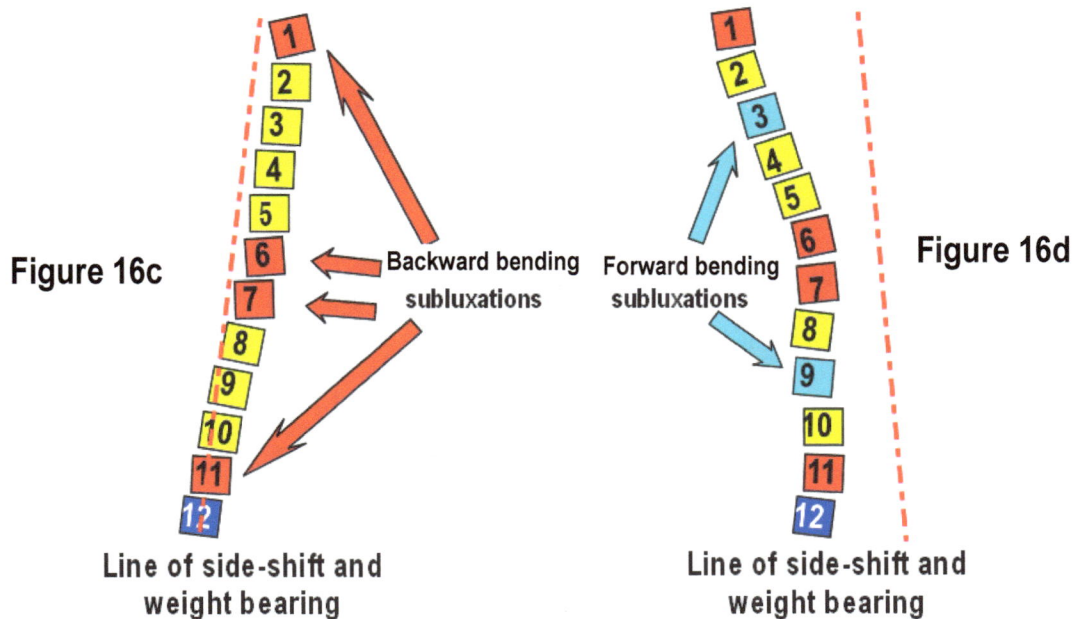

Figure 16c

Backward bending subluxations

Forward bending subluxations

Figure 16d

Line of side-shift and weight bearing

Line of side-shift and weight bearing

Figure 16c is an illustration of the points of maximum stress when a person backward bends and rotates right. *Pelvic side-shift is to the left.* Because T12 became locked as part of the lumbar vertebrae subluxations below, it is not considered as part of the thoracic extension pattern. Therefore the lowest free thoracic vertebra is T11.

By simple division, the maximum bending and stress is taken at the mid-point between T1 and T11, which is T6/T7, and the secondary areas of maximum stress are taken at the two ends, T1 and T11. Rotation with backward bending is not physiologically possible in the thoracic spine. Therefore, when rotation to the right in backward bending is forced, these four vertebrae will be the most likely sites for extension (impaction) subluxations.

These four subluxations will cause the person's thoracic spine to become locked-in backward bending and are locked in when the left sacroiliac joint subluxates. Therefore, when the person attempts to straighten the remaining free thoracic vertebrae will stretch apart in hyper-flexion. The maximum bending and stress is then taken at T3 and T9. Again it is a simple division, the mid point between T1 and T6 is T3 and the mid point between T7 and T11 is T9.

When the side-shift transfers to the right as shown in **figure 16d**, and it becomes locked in by the subluxated right sacroiliac joint, when the person straightens, T3 and T9 are forced to rotate to the right. The person will not be able to stand straight for long as the pull of the extension subluxations draws the thoracic spine backwards. When this happens T3 and T9 subluxate in flexion.

T6:
Extension Subluxation to the Left

This type of subluxation is caused when a person wants to backward bend and rotate their right arm behind them. The thoracic spine is physiologically incompatible with this movement and if forced, extension subluxations will follow.

To begin with, the person leans backwards as shown in **figure TSJ.** This closely approximates the inferior tips of the T6 facets with the lamina of T7. Pelvic weight bearing is taken on the left leg and ground resistance rises up the left side of the spine. This approximates the left hand facet of T6 with the lamina of the left T7 facet still further.

When pelvic side-shift sways to the left, as shown in **figure TSK,** T7 is also forced to side-shift to the left. The resistance of balance from above causes the T6 facets to side-shift to the right across the compacted convex facets of T7 to rotate to the left. The opposite direction the person wants to rotate.

This results in the left and right facets of T6 impacting against the lamina of T7. If the person then reaches out behind them to the right with their right arm, in such actions as putting a car seat belt on the inferior tips of the T6 facets become levered to the left, where they impact further into the lamina of T7.

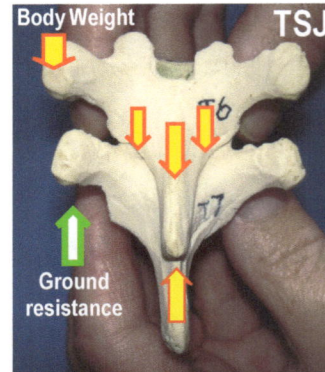

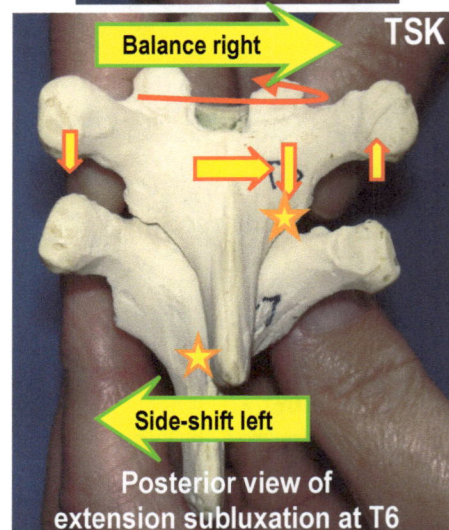

Posterior view of extension subluxation at T6

The ribs on either side fight to remain parallel and lock in the subluxation further, particularly on the right. The subluxation is so compacted that even as the person moves forward into the neutral position the right hand facets of T6 remain locked, bone against bone. These factors together typify this type of thoracic extension subluxation.

The T6 spinous process is approximated and to the right of the T7 spinous process. The right transverse process of T6 is anterior and separated in relation to the right transverse process of T7. The right hand T7 rib is separated from the right rib of T6 and the left side is approximated. T11, T7 and T1 will subluxate in exactly the same way as T3.

In this subluxation the ribs subluxate in the same torsions as those shown in **figures TSHa, TSHb** and **TSHc** illustrated on page 130 (T3). There is no spare movement. On the right, the rib is locked in expiration and on the left, inspiration.

T3:
Flexion Subluxation to the Right

The thoracic backward-bending extension subluxations at T11-T7-T6 are locked in by the subluxated sacroiliac side-shift to the left. T4 follows the line of T6 and is pulled downwards, rotated left and side-bent left, as shown in **figure TSL**.

This opens a gap on the left, between the facets of T4 and T3. From the backward leaning that caused the extension subluxations below, at some point the person will attempt to straighten by leaning forward. To do this they have to distribute their body weight more evenly on their pelvis. Weight is therefore taken on the right.

As they lean forward the facets of T3 rise up the facets of T4, as shown in **figure TSM**. Body weight and ground resistance rising up the right side of the spine approximate the facets on the right to a small degree.

When pelvic side-shift to the right takes place T4 follows in the same direction. However, the counter resistance of balance from above causes the facets of T3 to side-shift left across the facets of T4. In doing this T3 is rotated to the right and becomes locked in this position by the subluxated right sacroiliac joint. This is shown in **figure TSN**.

TSL

TSM
Body Weight
Ground resistance

TSN
Balance left
Side-shift right
Posterior view of flexion subluxation at T3

When the person relaxes because the subluxations in their back are predominantly locked in backward bending, the spine will lean backwards. This causes the left facet of T3 to move inferiorly and subluxate against the left T4 facet.

The ribs on either side fight to remain parallel and lock in the subluxation. In relation to the spinous process of T4, T3 is separated and to the left. And in relation to the left transverse process of T4, T3 is anterior and separated. The left T4 rib is separated from the left rib of T3 and the right is approximated. T9 will subluxate in exactly the same way as T3.

In this subluxation pattern the ribs subluxate with the same torsions as shown in **figures TSEa**, **TSEb** and **TSEc**, illustrated on page 129 (T6). On the right, the ribs becomes locked in inspiration and on the left, expiration.

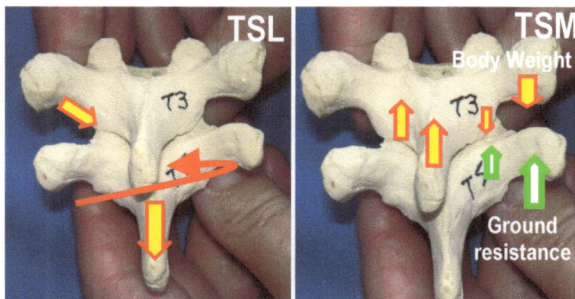

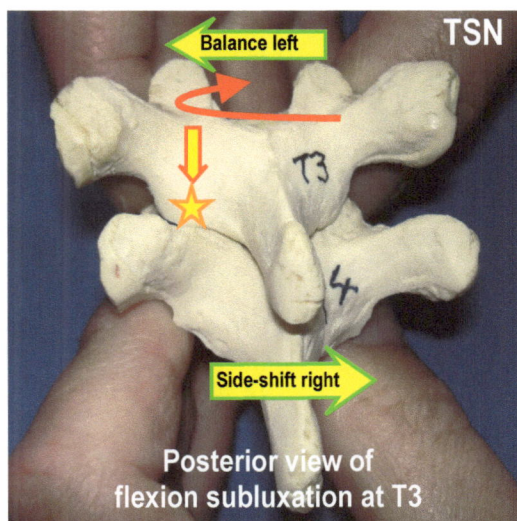

Thoracic L3-Left-Right Overview

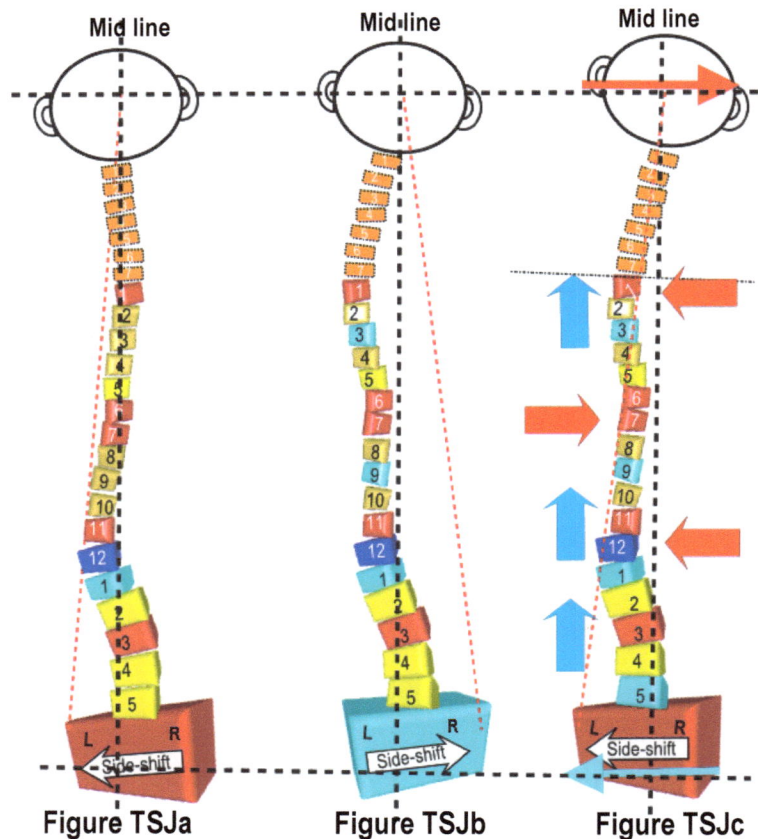

Figure TSJa   Figure TSJb   Figure TSJc

The above illustrations show how the thoracic vertebrae are affected by the forces that caused the L3-left-right subluxation pattern.

(Figure TSJa refers to **figure 16c**, and **figure TSJb** refers to **figure 16d** both on page 135).

Figure TSJa illustrates in three dimensions the thoracic vertebrae when side shift is to the left. T12 subluxated as part of the lumbar subluxation pattern. This means T11 is the lowest free thoracic.

Figure TSJb illustrates in three dimensions the change in the thoracic vertebrae when side-shift transfers to the right.

Figure TSJc illustrates in three dimensions the bowing compensations that are inflicted on the spine when the pelvis side-shifts to the left in an attempt to level the base.

Figure TSJc is typical of how a patient with the L3-left-right subluxation pattern presents.

L3-Left-Right Thoracic in 3D and Scapulae Displacement

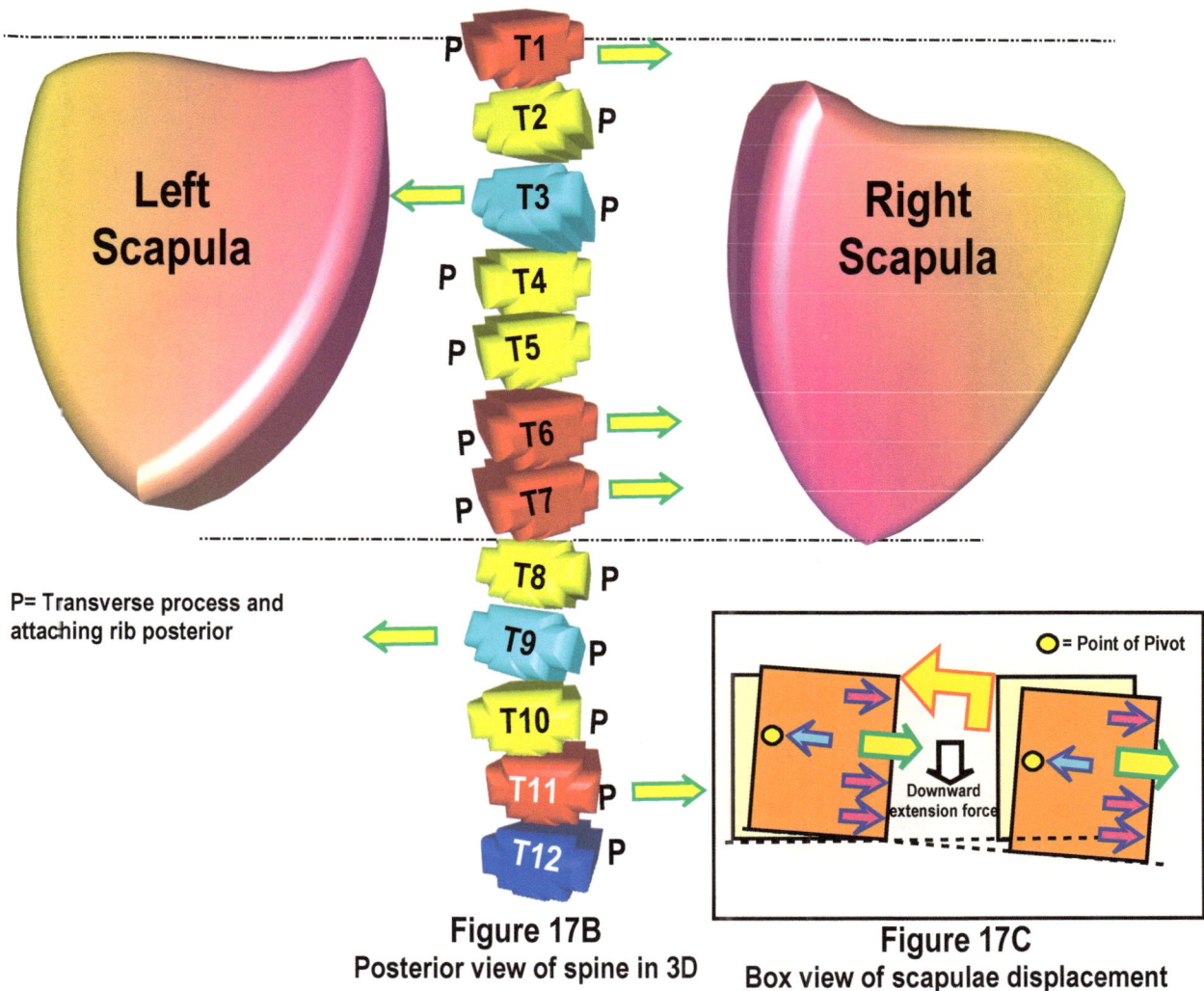

Left Scapula

Right Scapula

P T1
T2 P
T3 P
P T4
P T5
P T6
P T7
T8 P
T9 P
T10 P
T11 P
T12 P

P= Transverse process and attaching rib posterior

Figure 17B
Posterior view of spine in 3D

⬤ = Point of Pivot

Downward extension force

Figure 17C
Box view of scapulae displacement

Figure 17B is a continuation of **figure TSJc** on the previous page and shows the rotation and side-bending in more detail along with the effect this pattern has on the scapula bones.

The scapulae follow the angles and side-shift of the spine, as simplified and demonstrated in **figure 17C.** The points of pivot although not shown in the illustration (for the sake of simplicity), attempt to de-side-bend the scapulae. Note that the subluxation pattern draws both shoulders inferiorly, particularly on the right.

T11 follows the exaggerated rotation right of T12, though it is rotated left.

The free vertebrae between the subluxated vertebrae are pulled in all directions and locked in a state of torsion.

L3-Left-Right Thoracic Theory Outcome

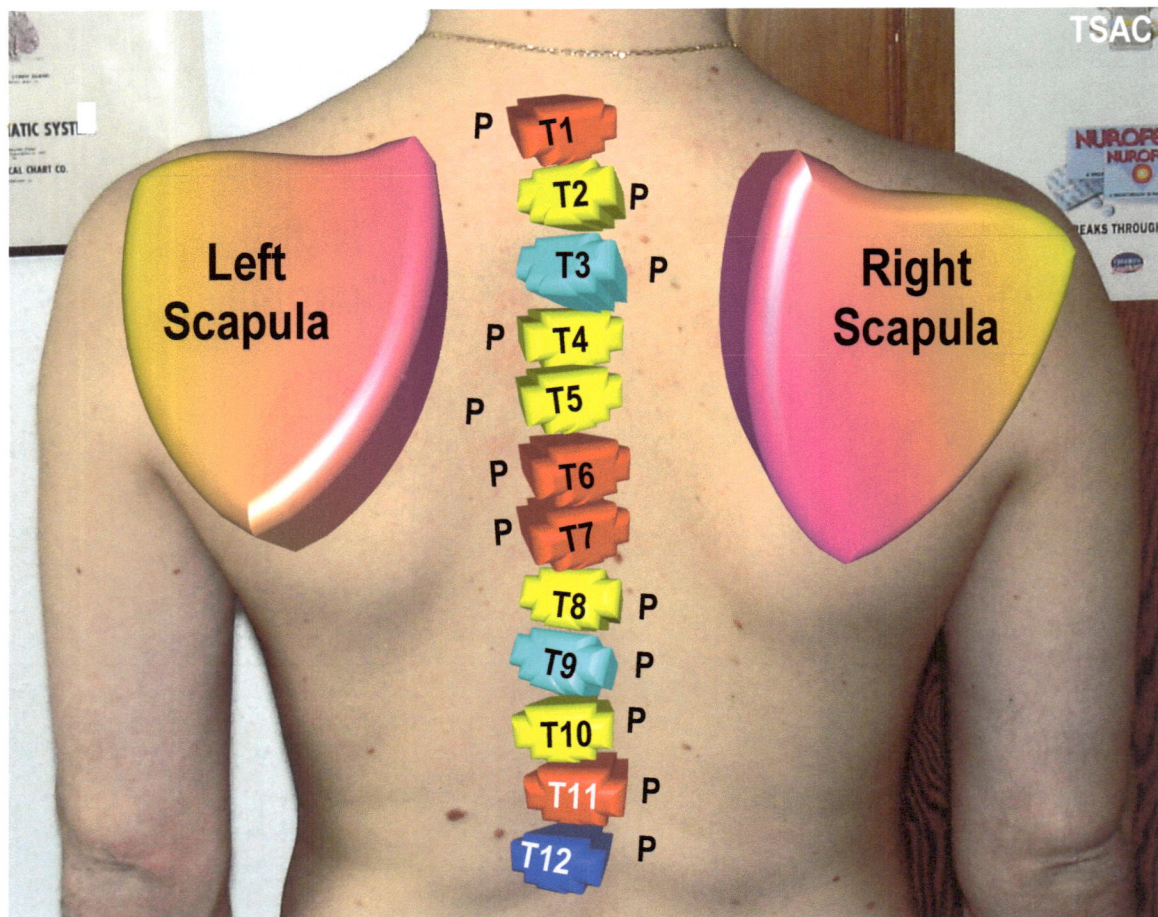

The above picture **figure TSAC** shows **figure 17B** on page 139 transposed onto a photograph of Matthew's back. It is not to scale.

The medial sides of the scapulae follow the curves and shapes of the vertebrae and ribs. For example if you look at the left side of T6/7, the transverse process is posterior which forces the attached rib posterior therefore, the medial inferior tip of the left scapula has no option other than to follow.

Chapter Thirteen
Subluxations of the Cervical Joints

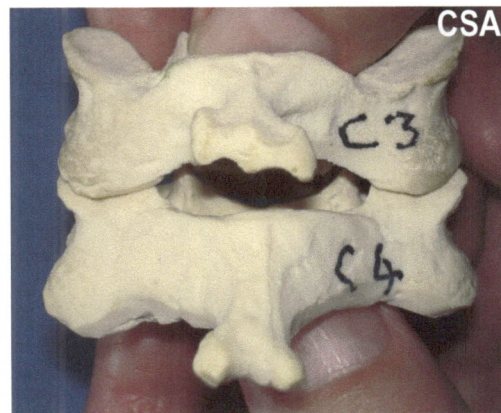

To recap on how C3 rotates to the right. Unlike the vertebrae below, the cervical vertebrae do not rely on side-shift for their movement. Instead they get their driving force from the surrounding muscles. This provides them with an independence of movement. See chapter seven for a more detailed account.

Figure CSA shows the C4-C3 joint in neutral, at the starting point.

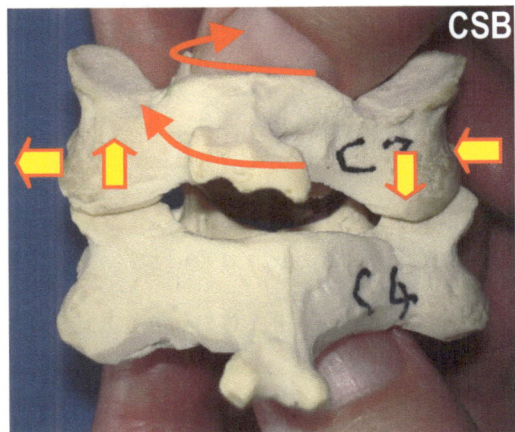

The neck muscles pull the right facet of C3 inferiorly, medially and posteriorly over the right C4 facet. On the left, the C3 facet moves superiorly, laterally and anteriorly. This action causes C3 to side-shift left and rotate and side-bend to the right in extension, as shown in **figure CSB.**

Cervical Theory:
L3-Right-Right Evolving Torsions

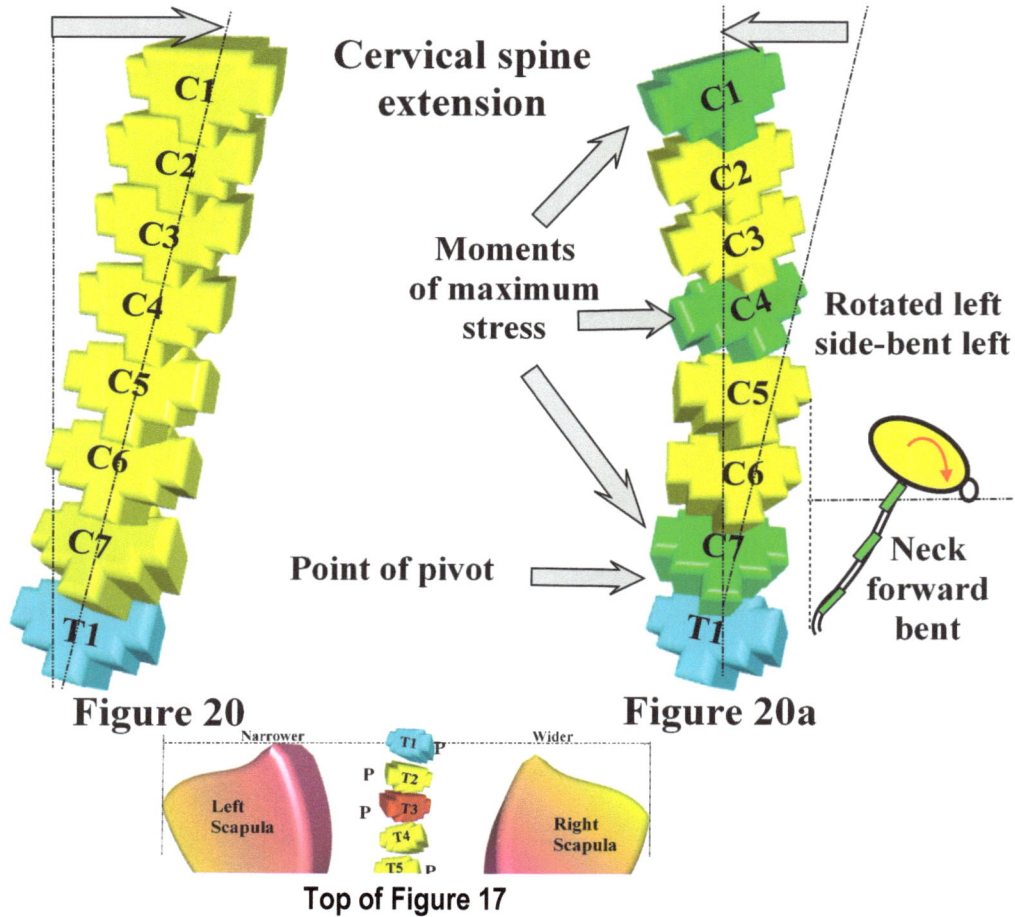

Cervical spine extension

Moments of maximum stress

Point of pivot

C1
C2
C3
C4
C5
C6
C7
T1

Figure 20

C1
C2
C3
C4
C5
C6
C7
T1

Rotated left side-bent left

Neck forward bent

Figure 20a

Narrower   Wider

T1 P
P T2
T3 P
T4
T5 P

Left Scapula

Right Scapula

Top of Figure 17

Figure 20 shows the vertical line that would follow on from the subluxated thoracic spine shown in **figure 17,** copied from page 132. The cervical vertebrae lean to the right and rotate right. The neck makes adjustments to counter the subluxation pattern below.

For survival, the eyes should be level and looking ahead, so with the aid of balance the skull attempts to maintain an upright position by rotating to the left.

Figure 20a shows the points of stress. Again it is a simple division of seven, with C4 in the middle taking the maximum bending and stress and the two ends, C1 and C7 taking the secondary stress.

Therefore, the Occiput-C1, C4 and C7 are forced to side-bend and rotate to the left, as shown in **figure 20a**.

142

Cervical:
L3-Right-Right Extension Subluxation

Figure CSC shows the C1-occipital joint in the starting position shown in **figure 20** on the previous page. C1 and the occiput are separated. In this position the right eye is lower than the left and the head is turned to the right.

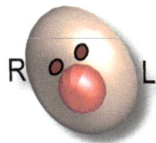

Figure CSCa shows the occipital bone rotating left as the person straightens their head and rotates left in an attempt to look forward. If the person does not straighten their head before rotating left, it is unlikely a subluxation will form. However, if the person does straighten their head first, which is the more likely occurrence, the occipital bone is forced to side-shift to the right. This derails the occipital facets from those of C1. If the person then rotates their head and forces it to the left, the joint subluxates.

Figure CSD shows the T1-C7 joint at the starting point, as illustrated in **figure 20**. **Figure CSDa** shows what happens at the T1-C7 joint when the person straightens their head and rotates left. In straightening, C7 side-shifts to the right across the facets of T1. This approximates the left facet of C7 with the left lamina of T1. When the person then rotates their head, the posterior part of left transverse process of C7 collides with the anterior surface of the left T1 transverse process, where it subluxates.

C5-C4 becomes trapped in the centre by the

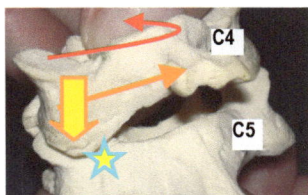

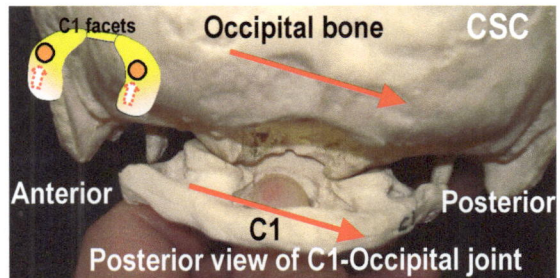
Posterior view of C1-Occipital joint

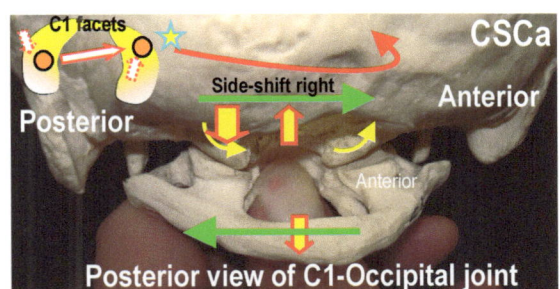
Posterior view of C1-Occipital joint

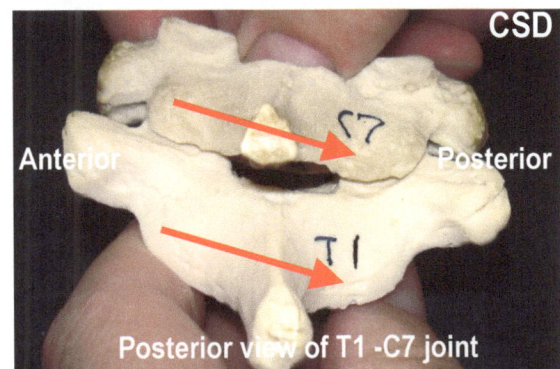
Posterior view of T1 -C7 joint

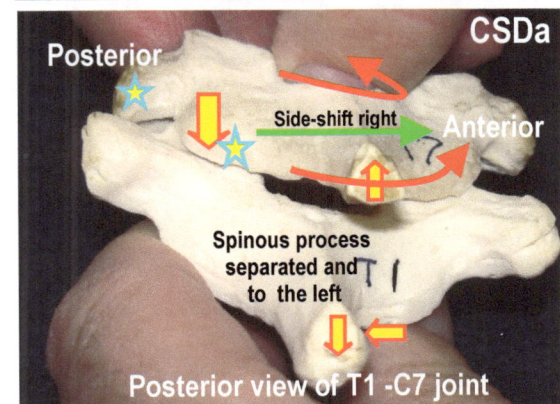
Posterior view of T1 -C7 joint

Cervical Theory:
L3-Right-Right Torsions

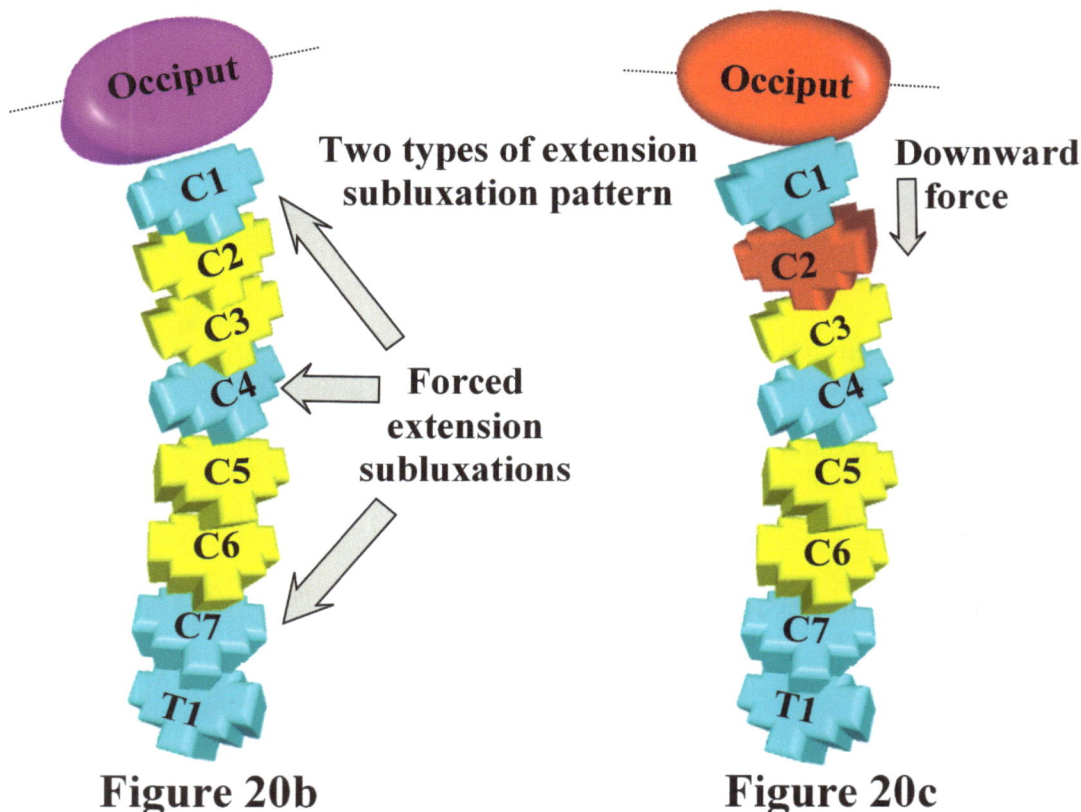

Occiput

C1

Two types of extension subluxation pattern

C2

C3

C4

Forced extension subluxations

C5

C6

C7

T1

Figure 20b

Occiput

C1

Downward force

C2

C3

C4

C5

C6

C7

T1

Figure 20c

Figure 20b shows the extension subluxations that occur at C5-4 and T1-C7 with the C1-occipital added. This causes the person to incline their head downwards and to the left as shown on the next page in **figure CSH**.

However, with these subluxations locked in place, if the person attempts to rotate their head to the right, as shown in **figure CSJ** on the next page, further complications arise. Rotating to the right causes the occipital bone to tilt backwards. The C1-occipital joint, therefore finds itself in a double lock subluxation.

When the occipital bone is forced to rotate right, a downward pressure is brought to bear on the right. The subluxated occipital bone and C1 have little room to manoeuvre and as a result C2 becomes compressed and in many cases subluxates in flexion, as shown above in **figure 20c**.

The L3-right-right patient can present with either or both of the neck patterns shown in illustrations **figure 20b** or **20c**.

Cervical Theory:
L3-Right-Right Outcome

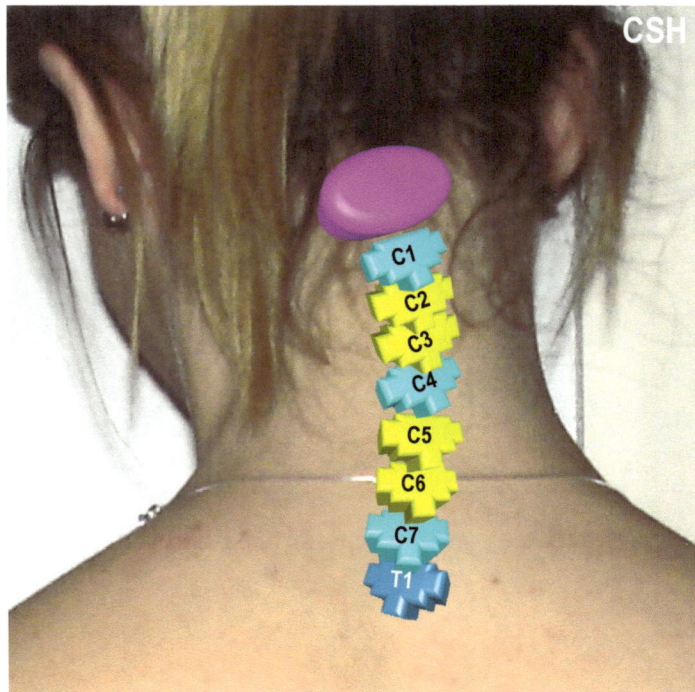

Figure CSH is a photograph of Lisa's neck with **figure 20b** illustrated on page 144, superimposed. Notice how the subluxation pattern inclines and rotates her head to the left.

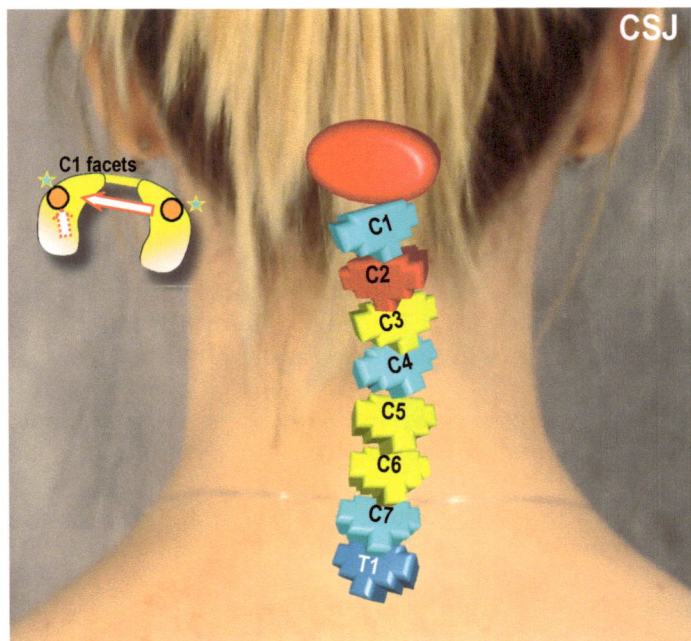

Figure CSJ shows a photograph of Lisa forcing her neck to rotate right in order to look straight ahead and level her ears.

In this photograph the subluxation pattern illustrated in **figure 20c** on page 144, has been superimposed.

To the casual observer it could be thought that she did not have a problem with her neck alignment.

145

Theory:
Cervical Flexion L3-Left-Right

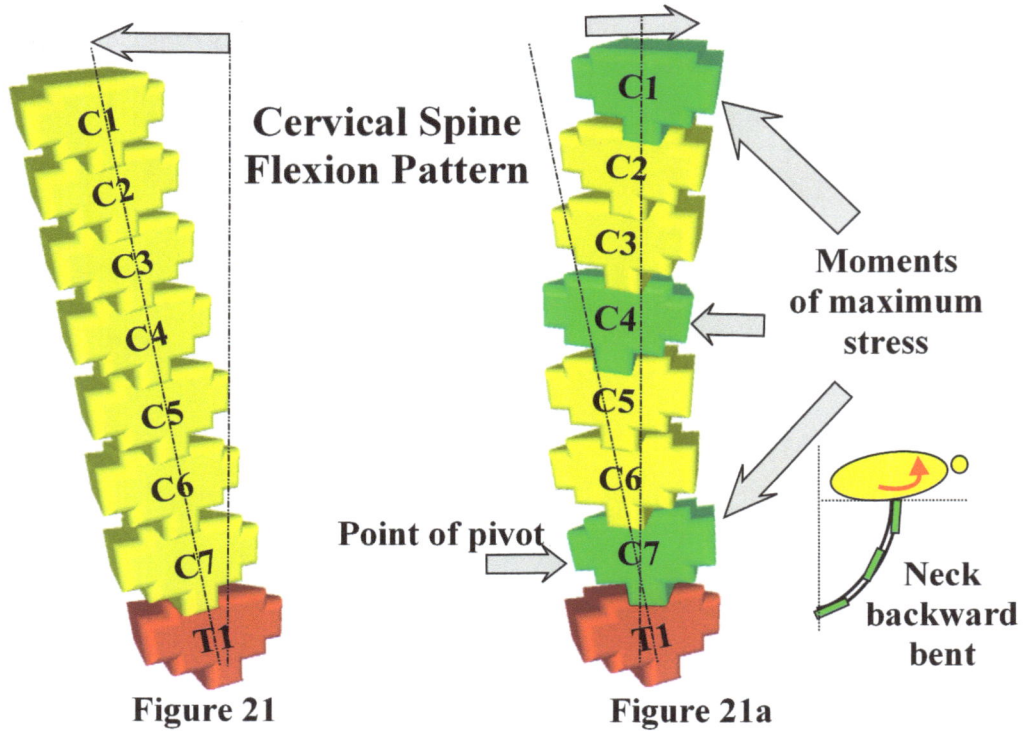

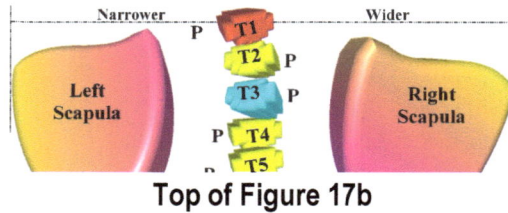

Cervical Spine Flexion Pattern

C1
C2
C3
C4
C5
C6
C7
T1

Figure 21

C1
C2
C3
C4
C5
C6
C7
T1

Moments of maximum stress

Point of pivot

Neck backward bent

Figure 21a

Narrower | Wider

T1
T2
T3
T4
T5

Left Scapula

Right Scapula

Top of Figure 17b

Figure 21 illustrates the line that would follow on from the subluxated thoracic spine shown in **figure 17b** on page 139. The cervical vertebrae lean to the left and rotate left. The neck makes adjustments to counter the subluxation pattern below.

For survival, the eyes need to be level and looking ahead and so with the aid of balance, the skull attempts to maintain an upright position by rotating to the right.

Figure 21a shows the points of stress. Again it is a simple division of seven, with C4 in the middle taking the maximum bending and stress and the ends, C1 and C7 taking the secondary stress.

Therefore, the Occiput-C1, C4 and C7 are forced to side-bend and rotate to the right, as shown in **figure 21a**.

146

Cervical:
in L3-Left-Right Flexion Subluxation

Figure CSC shows the C1-occipital joint in the starting position shown in **figure 21** on the previous page. C1 is positioned in backward bending. In this position the left eye is lower than the right and the head is rotated to the left.

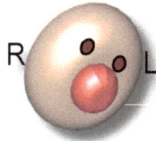

Figure CSEa shows the occipital bone rotating right as the person straightens their head and rotate right in an attempt to look forward. If the person does not straighten their head before rotating right, it is unlikely a subluxation will form. However, if the person does straighten their head initially, which is the more likely occurrence, the occipital bone is forced to side-shift to the left. This derails the occipital facets from those of C1. If the person then rotates their head and forces it to the right, the joint subluxates.

Figure CSF shows the T1-C7 joint at the starting point shown in **figure 21**. Extension with rotation in the cervical vertebrae is not possible. **Figure CSFa** shows what happens at the T1-C7 joint when the person straightens their head and rotates right, as shown in **figure 21a**, on straightening their head C7 side-shifts to the left across the facets of T1. This approximates the right facet of C7 with the right lamina of T1. When the person then rotates their head, the posterior part of the right transverse process of C7 collides with the anterior surface of the right T1 transverse process, where it subluxates. **C5-C4** becomes trapped in the centre by the downward force of

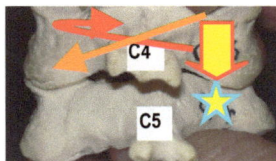

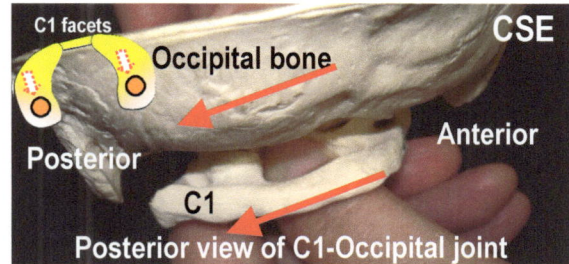

Posterior view of C1-Occipital joint

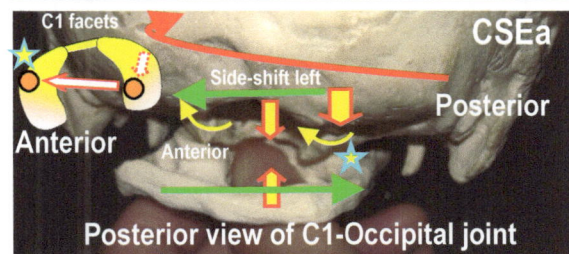

Posterior view of C1-Occipital joint

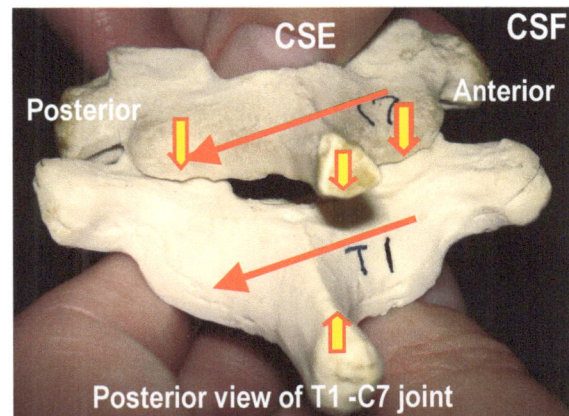

Posterior view of T1-C7 joint

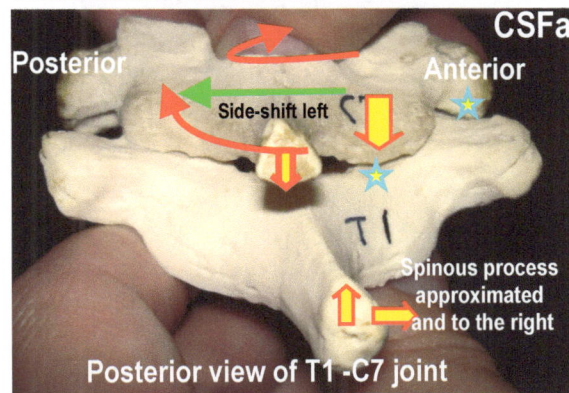

Posterior view of T1-C7 joint

Theory:
L3-Left-Right Evolving Torsions

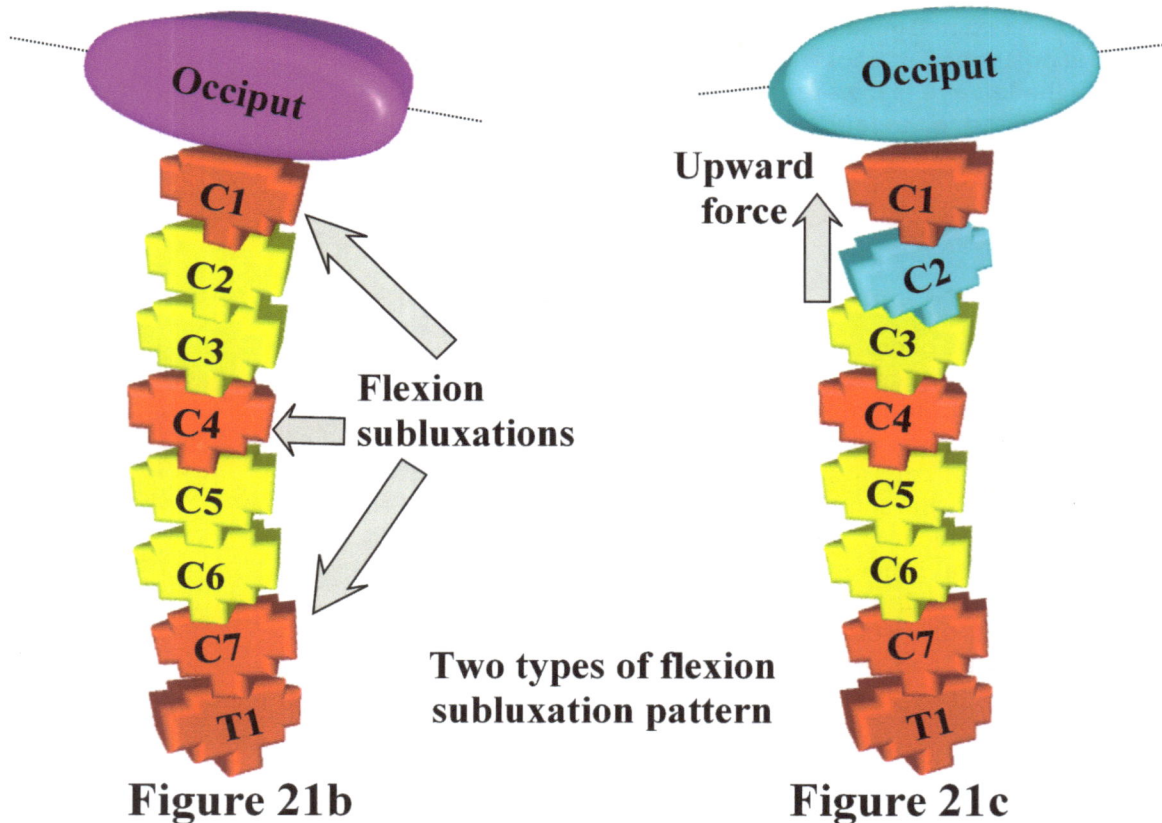

Figure 21b

Figure 21c

Flexion subluxations

Two types of flexion subluxation pattern

Upward force

Figure 21b shows the flexion subluxations that occur at C5-4 and T1-C7 with the C1-occipital added. This causes the person to incline their head upwards and to the right.

However, with these subluxations in place, if the person attempts to rotate their head to the left as shown in **figure 12c**, further complications arise. Rotating to the left causes the occipital bone to tilt downwards. The C1-occipital joint therefore finds itself in a double-lock subluxation.

If the occipital bone is forced to rotate left, an upward pressure is exerted on the left. The subluxated occipital and C1 joints pull the left side of the next vulnerable vertebra below C1 superiorly. As a result C2 is forced to subluxate in extension, as shown above in **figure 21c**.

The L3 left-right patient can present with either or both of the neck patterns shown in illustrations **figure 21b** or **21c**.

Cervical Theory:
L3-Left-Right Outcome

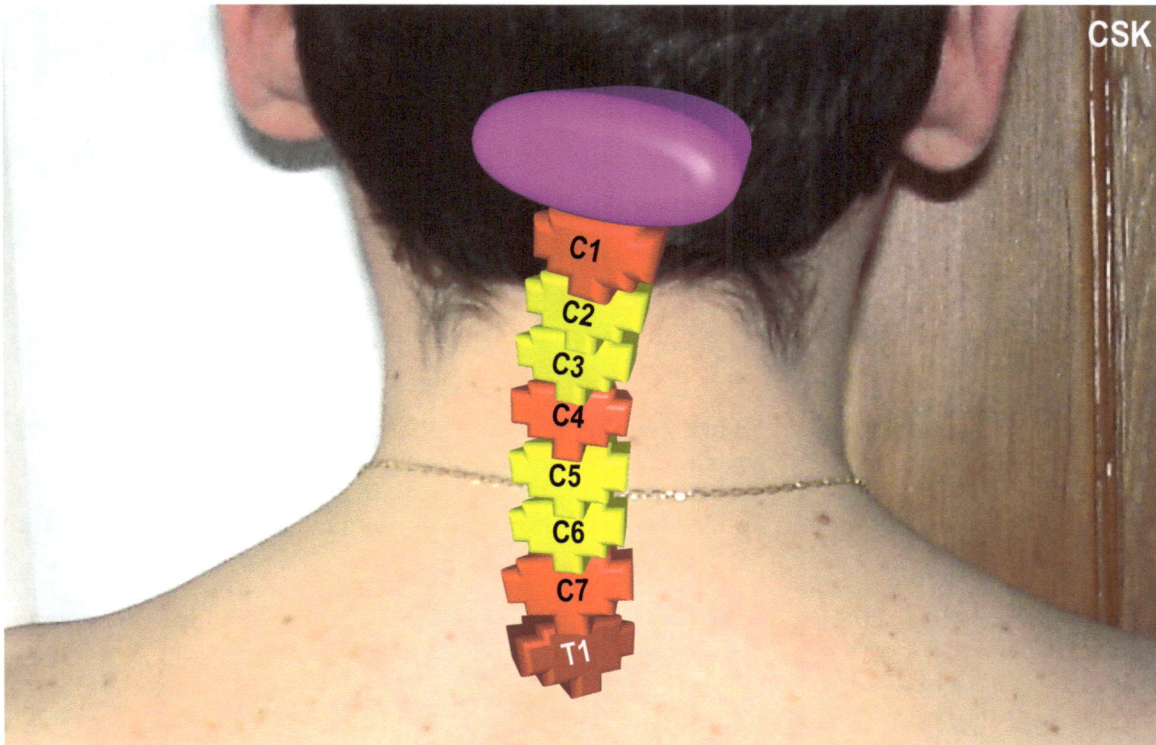

CSK

Figure SCK above is a picture of Matthew's neck with **figure 21b** on page 148, superimposed. Notice how his head rises and rotates to the right.

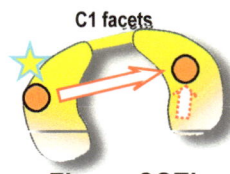

C1 facets

Figure CSEb

If Matthew were to turn his head left from the above position, the placement of the occipital facets acting on C1 would look like **figure CSEb**. Because the right occipital facet is not at the extremity of the C1 facet, the joint does not readily subluxate. Therefore, it is more usual for the person with the L3-left-right subluxation pattern to present as in **figure SCK**.

Conclusions:
Spinal Mechanics and Subluxations

As has been demonstrated, subluxations originating at L3 can create complex patterns through-out the body of self-tightening lever and counter-lever that distort and restrict body movement.

So what useful information can we extract from understanding spinal mechanics and how subluxations are created?

1) We know that when side-shift is locked in by subluxated sacroiliac joints that it is highly probable the thoracic vertebrae and ribs will become subluxated or worse still lesioned and hinder the breathing mechanism.

2) We know that when side-shift is locked in by subluxated sacroiliac joints, upward ground forces will cause the shoulders to become uneven and therefore the shoulder joints less efficient.

3) We know that the side-shift locked in by subluxated sacroiliac joints is likely to prohibit the neck from rotating fully.

4) We know that when side-shift is locked in by subluxated sacroiliac joints, the hips, knees and feet will in all likelihood be placed in positions of torsion. These torsions in turn, will act as precursors to excessive joint wear and tear.

5) We know that when side-shift is locked in by subluxated sacroiliac joints, manipulation of any of the joints above and most below will only be a temporary fix.

6) We know that the side-shift locked in by subluxated sacroiliac joints will in all likelihood prohibit some joints above and below from actually being manipulated, particularly the thoracic and neck joints.

7) We know that symmetry is attractive and a necessary component in natural selection. Nature is made up of symmetrical life forms and therefore a person with a distorted inefficient musculo-skeletal frame is likely to be disadvantaged.

8) We now know that the sacroiliac and spinal joints govern their own movements and that muscles play both a supporting and parallel role; not the governing role that was previously thought.

9) We know that backward bending of the thoracic spine with rotation to the right or left is not possible and that if it is forced, local subluxations and rib displacements are likely to occur.

10) We can conclude that reversing sacroiliac side-shift will enhance our chances of completing successful and more efficient manipulations.

Chapter Fourteen
From Spinal Mechanics
to Manipulation

At the heart of all non-traumatic subluxations whether they be in the neck, thoracic or lumbar, the subluxated sacroiliac joints always lock them in.

The four slimmed-down illustrations of the sacroiliac joint facets locked in subluxation are taken from their respective chapters. While they were worked out from breaking the laws of the 'Bayliss Sacroiliac Theory', if you compare the areas where the joints lock, it can be seen that the points of compaction (the rough) see page 156, bear an uncanny resemblance to a variety of previous sacroiliac theories illustrated approximately in **figure SA** and on pages 9 and 10.

It seems then, extremely likely that the past sacroiliac theories were not based on working sacroiliac joints; rather they were researched from subluxated joints. And what were presumed to be points of axis were in fact points of compaction.

The photographs on the following pages show Lisa and Matthew with all their subluxation pattern illustrations drawn in. The illustrations are not to scale.

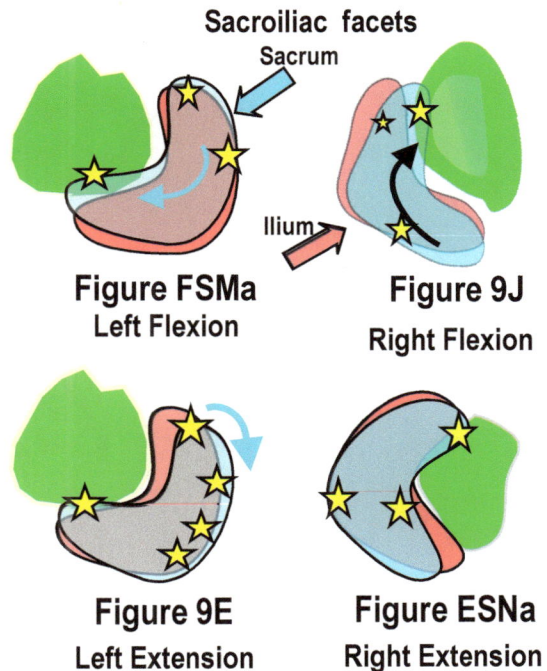

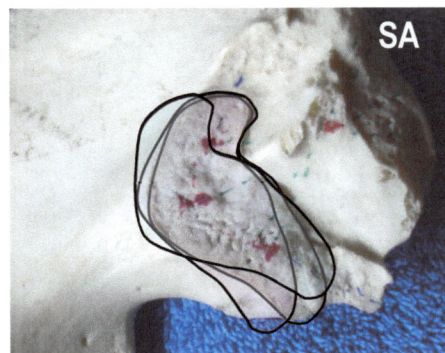

Sacroiliac facets
Sacrum

Figure FSMa
Left Flexion

Ilium

Figure 9J
Right Flexion

Figure 9E
Left Extension

Figure ESNa
Right Extension

SA

L3-Right-Right
Subluxation Pattern

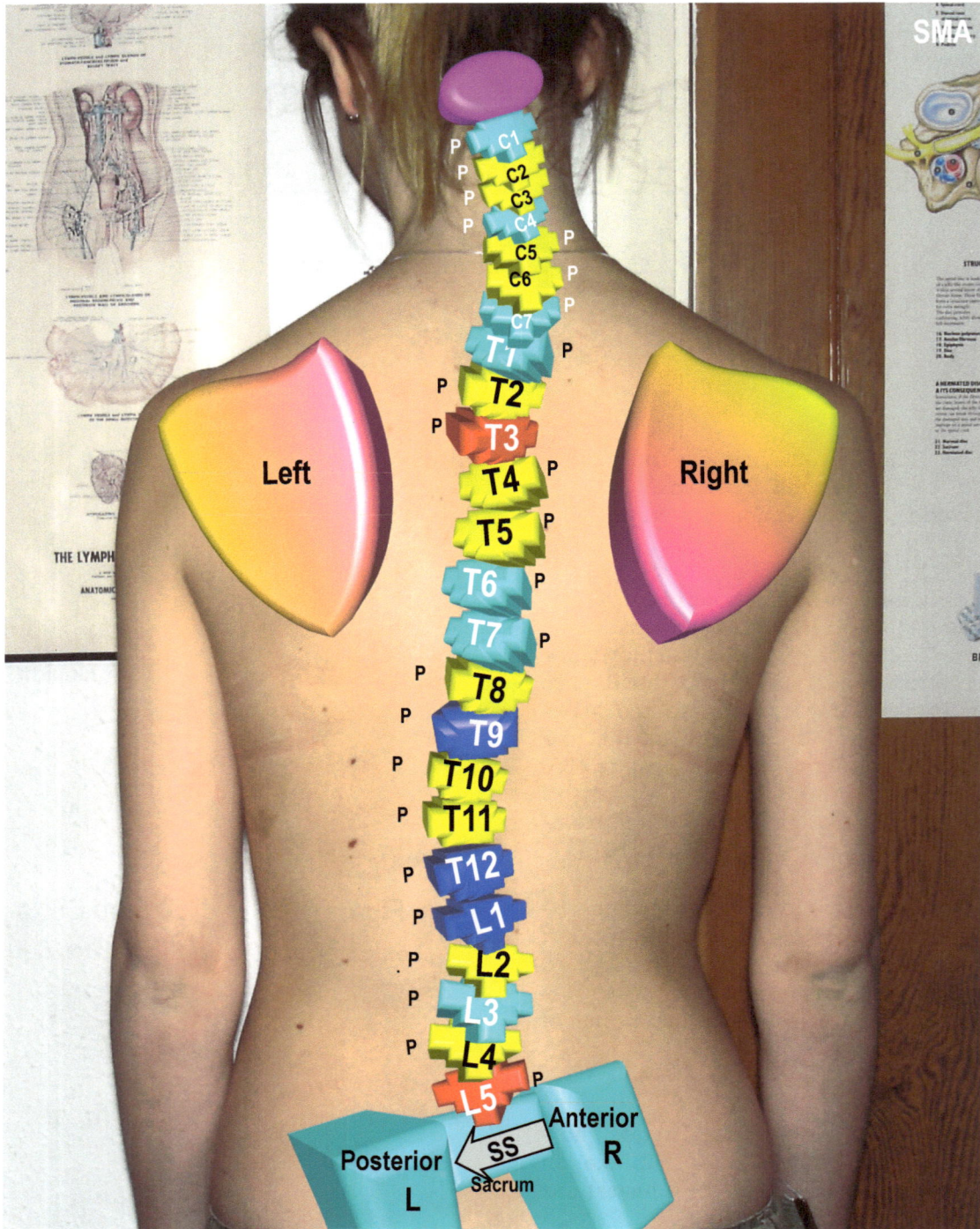

L3-Left-Right
Subluxation Pattern

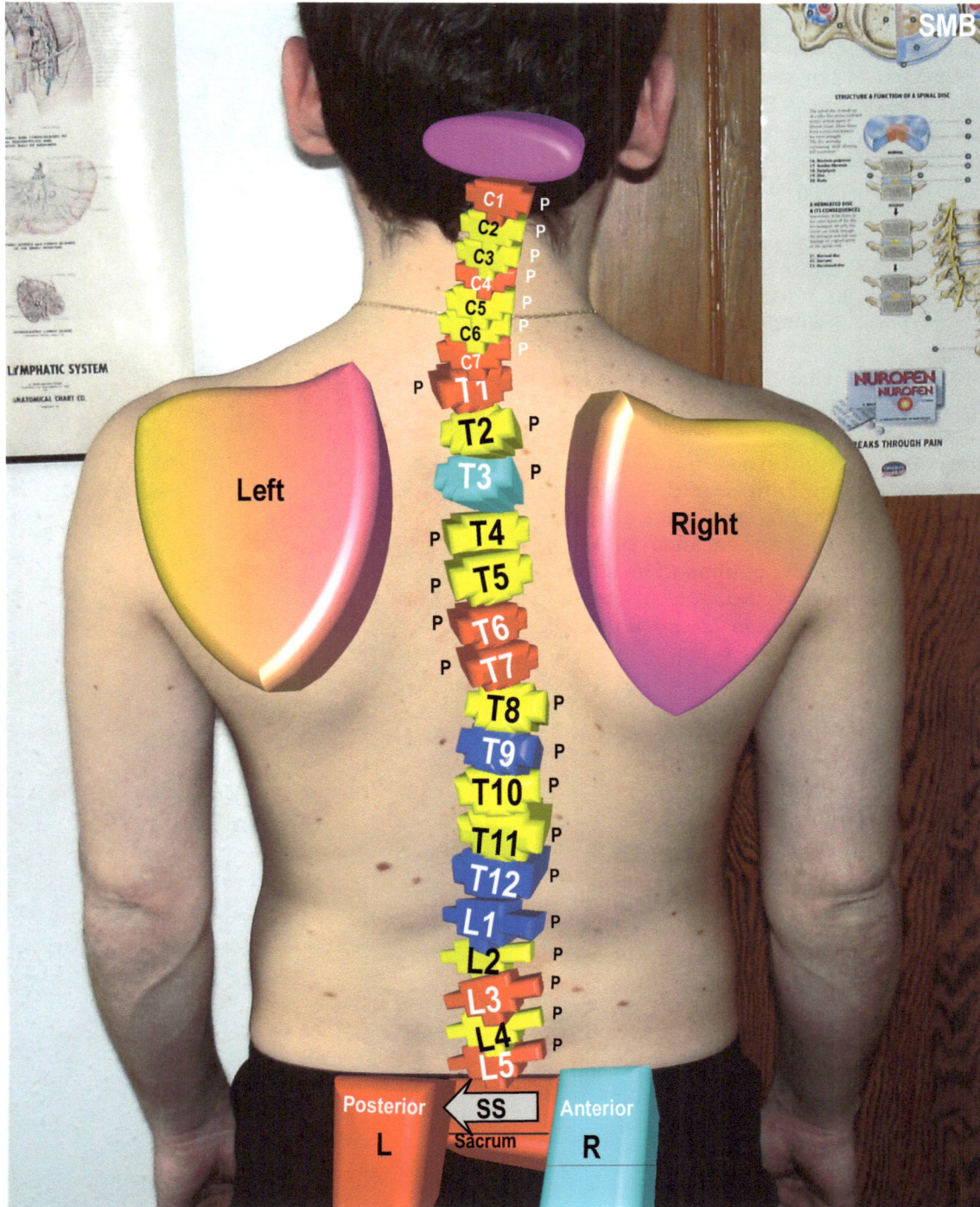

Why Manipulation?

Many professions claim to be able to treat back pain and each claims to have a measure of success. So what is special about manipulation as a valid treatment? **Figure SMC** is an illustration of a typical subluxated joint with the ligaments and muscles drawn in at the sides. Note that the muscles are stretched on the right and compressed on the left. As has been demonstrated in all the subluxation chapters, you can take a subluxation into the fixation but as described on page 90, it locks when you try to free it by taking the joint in the opposite direction.

Figure SMD shows what happens if an attempt is made to correct the joint by selective exercise, postural alignment or muscle release. If the muscles on the right are strengthened, and therefore tightened, the joint would be forced to side-bend to the right. To the casual observer the back may give the appearance of being straighter but the joint will continue to be subluxated and therefore weakened. Only now, it is less stable than before because of the additional side-bending.

If the left muscles are tightened, as shown in **figure SME,** the joint would side-bend to the left and compact the subluxation still further.

Figure SMF shows the same joint with the stretched muscle inflamed. If this were to be treated with steroidal or non-steroidal anti-inflammatory medication the inflammation would in all likelihood reduce. But the joint would still be locked, as shown in **figure SMC.** This is because anti-inflammatory-painkiller medicines cannot physically correct a subluxated joint that is physiologically locked in by surrounding joints, especially the sacroiliac joints which are continuously being reinforced by gravity during standing and walking.

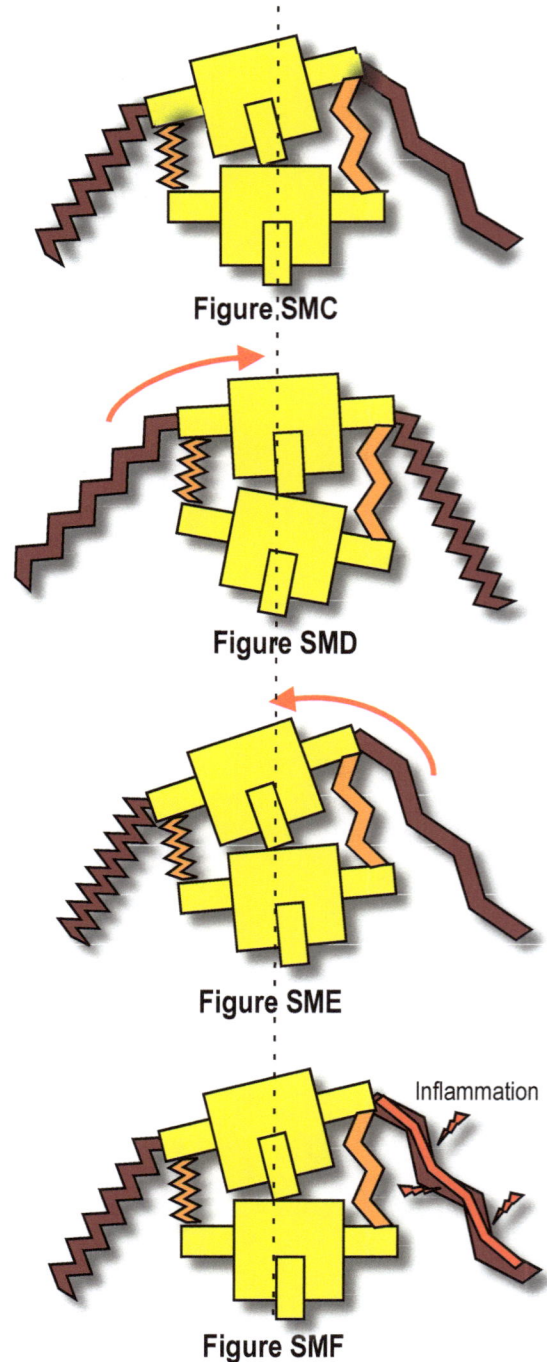

Figure SMC

Figure SMD

Figure SME

Inflammation

Figure SMF

Discussion about Manipulation

The manipulator's ultimate aim with patients should be to align their musculo-skeletal frame so that their patients stand erect, symmetrical and have as much mobility as possible.

Before a manipulative procedure is performed the muscles and soft tissue should be stretched and relaxed and all the spinal joints articulated. This is done to warm up the musculo-skeletal structures for the same reasons that an athlete warms up their muscles before an activity.

On the previous page changes made by muscle-based treatments were illustrated. Muscle treatments are important but their effect is superficial compared to the changes that take place after a manipulative procedure. Joint manipulation changes the internal structure of the body and the body has to come to terms with this change. Therefore, care should be taken by the patient not to over exert themselves or exercise excessively after a manipulative procedure. It is unclear how much recovery time should be allowed but the reasons for it are understood.

Figure SMC illustrates a joint in subluxation. The muscles and ligaments on the right are stretched and those on the right shortened. If this joint has been subluxated like this for some time the muscles and ligaments learn to adapt to this position.

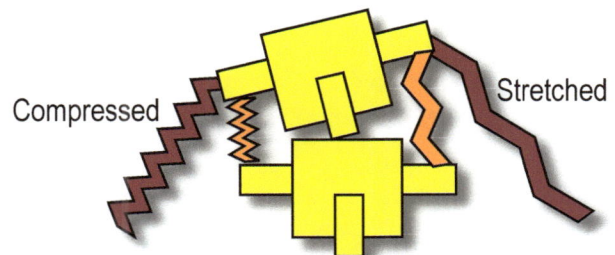

Compressed — Stretched

Figure SMC
Before Manipulation

So when the subluxation is corrected, as illustrated in **figure SMG,** the muscles and ligaments on the right become slackened off and those on the left stretched. It is this stretch on the left that can leave some patients feeling sore after a treatment. With the muscles and ligaments having to learn to adjust to their corrected position, the joint is temporally weakened.

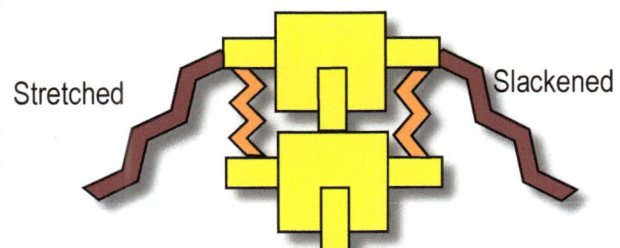

Stretched — Slackened

Figure SMG
After Manipulation

During a course of manipulative treatment, it is suggested that exercise should be light and repeated often.

From the subluxation chapters we learned that the subluxated sacroiliac joints lock in all the subluxations above and below. Therefore, the prime objective of the professional manipulator, where the cause is not due to recent direct local trauma, is to free the sacroiliac joints before any other joints, even if the patient has presented with what appears to be a very simple joint problem. This book does not cover the correction of the legs and feet, however, after the sacroiliac corrections, the torsions and subluxations that were inflicted on the knees and ankles must be corrected to create a stable foundation for the spine.

How the Sacroiliac Subluxation becomes Locked

Lumbar and sacrum working together

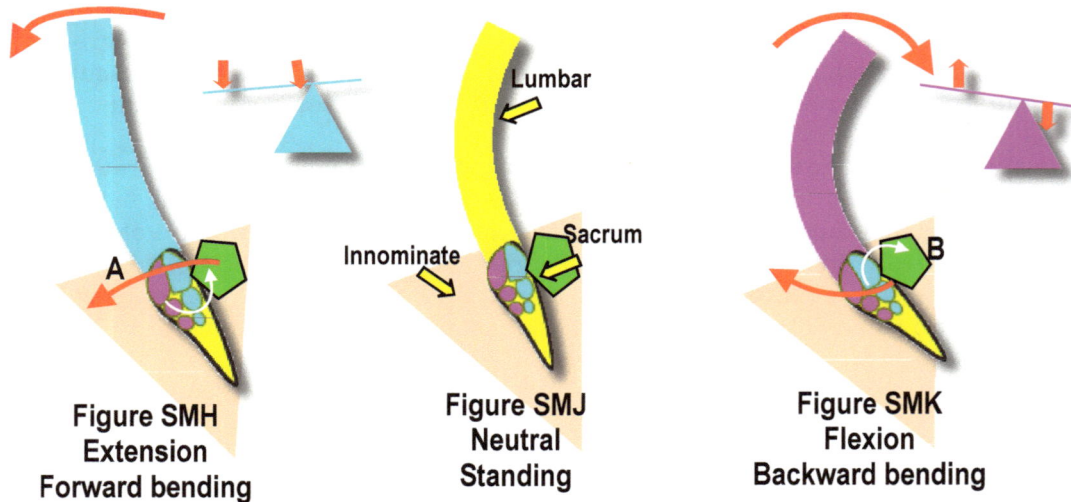

Figure SMH
Extension
Forward bending

Figure SMJ
Neutral
Standing

Figure SMK
Flexion
Backward bending

Although it is an obvious point, it needs to be reinforced that the sacrum moves as if it were an extension of the lumbar spine in the antero-posterior plane.   This is an important factor to have in your mind when manipulating the sacroiliac joints effectively.

Figure SMJ illustrates the sacrum and lumbar vertebrae in neutral and is shown for reference purposes only.

Figure SMH illustrates how the base of the sacrum arcs in an antero-inferior direction when the lumbar vertebrae are in extension.

Figure SMK illustrates how the base of the sacrum arcs in an postero-superior direction when the lumbar vertebrae are in flexion.

The areas that take the maximum impact and lock in the flexion and extension   sacroiliac subluxations are the areas between the iliac articular facets and the bony mass. There is no word for this area, so for clarity I have named it the 'Rough'. For recording purposes:

   '**REX**' *stands for* **R**ough **Ex**tension

   '**RFL**' *stands for* **R**ough **Fl**exion

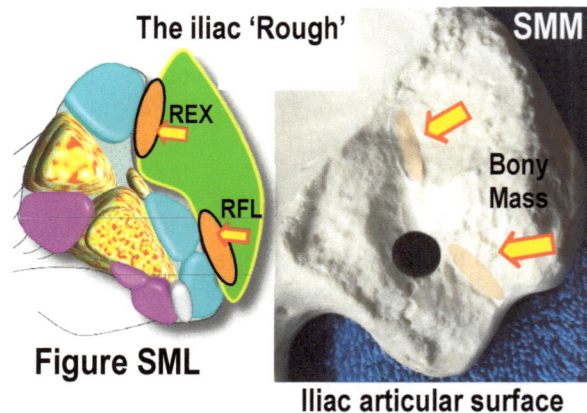

Figure SML

Iliac articular surface

156

Class 1, 2 and 3 Subluxations

The articular facets of the ilium and the sacrum are both covered by synovial membranes which makes the lubricated surfaces of the facets very slippery. This membrane is illustrated in **figure SMN.** With such a highly slippery surface it is unlikely that this is the area of the joint that becomes most fixated in a sacroiliac subluxation.

That is why the area termed as the 'rough' is the most probable site for locking to take place, especially as the forces during walking and standing reinforce the pressure on these two areas.

It can therefore be concluded that the main objective of the manipulator is to free this area, whilst at the same time correcting the alignment of the facets.

For this reason sacroiliac subluxations should be classified as; class 1. This means the locking is caused by bone against bone.

There three classes of subluxation:

Class 1 Bone locked against bone
Class 2 Bone locked partially against bone
Class 3 Bone locked by surrounding forces

Figure SMO is an illustration of the upper facets of a typical thoracic vertebra. The downward force created by the inter-costal muscles forces the inferior edge of the facet of the vertebra above against the bone below, in the rough. Thoracic subluxations of this type are therefore classified as; class 1.

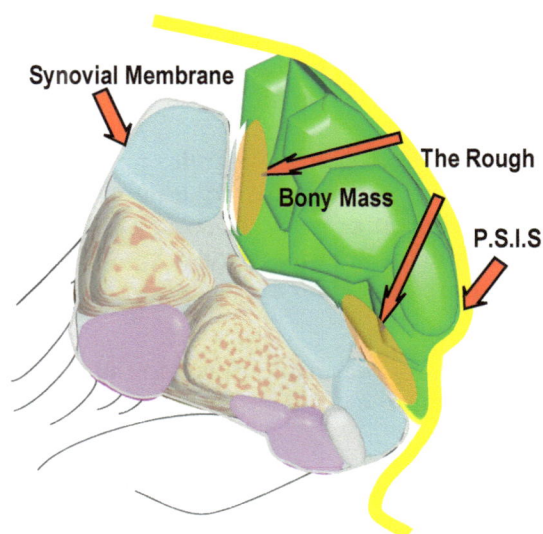

Figure SMN

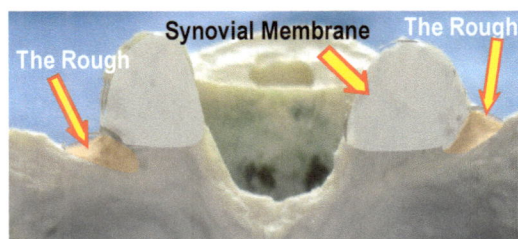

Figure SMO

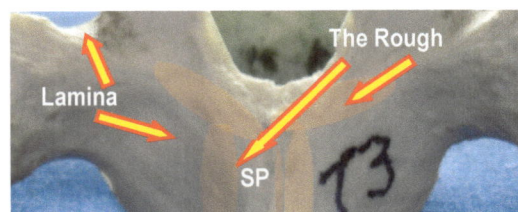

Figure SMP

Figure SMP illustrates the area on the lamina of a typical thoracic vertebra where the inferior edge of the facet of the vertebra above becomes locked in a typical extension (backward bending) subluxation. Because this is not a self tightening subluxation, it is classified as; Class 2.

Class 3 Subluxations

Figure SMQ illustrates the synovial membrane that covers the facets of a typical lumbar vertebra. As can be seen, the surface is smooth all over, therefore there is no 'rough'.

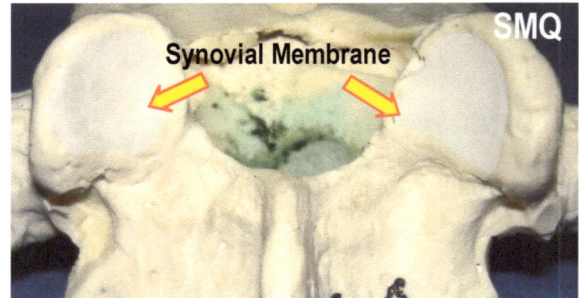

The lumbar subluxations of this type become locked in by the converging contorted forces from the sacroiliac and thoracic subluxations. For this reason, lumbar vertebra subluxations below L1 are classified as class 3.

For case history recording purposes subluxations of the spinal vertebrae and the sacroiliac joints can be classified as:

		INFORMATION ONLY
RFL	Iliac rough flexion subluxation...............	class 1
REX	Iliac rough extension subluxation...............	class 1
LFL	Lumbar flexion subluxation	class 3
LEX	Lumbar extension subluxation...............	class 3
TFL	Thoracic flexion rough subluxation........	class 1
TEX	Thoracic extension rough subluxation...	class 2
CFL	Cervical flexion rough subluxation.........	class 2
CEX	Cervical extension rough subluxation....	class 2

Because so many sacroiliac and spinal subluxations can now be corrected in one session, due to the small trauma footprint of PPT's, it would be an impossible task to record every joint that you have manipulated by its full title. Rather, use real world generalization terminology Ie:

PPT's- L's = lumbar's, **T's** = Thoracic's, **PPT's- C's** = Cervical's,
PPT's- S/I's = Sacroiliac, **PPT's- I/S** = Iliosacral

By putting in the type of subluxation pattern as a heading, I.e. L3-left-right = **LR** or L3-right-right = **RR**, the pattern of your manipulation plan should be instantly appreciated by colleagues.

Side-Shift

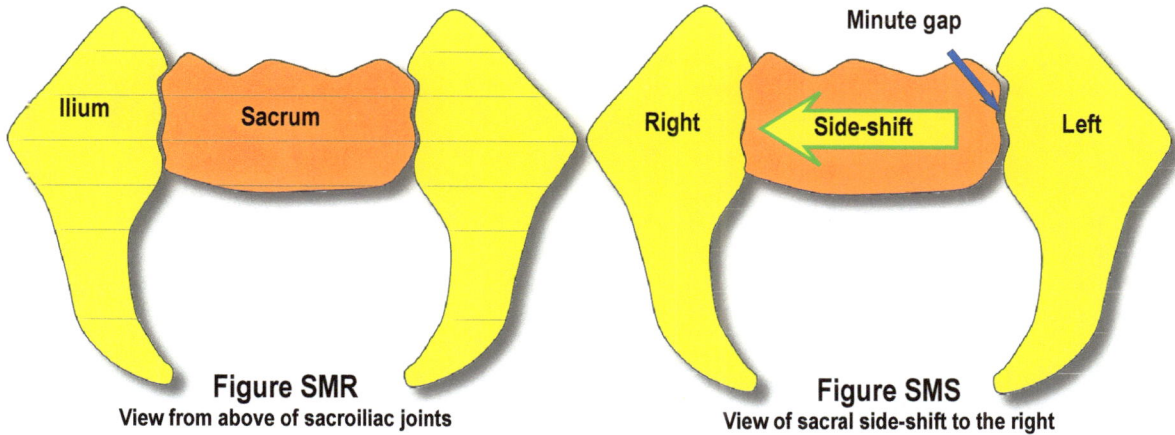

Figure SMR
View from above of sacroiliac joints

Figure SMS
View of sacral side-shift to the right

Sacral side-shift

Figure SMR shows the sacroiliac joints from above in neutral. The joints fit snugly on both sides

Figure SMS shows the sacroiliac joints when side-shift is to the right.   Note that a small gap opens up at the left sacroiliac joint that takes the tension out of the joint. Conversely, the right side of the joint becomes compressed. See chapter 4 on the walking action.

Side-shift

There is a distinct difference between side-bending and side-shift. Whilst this is a very obvious point, it has been illustrated in **figures SMT** and **SMU** as this is not a distinction that should be muddled up.

Another feature of side-shift is that the muscles to the opposite side to the side-shift which is to the left in **figure SMU**, become slackened. This can be useful to bear in mind when massaging or releasing tight and inflamed muscle groups.

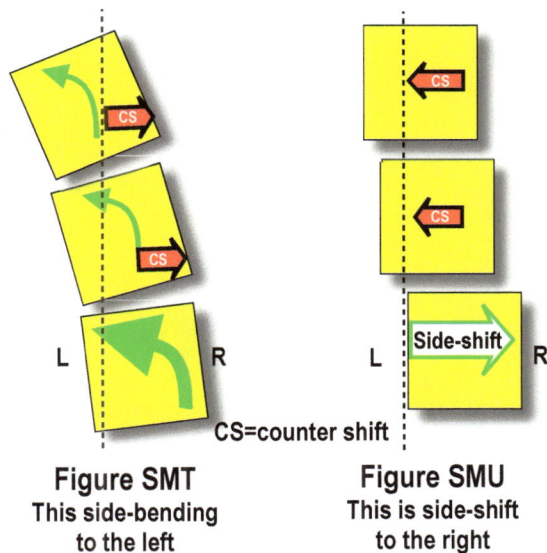

CS=counter shift

Figure SMT
This side-bending
to the left

Figure SMU
This is side-shift
to the right

Side-Shift Continued

Figure SMV illustrates the non weight bearing muscular skeletal frame, positioned in the mid-line. Any attempt to manipulate any joint of the body will meet with a counter resistance of opposing forces. Manipulative or releasing techniques therefore on any part of the musculo-skeletal frame would involve the use of considerable force. This force when passed on to the patient is often very uncomfortable, or worse still, painful.

Figure SMW illustrates the effect of transferring pelvic side-shift to the left, in a non weight bearing, knees flexed position.

It can be observed that the musculo-skeletal frame tightens up on the left when pelvic side-shift is to the left and loosens on the right. When force is applied from the left towards the right there is minimal resistance in the joints and tissue.

It is this simple physiological rule that allows manipulation directed from the left to the right to be applied to the spinal joints and muscles with relative ease. Further, joints that are not under normal bilateral tension due to the pelvic side-shift to the left are more easily managed. Therefore, the following areas on the right side of the body can be manipulated or balanced with comparative ease.

All muscles and fascia on the right.
Cranium (as part of cranial osteopathy).
Lower limb: Hip, knee, ankle and foot etc.
Posterior torso: Sacroiliac, spine, scapula and clavicle etc.
Anterior torso: Clavicle and manubrium, sternum etc
Upper limb: Shoulder, elbow and wrist..

Caution

In our example, caution should be exercised on the right side of the body, as the soft tissue and joints on the right have minimal protection against excessive force.

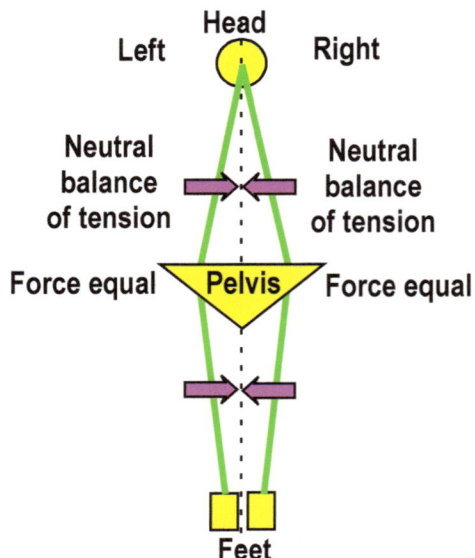

Figure SMV
This is a non weight bearing body frame
with the pelvis in the mid line

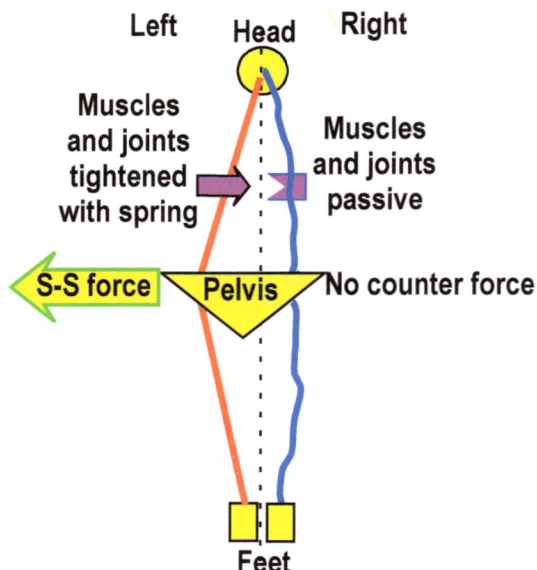

Figure SMW
This is a non weight bearing body frame
with pelvic side-shift to the left

Applying Side-Shift

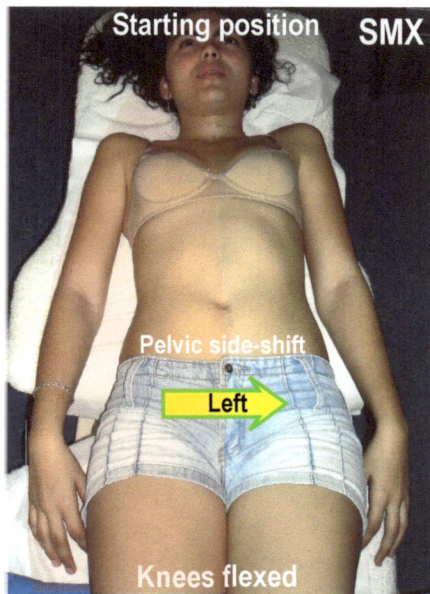

Starting position — SMX
Pelvic side-shift — Left
Knees flexed

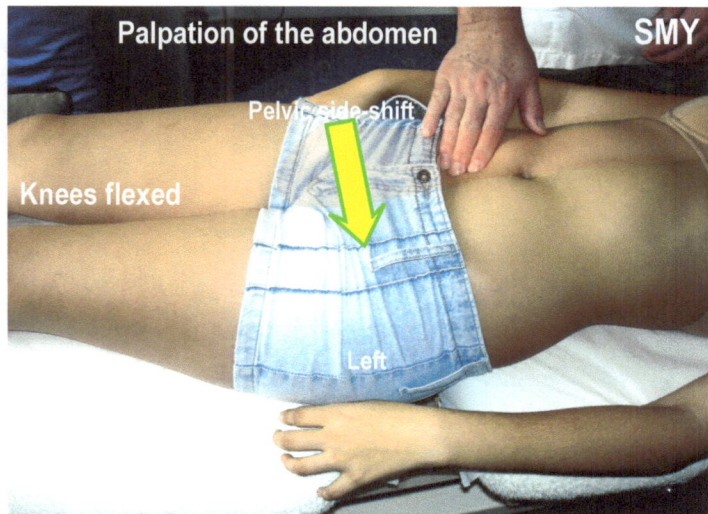

Palpation of the abdomen — SMY
Pelvic side-shift
Knees flexed
Left

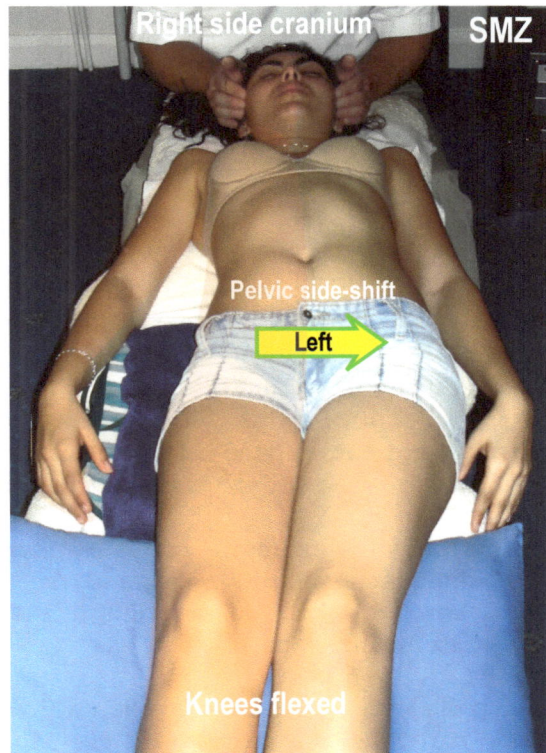

Right side cranium — SMZ
Pelvic side-shift — Left
Knees flexed

Position: When treating the anterior right side of the body, as shown in **figure SMX,** it makes a significant difference if the pelvis is side-shifted to the left. This is because the position takes much of the stress out of the soft tissue on the right. See the previous page for an explanation. The couch should be level. **Care should be taken to ensure that the pelvis has a soft surface. This is to avoid destabilizing the sacroiliac joints.**

Medical Palpation: In making medical abdominal examinations on the right as shown in **figure SMY,** visceral definition is more clearly defined if the patient lies with their knees partially flexed and with their pelvis side-shifted to the left.

Cranial Osteopathy: Cranial bones on the right are made more malleable when the knees are flexed and the pelvis is side-shifted to the left, as shown in **figure SMZ.** Side-shift should not be taken to the limit when treating with cranial techniques.

Side-Shift:
Power Massage and Muscle Release

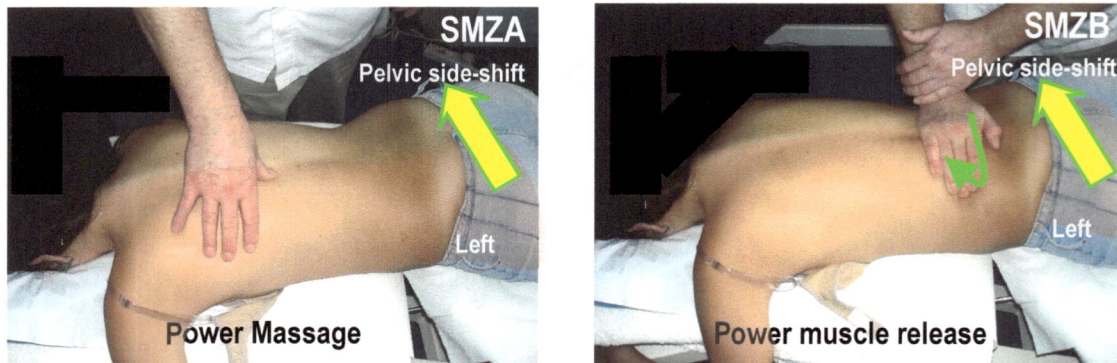

Power Massage

Figure SMZA shows the patient position to receive a power massage to the left side torso/buttock and leg muscles. The knees, though not shown, are flexed by placing a cushion under the patient's shins, with the pelvis side-shifted to the right. The position takes the tension out of the left side muscles; therefore less effort is required for the massage. As with all the soft tissue on the left in this position, the muscles become more easily defined.

Figure SMZB shows the lumbar being treated by power muscle release technique on the left. The patient position is the same as in the in **figure SMZA**. The muscles have little resistance in this position therefore even minimal force will achieve a lot.

Muscle stretch

Sometimes muscles need to be stretched to release them. With the help of pelvic side-shift this can be achieved with added power and less effort. With the patient in the same position as shown in **figure SMZA,** the muscles on the right are put under stretch and torsion by the pelvic side-shift to the right. If the distal end of the couch is lowered the patient's legs will be forced into forward bending. This will automatically stretch all muscles on the right side of the body. This position together with the side-shift puts considerable stretch on all of the muscles on the right and that is before the patient has even been touched.

There is already an extensive range of information on massage, muscle release and muscle stretch techniques available in the media's; therefore, there is no need to elaborate on these. The purpose of this book is to highlight the benefits of having a thorough understanding of synergetic spinal mechanics.

By placing the knees in a flexed position with the pelvis side-shifted the body is made vulnerable, therefore, care must be taken not too use excessive force. Pelvic side-shift should not be taken to its maximum.

Co-Operative Supine Techniques: CST's

CST's is the name given to techniques where the patient lies in a supine position and co-operates in some way, whilst their body is destabilized by pelvic side-shift and knee flexion. The starting position is shown in **figure SMX.** Below are photographs of examples of the many assessment, articulation and manipulative procedures that can be made easier and more efficient by this position. The purpose for adding the pelvic side-shift is that it isolates the joints, so that palpation and manipulation is not encumbered and made more difficult by soft issue tension.

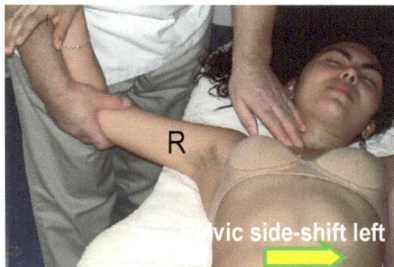

Clavicle articulation

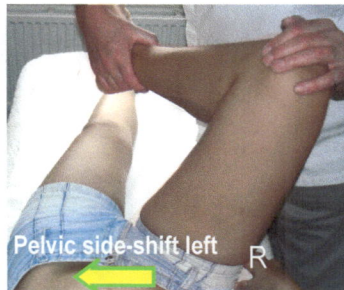

Hip articulation

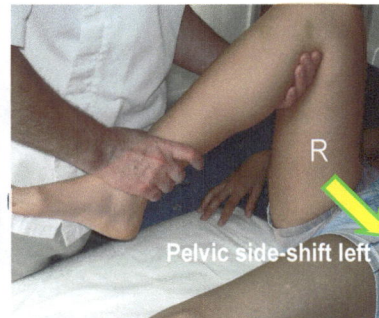

Knee assessment

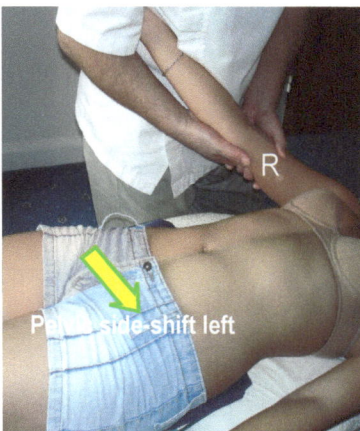

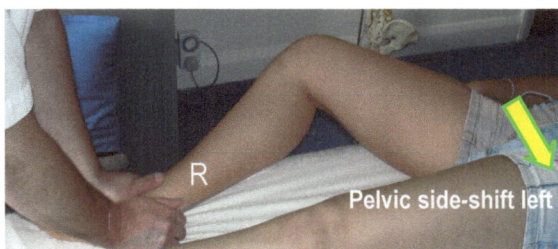

Elbow manipulation

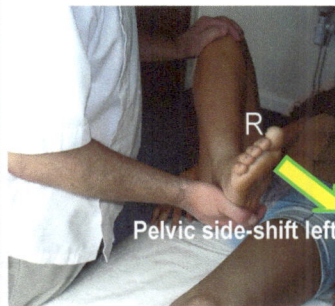

Hip assessment

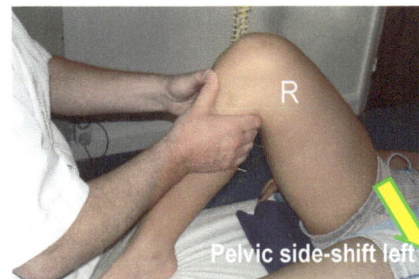

Knee assessment

Ankle manipulation

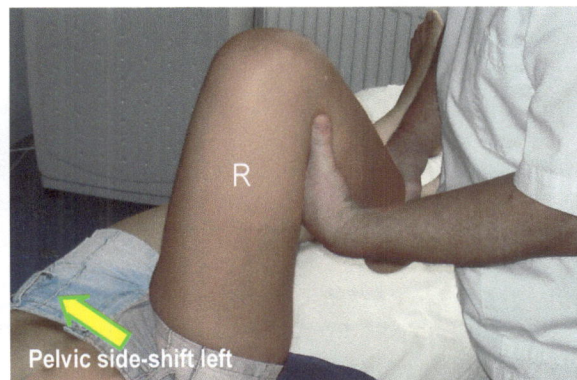

Knee manipulation

The Forces that Compound and Create Thoracic Extension Lesions

When correcting an extension Osteopathic lesion in the thoracic area, the following side-shift, forward and backward bending pattern forces must be retraced in order to realign the joint back into neutral. See chapters 8, 9,10 and 11 and specifically page 90 to understand the mechanics behind the flow chart below. Practical application of the movements is illustrated on the following page.

Note: The illustration is greatly exaggerated, in reality the difference from start to lesion is a few millimetres at most. It is for this reason that Osteopathic lesions are hard to differentiate when examining X-rays.

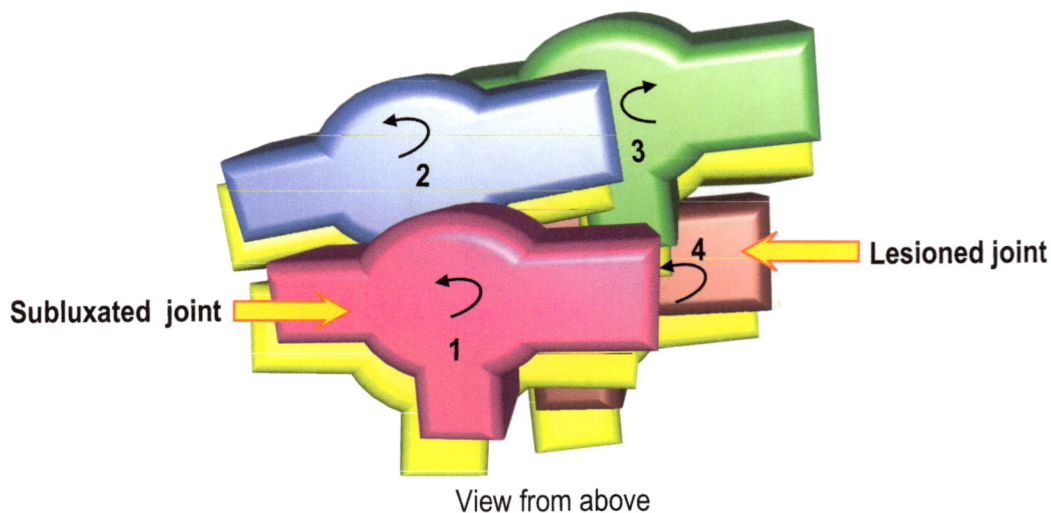

View from above

Using T3-4 as an example, T3 is forced into the rough (see pages 130 and 157) where it subluxates with rotation and side-bending to the left. The following explanation details the stages that compound a thoracic extension subluxation and make it into an Osteopathic lesion.

1. The extension side-bending subluxation arcs both T3 and T4 anteriorly. (Pelvic side-shift left)

2. When the person leans forward both T3 and T4 which are locked together, become levered in the same direction. This takes them fractionally further anteriorly and rotates them to the left.

3. When pelvic side-shift transfers to the right, T3 and T4 acting as one, become side-shifted and dragged to the right. This has the effect of levering them slightly further anteriorly whilst at the same time rotating them to the right.

4. Finally when the person straightens or back-ward bends and side-shifts their pelvis to the left T3 and T4 acting as one become levered posteriorly and attempt to rotate left. This really tightens the joint and digs T3 further into the rough of T4 and makes it impossible for the joint to move posteriorly. It is this accumulation of mismatched and conflicting forces that causes T3-T4 to become so rigidly fixated and positioned anteriorly.

It is worthy of note that most L3-R-R and L3-L-R people habitually side-shift and stand singularly on their left leg and this reinforces all of the left thoracic lesions.

164

How to Unlock Thoracic Extension Lesions
Example: T3 Rotated and Side-Bent Left

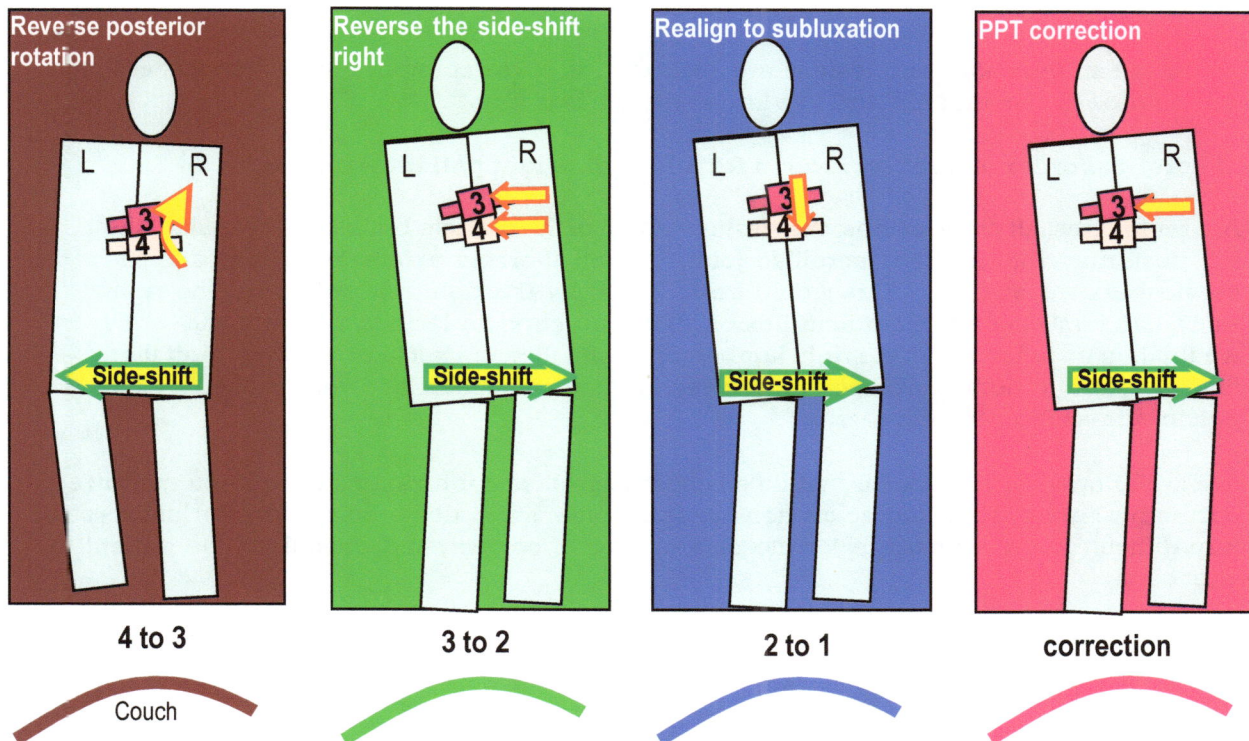

Reverse posterior rotation	Reverse the side-shift right	Realign to subluxation	PPT correction
4 to 3	**3 to 2**	**2 to 1**	**correction**
Couch			

The above show how to practically unlock the illustration on the previous page. While T3 is shown, the principal applies to the correction of all backward bending lesions rotated and side-bent to the left in the thoracic spine.

In all of these manoeuvres the distal and proximal ends of the couch need to be lowered to apply thoracic flexion and stretch to the spine. The Manipulator stands to the right of the patient.

Reverse posterior rotation

Place the patient in a prone position with their pelvis side-shifted to the left. Now gently de-rotate <u>both</u> T3 and T4 very slightly to the right in a superior arc. This reverses force 4-3.

Reversing the side shift

Ask your patient to side-shift their pelvis to the right and then ease <u>both</u> T4 and T3 to the left. This reverses force 3-2.

Realign to original subluxation

The pelvic side-shift should still be to the right. Now ease <u>both</u> T4 and T3 inferiorly. This reverses force 2-1.

Finally PPT Manipulation

Finally keeping the pelvic side-shift to the right make a gentle PPT push to the left against the right side of the T3 transverse process, as described in detail on page 178, to remove the subluxation.

If this procedure is followed both the lateral and anterior curves should be removed.

Order of Adjustment

The order the subluxations and lesions are corrected is of great importance. Theoretically, the order should be 'last in first out' and to a large extent this is true.

The theoretical order of joint correction for a L3-right-right patient would be:

> All trauma ribs, all anterior ribs, the sternum, both of the clavicle bones, the scapulae, the left posterior ribs, the left sacroiliac joint, the left thoracic extension lesions and the cervical lesions on left. This would be followed by the right posterior ribs, the right sacroiliac joint, the right thoracic flexion and then cervical lesions/subluxations. This would then be followed by the right lumbar joints and then the left lumbar joints. And then finally, return to both sacroiliac joints to realign any anomalies that were caused by the pelvic side-shift during the session.

My research however, has shown that unless both sacroiliac subluxations have been mobilized and correctly aligned, some thoracic extension subluxations and all thoracic extension lesions can be very difficult if not impossible for the manipulator to correct, and painful for the patient to experience.

A practical solution to this dilemma is to keep the order above with the exception that both sacroiliac joints should be mobilized and correctly aligned at the start of the treatment*.

It is probable that a joint correction might need repeating. This is because some joints particularly in the thoracic region due to reasons such as direct trauma and gravity misdirection can become locked in by their adjoining joints in a 'catch 22' counter lock. For example, some rib subluxations/lesions can become so tight and distorted that it makes it impossible to move the adjoining vertebrae. In these cases you have to toggle between the two areas several times to free the joints.

A lot of joints get manipulated within a single treatment session. This is because our goal is posture re-alignment, symmetry and synergetic mobility and not just clicking a few selected spinal and sacroiliac joints here and there to get the patient out of pain.

After the first session, with a healthy patient you should expect to see a considerable improvement to the symmetry and mobility of the spinal and sacroiliac joints etc. However, your job is not finished yet because, once the patient gets off your couch and goes about their daily business gravity will take its toll. This can be a useful diagnostic tool, because when the patient returns you will be able to identify more clearly the underlying causes and consequences of their subluxation/lesion pattern.

PPT's, PST's and CST's have opened up new possibilities in how much can be achieved in one single treatment session. It should be possible using these techniques to take posture realignment, symmetry and synergetic mobility to new levels of excellence.

---

* This book does not cover the lower extremities in any depth however; the hips, knees, ankles and feet must be in mobile alignment before any work is carried out above. This is so that the sacrum when freed can function as a level mobile base for the spine.

Chapter Fifteen
PPT
Spinal Manipulation

Anyone can manipulate a joint if they have the strength and a small degree of know-how. In fact, I have witnessed in Turkey, waiters practice their thoracic, lumbar and neck techniques on holiday makers as a sort of perverse after-dinner entertainment. And some are very good at what they do. So what separates the professional manipulator from these natural manipulators?

The answer comes in four parts:

1) Safety. Manipulation should only be carried out by fully trained professionals who have undergone lengthy medical training and are fully conversant with the dangers of incorrect diagnosis.

2) A subluxation pattern can be likened to a piece of string tied in lots of knots. In order to untangle the string, the knots must be untied in the sequence they were tied otherwise the tangle becomes even more complicated. The professional manipulator has to have a good working knowledge of the sequence in which the subluxations were created.

3) Gapping a joint is not good enough. The forces that are applied to free a subluxated joint must be administered in the precise reverse order in which the joint became locked. The satisfying sound of a clunk is not evidence that a joint has been correctly re-aligned.

4) All the corrupt side-shift must be removed, otherwise the benefit of the corrections will only be temporary.

Manipulation is an exact science where the laws of physics must be obeyed.

The techniques that follow are by no means the definitive way to correct particular types of subluxations. However, they do illustrate the logic behind each technique. This book attempts to fill in the gaps that have been missing from previous accounts of how the spinal joints articulate and subluxate. By adding the previously missing factors into manipulative techniques, it should now be possible to gain a higher degree of success.

Helping people to get out of pain should not be the only criterion of the professional manipulator. Like a nut and bolt, the nut that is correctly aligned on the thread and mobile, is more functional than a nut that is cross-threaded and jammed.

The Principles of Manipulation

To free a spinal or sacroiliac joint <u>all</u> the forces that created the subluxation must be reversed with the corrective thrust applied to the area of the bone that created the subluxation.

To recap on the forces that create a subluxation:

Rotation movements are the precursor to joint subluxations when the knees are kept straight and weight-bearing is on the same side as the pelvic side-shift. The subluxation is caused at the point where either forward bending changes to backward bending or backward bending to forward bending, without change to the weight bearing or direction of side-shift.

From this it can be deduced that there are rules that need to be applied during spinal manipulative procedures.

1) The patient's safety is your prime concern. So make sure your case history, clinical tests and palpation confirm it is safe to manipulate.

2) The body should not be weight-bearing.

3) The knees should be flexed for all sacral and spinal corrections.

4) Position the side-shift of the pelvis so that it is to the opposite side to that created in the subluxation patten.

5) Forward bend, neutralize or backward lean the torso in the opposite direction to that which the person was changing to at the moment of subluxation.

6) The corrective thrust must be to the area of the bone that created the subluxation.

7) The direction of the thrust must be the reverse of that which caused the subluxation.

8) The order in which the subluxations were created must be reversed in the precise order in which they were created.

Warning: Incorrect use of the above powerful forces can exaggerate a subluxation.

When analysing the position of pelvic subluxations/lesions on a prone patient, make sure that the A.S.I.S on both sides are an equal distance from the couch. This provides a 'constant' in your analysis and that any bony discrepancies are made more obvious at the posterior part of the sacroiliac joints. Also make sure that the patient is lying straight and in the middle of the couch with their knees mildly flexed and the angles of their feet matching.

It took a long time and effort to write the chapters on spinal mechanics and how subluxations are caused. The information is relevant, therefore, always refer to the chapters about the causes of each subluxation and become an expert manipulator not a mimic.

PPT Manipulation:
General

PPT stands for <u>P</u>assive <u>P</u>rone <u>T</u>echnique and I discovered PPT manipulation simply by reversing the forces that created subluxations. The idea of passive came from one of my patients, he asked me if I would do that 'passive' technique on him again. And that was how the passive part of the name came about. The 'prone' part came from the fact that the patient adopts a relaxed prone position on the couch.

PPT's are genuine noiseless manipulations. When joints subluxate they do not make any sound, and therefore, they should make no sound when they are corrected.

Because PPT's have such a small trauma footprint on the body all the joints from the iliosacral to the uppermost thoracic can be manipulated many times in one treatment session without destabilizing the back or causing undue distress to the patient. This provides the professional manipulator with the potential to get their patients backs straighter, more mobile and in a quicker time than was ever possible before.

PPT's work by reversing <u>all</u> the forces that created them. Minimal amounts of movement and energy are needed to be effective and great care must be taken to avoid excessive thrusts when the joints are at their most vulnerable. The first time you apply PPT's you will be amazed at how easy it is to correct even the most stubborn joint. You just feel the joint slipping back into place under your fingers.

Because muscles are rarely mentioned in this book it does not mean that they should be ignored. In fact correct application of their function can be very useful to enhance technique.

In **figure one** Marielle can be seen awaiting PPT manipulation. It can be seen that her right arm is parallel with her torso and that her left arm is raised.

If we observe the upper part of her body we can see that this posture relaxes her shoulder and muscles on the right. Whilst conversely, her raised arm stretches and pulls her left shoulder and muscles. Therefore, when the PPT push is made against the right side of the spinous process, the muscles on the left side will help to spring the joint back into place*. If we now observe her lower back area, the muscles again help us with our PPT's. With the left arm raised the whole of her left side musculature is pulled upwards, which lifts the iliac crest. This can help when it would be beneficial for the ilium to be raised.

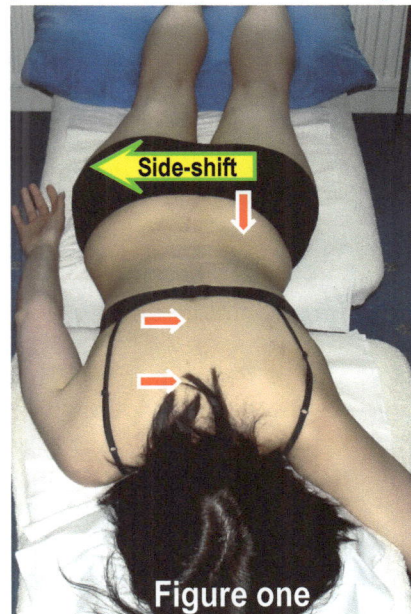
Figure one

The position of the arms are not shown in the photographs that follow for purposes of clarity.

* There is also a case for keeping both arms at the sides of the torso so that the spine and rib cage are kept in neutral, thus maintaining mid-line alignment of the spine.

Recap: Side-Roll Technique:
Left Posterior Ilium

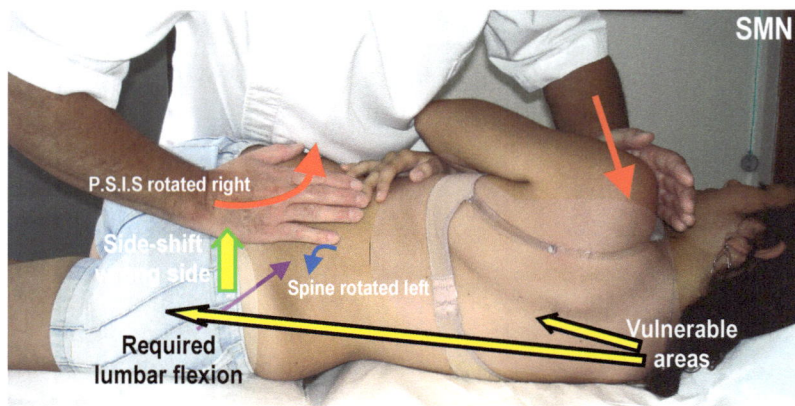

SMN

P.S.I.S rotated right

Side-shift
to my side

Spine rotated left

Required
lumbar flexion

Vulnerable
areas

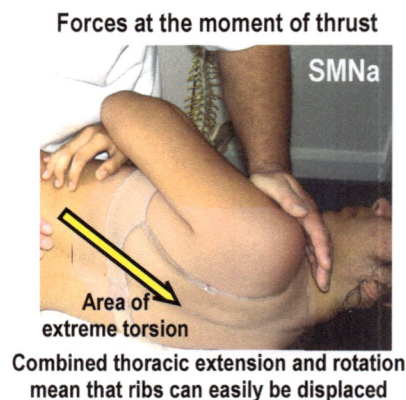

Forces at the moment of thrust

SMNa

Area of
extreme torsion

Combined thoracic extension and rotation
mean that ribs can easily be displaced

Side-Roll

For all the unwanted stresses and torsions this classical technique places on the upper body, it remains a valid way of correcting an iliosacral subluxation. Manipulators have speculated over the angle of the legs and how to stabilize the upper body to lessen the trauma to the thoracic vertebrae and ribs, and on the angle of thrust to obtain the optimum effect. **Figure SMN** is a photograph of Rafaela having her left sacroiliac joint manipulated in the basic side-roll position. The left ilium is often referred to as the posterior innominate because of its position relative to the anterior base of the sacrum.

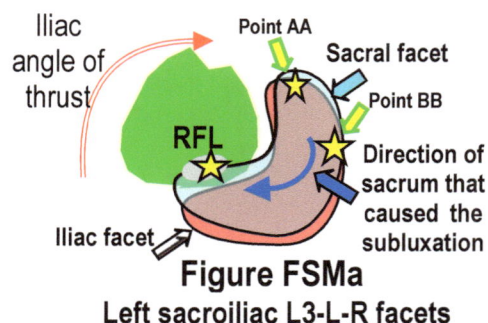

Iliac
angle of
thrust

Point AA

Sacral facet

Point BB

RFL

Direction of
sacrum that
caused the
subluxation

Iliac facet

Figure FSMa
Left sacroiliac L3-L-R facets

Evaluation of this technique:

The side-shift is to the left which tightens the left sacroiliac joint and destabilizes the right. This means that at the moment of thrust the manipulator runs a high risk of thrusting the right side of the sacrum anteriorly. Luckily this is a positive side-effect as we want the right side of the sacrum to move in that direction. As we have established, the pivot points of maximum impaction are at the '**RFL**', '**AA**' and '**BB**', as shown in **figure FSMa.** The angle of the left flexed leg levers the P.S.I.S in an inferio-posterior direction which is opposite to the intended direction of thrust? The weight of the flexed left leg, angled over the side of the couch, levers the posterior part of the iliosacral joint apart by compressing points **AA** and **BB**. The 'locked in' rotation of the spine to the left, together with the flexion of the lumbar, lever the base of the sacrum posteriorly and into a position that should favour the alignment of the facets. The manipulative technique itself starts with the left P.S.I.S being separated away from the sacrum, using points **AA** and **BB** as a fulcrum, followed by a high velocity thrust with an antero-superior trajectory. As this is a gapping technique there is an audible click.

However, mobility tests after manipulation indicate that the left sacroiliac facets, whilst palpably looser, may not be fully seated and could still be semi-restricted at the '**RFL**'.

Bayliss PPT:
Left Posterior Ilium

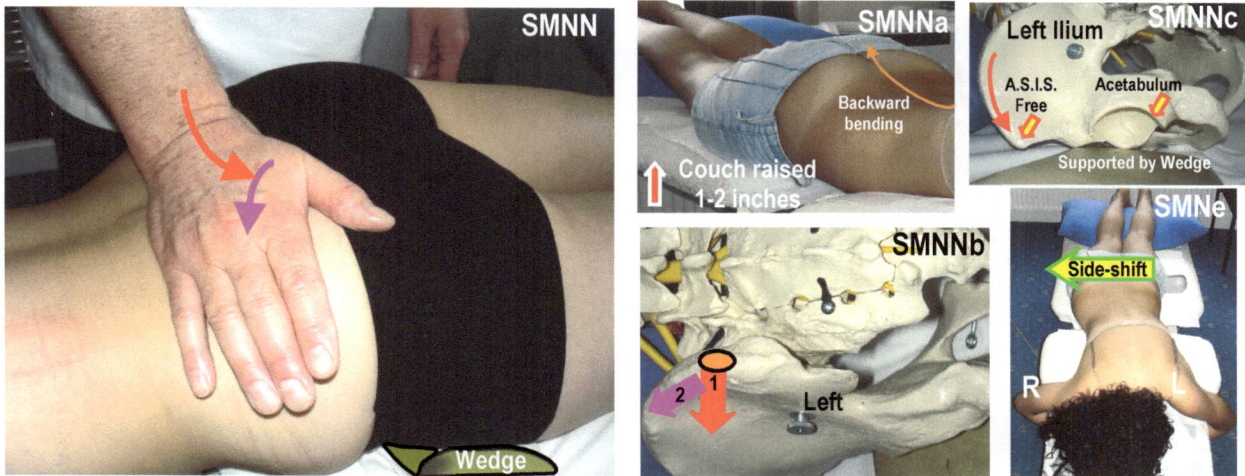

This iliosacral technique for a posterior innominate takes very little effort on the part of the practitioner and the patients find it a relatively comfortable procedure to have performed on them. The big plus point about all PPT procedures, and this one is no exception, is that the relaxed prone body does all the hard work, and the thrust is little more than a gentle push than a jerk.

Technique:
Generally, this technique should be the first manipulation carried out. The patient adopts a prone position with their pelvis located on the distal part of the couch and their right arm optionally at their side. The distal part of the couch is raised 1-2 inches so as to induce mild backward bending in their lower back. A cushion is placed under the patient's shins to create flexion of their knees which has the added dividend of patient comfort. The manipulator stands to the right of the patient, adjacent to their pelvis, and asks the patient to take their lower body weight on their knees and to raise their pelvis a few inches. The manipulator then manually side-shifts the pelvis to the right and the patient relaxes back onto the couch, as shown in **figure SMNe**.

The manipulator then moves down the couch to be level with the patients thighs and makes two separate movements 1) They place the hypothenar eminence of their right hand against the medial side of the P.S.I.S and push laterally. This separates the posterior part of the iliosacral joint and compresses points **AA** and **BB** shown in **figure FMSa** on the previous page. 2) They then gently push the P.S.I.S in an antero-superior direction along the line of the iliac crest. There is no click, just a feeling of 'give'. Care should be taken not to press too hard. The joint aligns with very little effort and movement .

So how does the technique work?
The side-shift to the right causes the left side of the sacroiliac joint to become malleable. The backward-bent angle of the lumbar spine levers the base of the sacrum posteriorly. The wedge under the left acetabulum/femoral head lifts the ilium and the A.S.I.S off the couch and provides a point of pivot for the A.S.I.S to rotate anteriorly, see **figure SMNNc** above. After manipulation the sacroiliac joint, though more mobile, is unlikely to be fully aligned. The technique on the next page should follow on to complete the alignment of this joint.

171

Bayliss PPT:
Left Posterior Sacroiliac

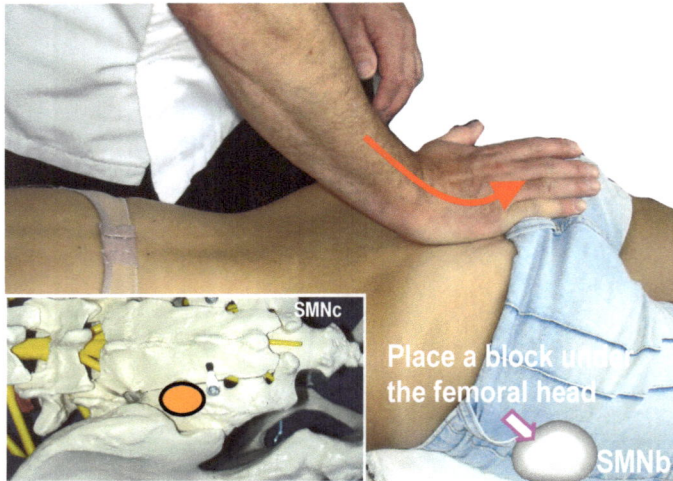

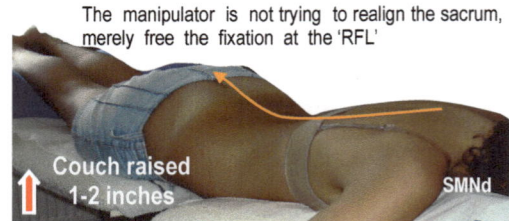

The manipulator is not trying to realign the sacrum, merely free the fixation at the 'RFL'

Couch raised 1-2 inches

SMNd

SMNc

Place a block under the femoral head

SMNb

There is no tension placed on the thoracic spine or ribs. Even the most tense patient remains passive which allows the manipulator to have full control of the procedure and timing.

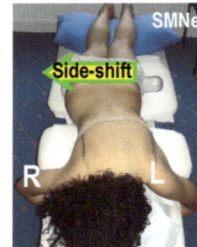

SMNe

Side-shift

R L

This posterior sacroiliac technique takes very little effort on the part of the practitioner and patients find it a fairly comfortable procedure to have performed on them. The big plus point of this procedure is that the relaxed prone body does all the hard work, and the thrust is little more than a gentle push than a jerk.

Technique:

Where applicable, this technique should be carried out after the 'left side-role' or preferably the 'Bayliss PPT posterior ilium technique'. The patient adopts a prone position on the couch with their pelvis located on the distal part of the couch and their right arm at their side.. The distal part of the couch is raised 1-2 inches so as to induce mild backward bending in the lower back. A cushion is placed under the patient's shins to create flexion in the knees, with the added dividend of patient comfort. The manipulator stands to the right of the patient, adjacent to the pelvis, and asks the patient to take their lower body weight on their knees and raise their pelvis a few centimetres. The manipulator then manually side-shifts the pelvis to the right and the patient relaxes back onto the couch. The side-shift destabilizes the left side of the sacroiliac joint. All that is necessary now is for the manipulator to place the hypothenar eminence of their right hand on the sacrum above the '**RFL**' and gently push down in a antero-inferior direction. There is no click, just a feeling of 'give'. Care should be taken not to press too hard.

So how does the technique work? The side-shift to the right causes the left side of the sacroiliac joint to become malleable. The backward bent angle of the spine levers the base of the sacrum posteriorly. Whilst the raised legs lever the crest of the ilium anteriorly. This creates two opposing long levers in the directions necessary to release the joint. The antero-inferior push directly towards the '**RFL**', as shown in **figure SMNb** and **figure SMK** on page 156, releases the impaction. This, combined with the long levers, causes the posterior sacroiliac 'E' facets to correctly realign in neutral.

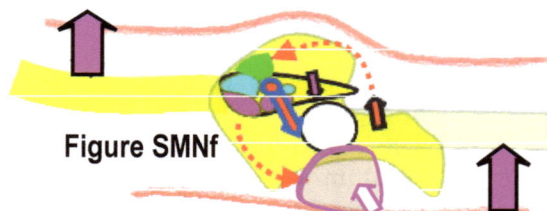

Figure SMNf

Important: Place a wedge under the femoral head to add stability and act as a pivot

Recap: Side-Roll Technique: Right Anterior Ilium

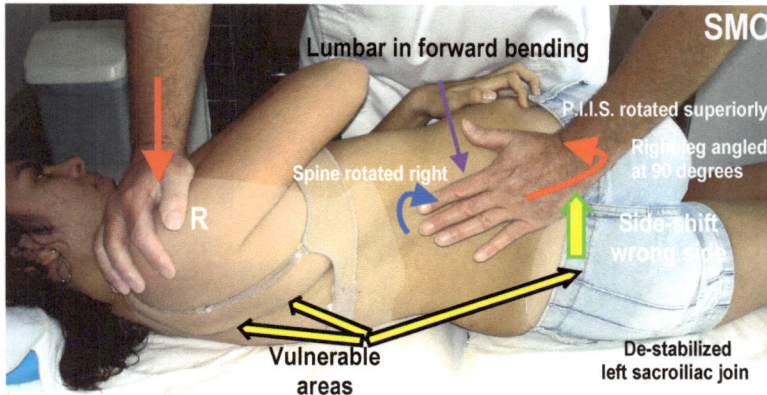

Figure SMO labels: Lumbar in forward bending · SMO · P.I.I.S. rotated superiorly · Spine rotated right · Right leg angled at 90 degrees · R · Side-shift wrong side · Vulnerable areas · De-stabilized left sacroiliac join

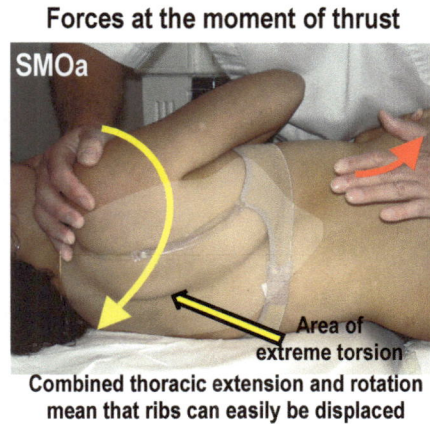

Forces at the moment of thrust · SMOa · Area of extreme torsion
Combined thoracic extension and rotation mean that ribs can easily be displaced

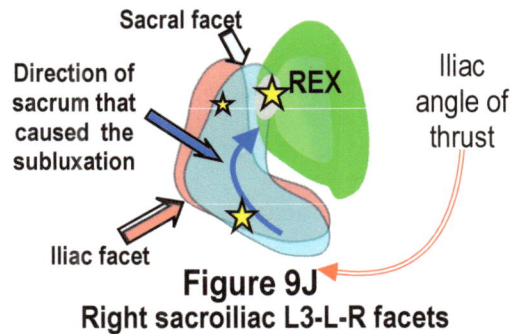

Sacral facet · Direction of sacrum that caused the subluxation · REX · Iliac angle of thrust · Iliac facet

Figure 9J
Right sacroiliac L3-L-R facets

Right Side-Roll

The above photograph **figure SMO,** shows a right anterior subluxation being manipulated. This subluxation gets its name from the anterior position of the ilium in relation to the posterior base of the sacrum.

This is an iliosacral technique. In both the L3-left-right and L3-right-right patterns the anterior subluxation is sacroiliac. **Figure SMO** is a photograph of Rafaela having her right sacroiliac joint manipulated in the side-roll position. The thrust is made in an antero-superior direction against the superior aspect of the right iliac P.I.I.S. To gain a good purchase the manipulators right hand has to rotate the shoulder to the left.

Evaluation of this technique:

The side-shift is to the right which tightens the joint to be manipulated on that side at the expense of destabilizing the recently-manipulated left sacroiliac joint. This has the implication that a high velocity thrust performed on the right ilium could undo what has just been achieved on the left. Further, the spinal rotation to the right levers the base of the sacrum on the right side posteriorly, which is the opposite direction needed to release the subluxation. This spinal rotation is likely to further destabilize the left side of the sacrum by levering it anteriorly against the ilium.

Almost redeeming, the right side of the sacrum at the base is blocked by the forward bending caused by the acutely angled overhanging right leg. The overhanging leg also has the advantage of levering apart the point of impaction 'REX' in **figure 9J**.

Recap: Chicago Technique:
Right Anterior Ilium

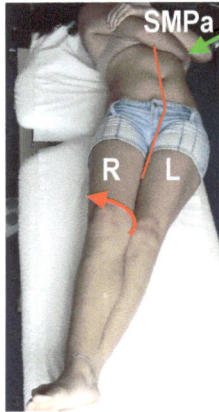

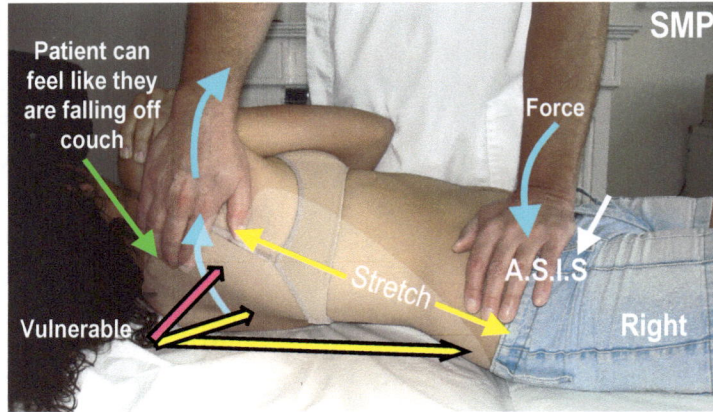

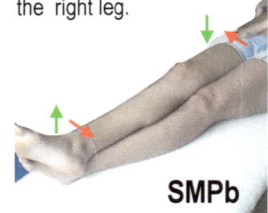

Right Chicago

The 'Chicago' technique is a popular procedure with many manipulators who correct the right anterior sacroiliac subluxation. Theoretically, this is a technically superior type of manipulation to the right side-roll, because the thrust is aimed through the '**REX**'.

Having said this, it is an uncomfortable technique because it contorts the patient's body in so many directions. This, together with the shearing thrust that is applied over the sensitive A.S.I.S in my experience makes this technique unpopular with patients.

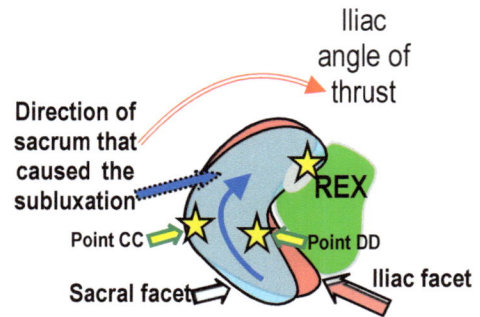

Figure ESNa

Right sacroiliac L3-R-R facets

Figure SMP is a photograph of Rafaela having her right sacroiliac joint manipulated in the 'Chicago' position. The thrust is made in an arcing postero-superior direction over inferior aspect of the right A.S.I.S.

Evaluation of this technique:
This is a sacroiliac subluxation being corrected by an iliac thrust and therefore risks further distortion of the sacroiliac joints. The spinal rotation to the left offers an opposing sacral counter force, so the technique should work. There is some unintentional side-shift to the left which is ideal, but this comes in the guise of unwanted and excessive side-bending applied to the lumbar spine and legs. The side-bending over compacts the upper half of the right sacroiliac joint and locks bone against bone at the '**REX**' shown in **figure ESNa**, which is the point the technique attempts to free. The knees are straight and, because of this, they tighten the pelvic muscles and make it harder to manipulate. A considerable amount of force is needed to make the thrust and if successful it make an audible click.

Bayliss PPT:
Right Anterior Sacroiliac

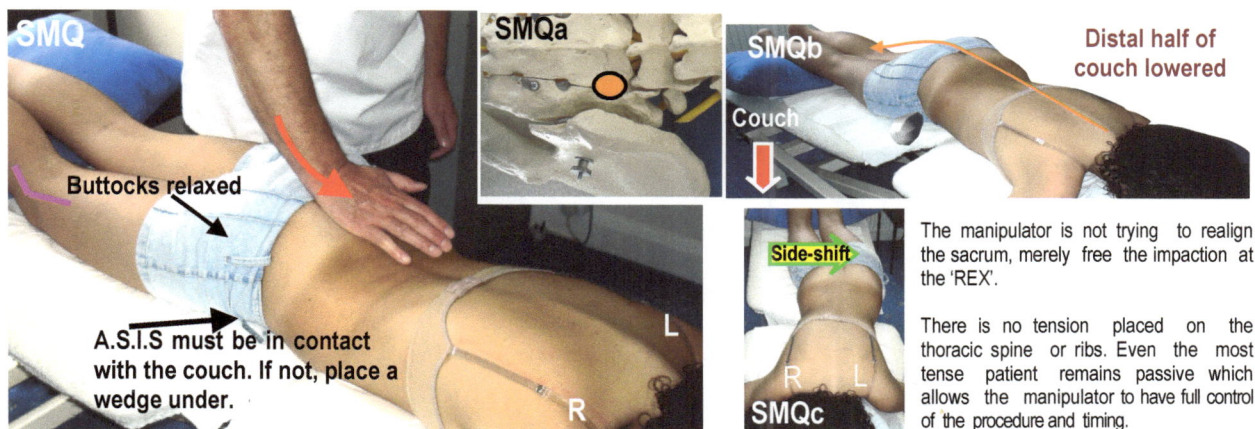

Buttocks relaxed

A.S.I.S must be in contact with the couch. If not, place a wedge under.

SMQa

SMQb

Couch

Distal half of couch lowered

Side-shift

SMQc

The manipulator is not trying to realign the sacrum, merely free the impaction at the 'REX'.

There is no tension placed on the thoracic spine or ribs. Even the most tense patient remains passive which allows the manipulator to have full control of the procedure and timing.

Technique: This technique is used to correct a right anterior sacroiliac subluxation resulting from the L3-left-right pattern subluxation. The patient adopts a prone position with their pelvis located on the distal part of the couch, such that when the distal half of the couch is lowered, forward bending is introduced in the lower back. The right arm should be placed at the side of the torso. A cushion is placed under both of the patient's anterior shins to create flexion in the knees.

The manipulator stands to the left of the patient adjacent to the pelvis and asks the patient to take their lower body weight on their knees to raise their pelvis a few centimetres. The manipulator then manually side-shifts the pelvis to the left and the patient relaxes back onto the couch. The side-shift destabilizes the right side of the sacroiliac joint. All that is necessary now is for the manipulator to place the hypothenar eminence of their right hand on the sacrum above the '**REX**' and gently push down in a supero-anterior direction. There is usually no audible click, just a feeling of 'give'.

So how does the technique work? The side-shift to the left causes the right side of the sacroiliac joint to become malleable. The forward bending of the spine levers the base of the sacrum anteriorly, whilst the forward bending of the legs rotates the ilium posteriorly. This creates two opposing long levers in the directions necessary to release the joint. The antero-superior push directly over the '**REX**', as shown in **figure SMQa** above, releases the impaction. This, combined with the long levers of the spine and legs, causes the posterior sacroiliac 'F' facets to realign in neutral, as illustrated in **figure SMQd** below, and **figure SMH** on page 156.

This is a highly specific long-lever technique. Because the left side of the sacroiliac joint was not placed in torsion, it is unaffected by the correction on the right.

Iliosacral involvement

Because there is weight bearing on the right leg there could be an element of iliosacral subluxation present. Therefore, apply the posterior iliosacral technique shown on page 172 lightly to the right ilium before performing the above. On this side the distal end of the couch should be lowered.

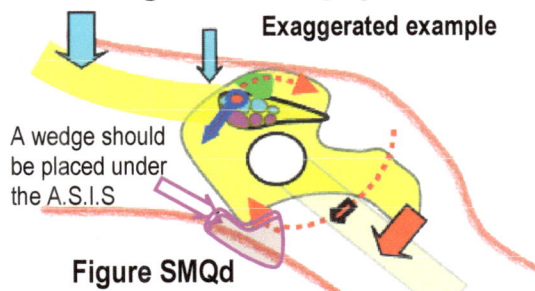

Exaggerated example

A wedge should be placed under the A.S.I.S

Figure SMQd

Recap: Thoracic Dog Technique

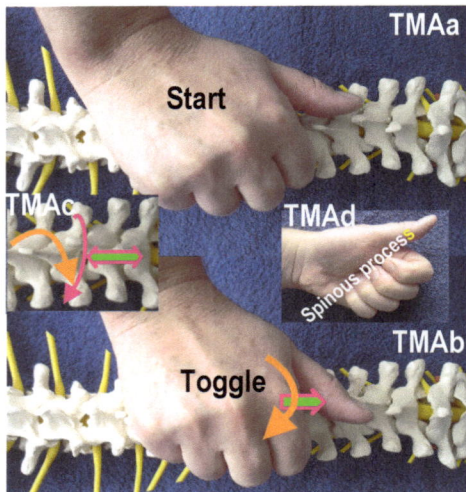

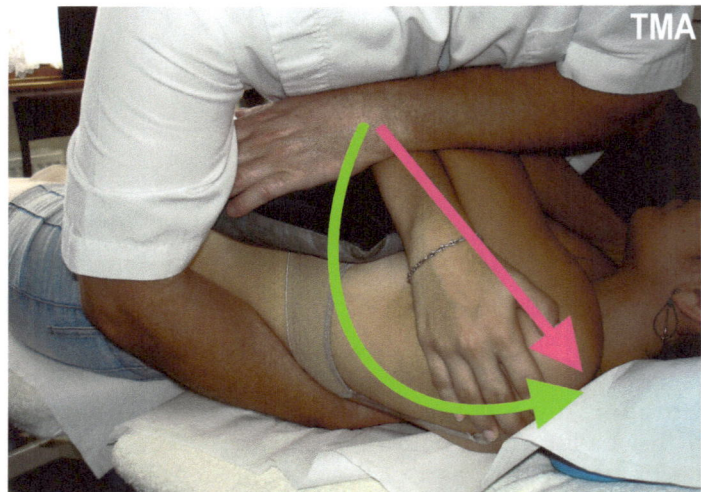

If you ask any professional manipulator, they would probably say that this is the technique they do the best. But patients would disagree. They get the manipulators fist in their back, right in that 'sensitive bit', which is very uncomfortable, followed by the manipulator bearing down on their arms and half knocking the wind out of them. And to boot, as this is not an efficient technique, the subluxated vertebrae does not always move, so the patient gets the pain of the manipulators knuckles right on the bone in that 'sensitive bit'.

So let us analyse the 'Dog' technique. **Figure TMA** is a photograph of Rafaela having her thoracic joint manipulated in the 'Dog' position. The manipulator locks the spinous process of the thoracic vertebra below the vertebra to be released within the knuckles of their fist, as shown in **figure TMAd**. There are two ways to thrust; either through the long bone of the arms, as shown by the magenta arrow to correct a flexion subluxation, or by scooping the arms towards the shoulders to correct an extension subluxation, as shown by the green arrow.

Some manipulators will place their locking fist under the vertebra being manipulated and de-rotate, de-side-bend, de-flex and de-extend as they think appropriate at the moment of thrust. This is shown in **figures TMAa** and **TMAb**.

Evaluation of this technique:

Even though this technique uses the long lever of the arms it still relies on quite a large degree of force to gap the joint. Because the manipulator cannot see the joint that they are manipulating, they rely on memory and reverse palpation to get their bearings. By default this makes the technique less than precise, especially where there are clusters of extension and flexion subluxations in very close proximity camouflaging the other. There is an audible click.

Recap: Thoracic Toggle Technique

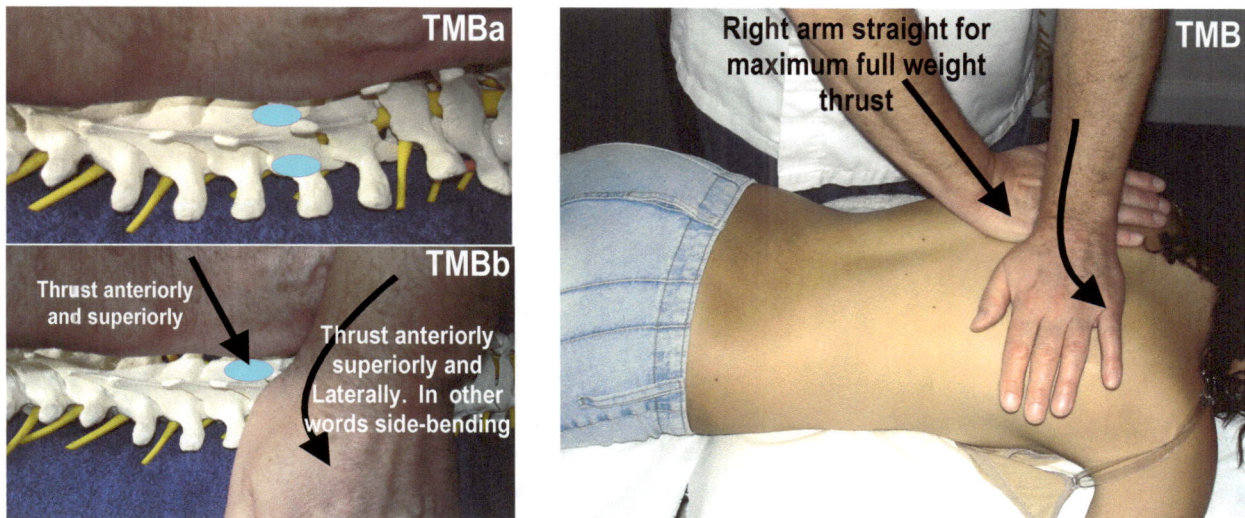

TMBa

TMBb

Thrust anteriorly and superiorly

Thrust anteriorly superiorly and Laterally. In other words side-bending

Right arm straight for maximum full weight thrust

TMB

The 'Toggle' technique is favoured by some because the manipulator can clearly see the joint they intend to release and have room to work. It is therefore a highly specific technique. The patient is placed in a comfortable prone position, which takes a lot of the anxiety out of the procedure for the patient. However, because this is a short lever technique, considerable force is needed to gap the joint.

So let us analyse the 'Toggle' technique. **Figure TMB** is a picture of Rafaela having her thoracic joint manipulated in the 'Toggle' position. The manipulator places their right hyper-thenar eminence over the transverse process of the thoracic vertebra to be manipulated. They then place the thenar eminence of the other hand against the right side of the spinous process of the same vertebra. The thrust is made by pushing the transverse process superiorly and anteriorly with the one hand whilst the other side-bends the spinous process to the right in a heavy toggling action.

Some manipulators leave out the side-bending and thrust both hands in a anterior-superior direction on the left to simply gap the joint.

Evaluation of this technique:

The downward force on the transverse process can be very painful for the anterior rib cage if the couch is not padded enough, especially when some manipulators use the full weight of their body in a body drop focused in the line of drive. If de-side-bending or de-rotation are emphasized during the high velocity thrust, bone is pushed against bone. Of course brute force produces a gapping but because the side-shift has not been neutralized, the joint will in all likelihood come out of place once the body becomes weight-bearing again. This can also be said for the 'Dog' technique.

Bayliss PPT:
Thoracic Rotated Left in Extension

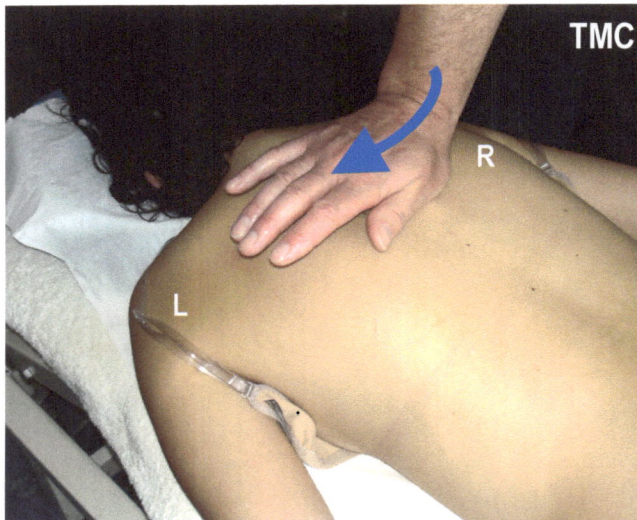

TMC

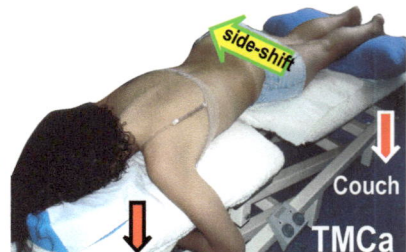

side-shift

Couch

TMCa

Figure TMCb Shows T3 rotated to the left.

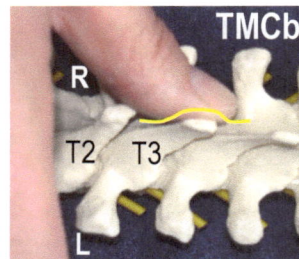

TMCb

R

T2   T3

L

The side of the subluxated spinous process is palpated using the pad of the thumb. The thrust could be made with the thumb. Ensure that T3 is in extension and not flexion.

This thoracic technique takes very little effort on the part of the practitioner and the patients find it an easy and fairly comfortable procedure to have performed on them. The beauty of this procedure like those of the sacroiliac joints is that it uses the body as a long lever of to do all the hard work and the thrust is little more than a gentle push.

This is such a gentle technique that in many cases the patient does not even know they have been manipulated. With such a low trauma impact post-manipulative recovery should be speedy. A positive aspect of this technique is that the manipulator can see exactly what they are doing and can therefore theoretically achieve much higher degrees of accuracy.

Technique:

The patient adopts a relaxed prone position on the couch with their pelvis side-shifted to the right with the distal and proximal sections of the couch lowered. See **figure TMCa.** Though not shown the right arm could optionally be placed on the couch parallel to the torso .

The manipulator stands to the right of the patient and moves adjacent to the thoracic vertebra to be manipulated. In this case T3 is locked in extension and awaiting manipulation. Having located the subluxated joint with the pad of their thumb against the side of the spinous process, see **figure TMCb**, the manipulator uses the pad of their thenar eminence to make a gentle side-ways push against the spinous process. Again the reason for using the pad of the hand is purely for patient comfort. The manipulator's hand experiences a slight feeling of 'give', which is the joint slipping back into place. There is no click or thud. This technique is used on all thoracic vertebrae subluxated in extension that are rotated to the left. This means that vertebrae as high as T1 to the convoluted rotations of T12 can also be manipulated using this simple technique.

Bayliss PPT: Left continued

So how does the technique work?

This is a highly specific technique using the long lever of the relaxed body to do the heavy work.

The way the joints get their driving force is similar to the way a pendulum creates the momentum to turn the cog wheels of a clock. A further explanation of this is in chapter one.

In **figure TMCc** it can be seen that T4 and the vertebrae below are being levered to the right. This side-shift to the right is drawn from the force of the destabilized pelvis shown in **figure TMCd.**

The destabilization of the pelvis on the left takes all the tension out of the spine on the left, all the way up to the neck. It is this lack of tension that enables all of the thoracic vertebrae, and for that matter all of the lumbar vertebrae, to be manipulated with minimal force.

The flexed legs, as shown in **figure TMCe,** pull the vertebrae below T3 in an inferior direction, which opens the thoracic facets.

With T4 and all the vertebrae below side-shifted to the right and the legs flexed and levering the joint T3-T4 open, all the hard work is done. All the manipulator has to do is gently push the spinous process of the destabilized T3, to the left.

Caution should be exercised. Do not to use excessive force. If the T3 joint does not side-shift with minimal force, suspect that it is either lesioned or locked in flexion or that the attaching ribs are subluxated in such a way as to block the movement.

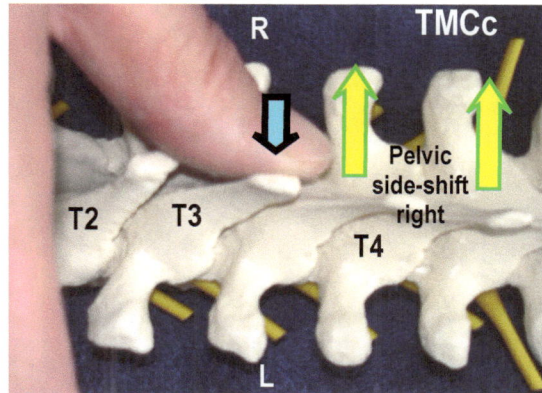

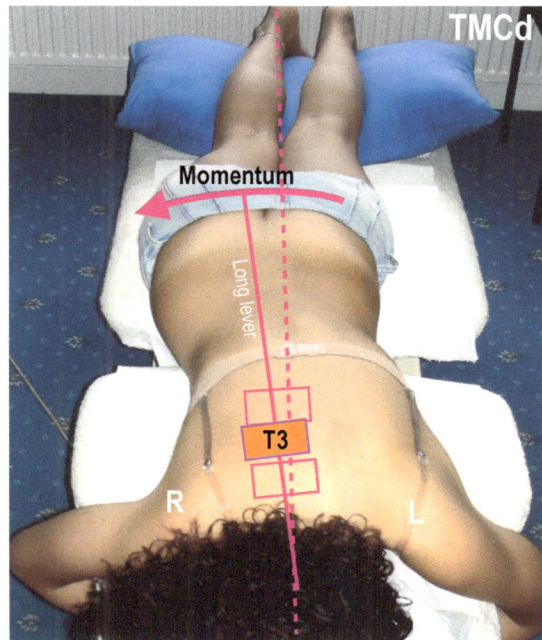

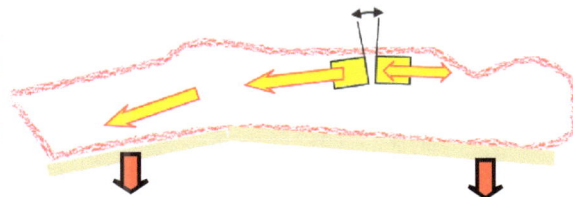

Figure TMCe
Person lies prone with their legs flexed

Bayliss PPT:
Rotated Right in Thoracic Flexion

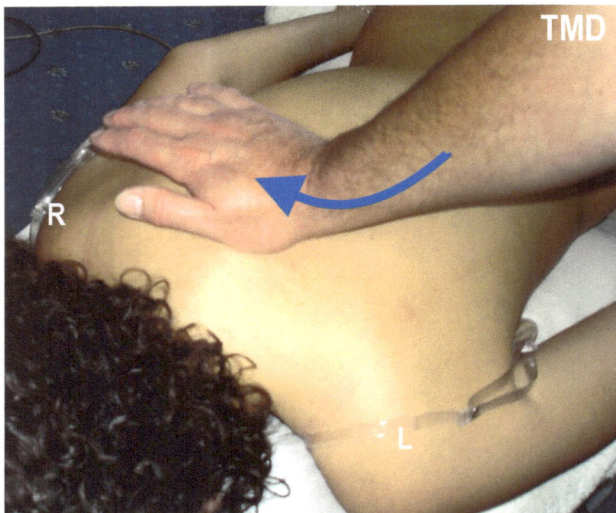

Figure TMDb
Shows T3
rotated to
the right.

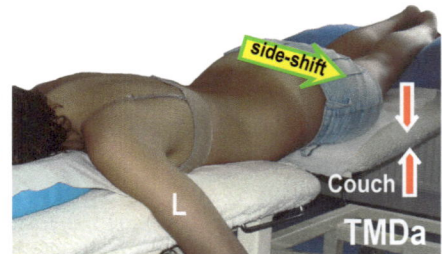

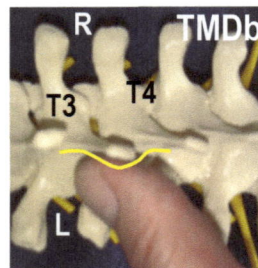

The side of the subluxated spinous process is palpated using the pad of the thumb. The thrust could be made with the thumb. Ensure that T3 is in flexion and not extension.

This thoracic technique takes very little effort on the part of the practitioner and the patients find it an easy and fairly comfortable procedure to have performed on them. Again the beauty of the procedure is that it uses the long lever of the body to do all the hard work and the thrust is little more than a gentle push.

This is such a gentle procedure that in many cases the patient does not even know they have been manipulated. The manipulator can see exactly what they are doing and can therefore theoretically achieve a much higher degree of accuracy.

Technique:

The patient adopts a relaxed prone position on the couch with their pelvis side-shifted to the left with the couch level. See **figure TMDa**. Though not shown the left arm could optionally be placed on the couch along side of the torso.

The manipulator stands to the left of the patient and moves adjacent to the thoracic vertebra to be manipulated. In this case T3 is locked in flexion and awaiting manipulation. Having located the subluxated joint with the pad of their thumb against the side of the spinous process, see **figure TMDb,** the manipulator then uses the pad of the thenar eminence to make a gentle side-ways push against the spinous process. The manipulator's hand experiences a feeling of 'give', which is the joint slipping back into place. There is no click or thud. This technique can be used on all the thoracic vertebrae subluxated in flexion and rotated to the right. This means that vertebrae as high as T1 and the convoluted rotations and side-bending of T12 can also be manipulated using this simple and accurate technique.

Bayliss PPT: Rotated Right in Thoracic Flexion Continued

So how does the technique work?

This is a highly specific technique using the long lever of the relaxed body to do all the heavy work.

In **figure TMDc** it can be seen that T4 and the vertebrae below are being levered to the left. This side-shift to the left is drawn from the force of the destabilized pelvis shown in **figure TMDd.**

The destabilization of the pelvis to the right takes all the tension out of the spine, on the right, all the way up to the neck. It is this lack of tension that enables all of the thoracic vertebrae, and for that matter all of the lumbar vertebrae, to be manipulated with minimal force.

The neutral angle of the legs as shown in **figure TMDe** is enough to extend the thoracic vertebrae and bring the facets together. Be wary of adding height to the distal half of the couch otherwise the thoracic joints will become too compacted to be corrected.

With T4 and all the vertebrae below side-shifted to the right and the extended legs approximating the T3-T4 joint, all the hard work is done. All the manipulator has to do is gently push the spinous process of the destabilized T3, to the right.

Caution should be exercised. Avoid excessive force. If the joint does not side-shift with minimal force, recheck your diagnosis and suspect that the joint is locked in extension, the spinous process is not symmetrical or that the attaching ribs are subluxated in such a way as to block the movement.

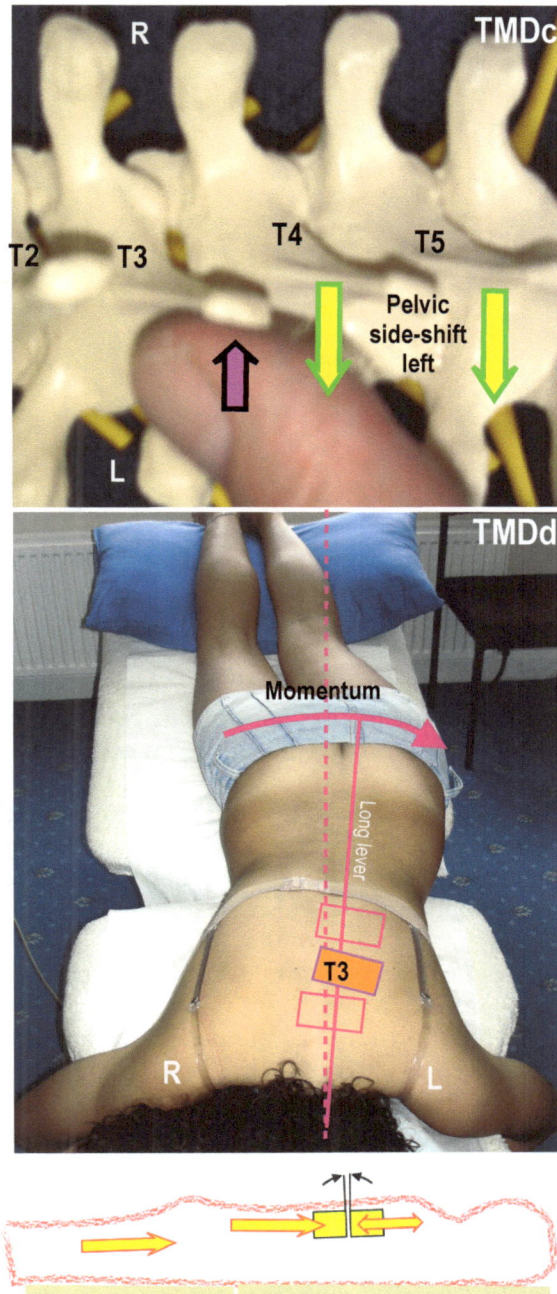

Figure TMDe
Person lies prone with their legs extended

Lumbar Side-Roll
L3-Right-Right: L3-Left-Right

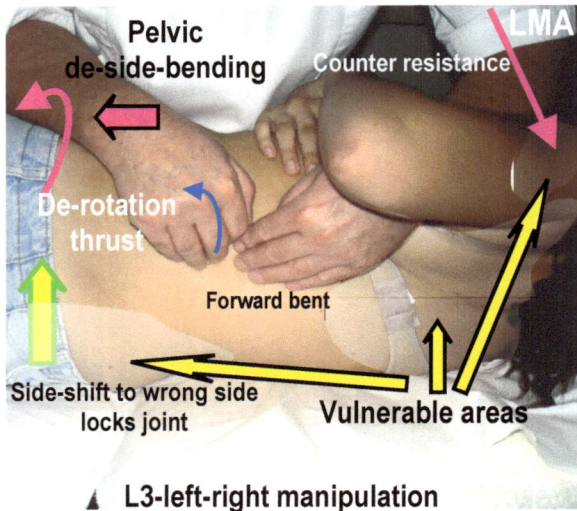

Pelvic de-side-bending
Counter resistance
LMA
De-rotation thrust
Forward bent
Side-shift to wrong side locks joint
Vulnerable areas

▲ **L3-left-right manipulation**

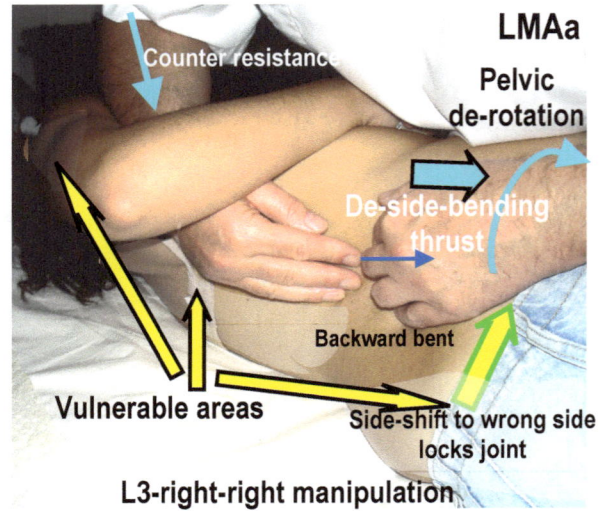

Counter resistance
LMAa
Pelvic de-rotation
De-side-bending thrust
Backward bent
Vulnerable areas
Side-shift to wrong side locks joint

L3-right-right manipulation

The side-roll techniques are the standard traditional method of correcting lumber vertebrae subluxations. However, these techniques have some disadvantages that bring their effectiveness into question.

So let us analyse the reasons why their effectiveness is in question. The two photographs above illustrate Rafaela having her lumbar vertebra manipulated in the de-rotation and de-side bending side-roll positions. The L3-left-right correction and the L3-right-right correction.

In **figure LMA**, L3 is side-bent left and rotated right in flexion. The left shoulder is rotated right and pinned down. The lumbar is forward bent to counter the lumbar flexion. Side-bending comes from the pelvis, so the iliac crest of the pelvis is levered inferiorly. The manipulative thrust is applied using the overhanging left leg as a lever and concentrating the de-rotation force at L3.

In **figure LMAa**, L3 is rotated right and side-bent right in extension. The right shoulder is rotated left and pinned down. The lumbar is backward bent to counter the lumbar extension. Rotation comes from the pelvis, so the pelvis is rotated left, aided by the overhanging right leg. Forces are concentrated at L3 and the manipulative thrust is applied by pushing inferiorly on the right ilium in order to de-side-bend L3.

Evaluation of this technique:

Side-roll manipulations can be uncomfortable for the patient, the higher up the lumbar the more uncomfortable and stretched the patient feels. This can make patients tense and therefore harder to handle. The side-shift is to the wrong side and tightens the joint to be manipulated rather than loosens it, while at the same time the position de-stabilizes the opposite side. Because this is a long lever technique the upper shoulder is used to gain leverage which, even with the best of intentions, puts considerable torsion on the thoracic vertebrae and ribs, especially at the moment of thrust.

Bayliss Basic Lumbar PPT:
L3-Left-Right

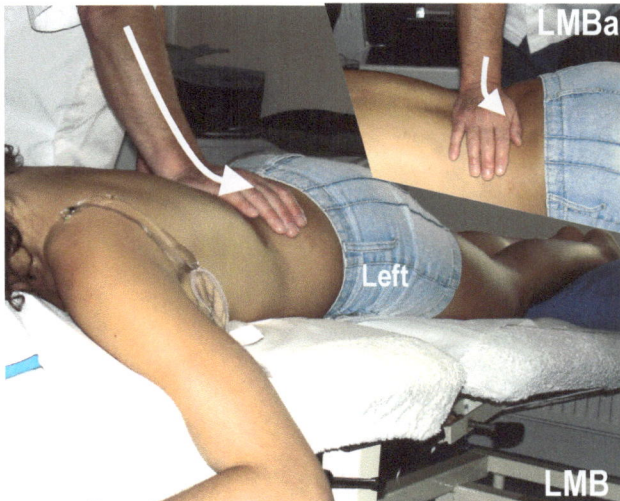

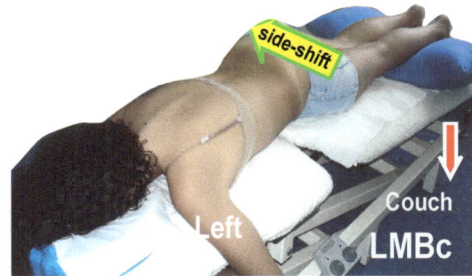

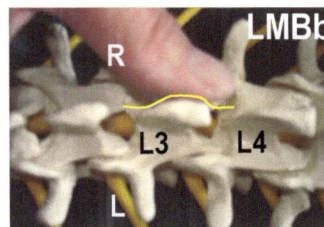

The side of the subluxated spinous process is palpated using the pad of the thumb. The thrust could be made with the thumb. Ensure that L3 is in flexion and not extension.

This is a long lever technique and is very similar to the technique used for correcting the thoracic vertebrae.

Technique:

The patient adopts a relaxed prone position on the couch with their pelvis side-shifted to the right with the distal part of the couch lowered. See **figure LMBc**. Though not shown the right arm could optionally be placed on the couch parallel to the torso. The manipulator stands to the right side of the patient, adjacent to the lumbar vertebra to be manipulated. In this case L3 is subluxated with rotation to the right in flexion, awaiting manipulation.

The subluxated joint is located by running the pad of the thumb against the side of the spinous process, see **figure LMBb**. The manipulator then uses the pad of their thenar eminence, as shown in **figures LMB** and **LMBa** to make a gentle sideways push to the left against the side of the spinous process. The manipulator's hand experiences a feeling of 'give', which is all that is needed for the joint to slip back into place. Usually there is no click or thud. This technique is used to correct the lumbar vertebrae between L2-L5 that are rotated to the right.

How does the technique work?

The lowered legs, as shown in **figure LMBf**, pull on the lumbar vertebrae and extend (forward bend) the joints and therefore prize apart the facets. With the sacroiliac and all the vertebrae below side-shifted to the right and the flexed legs levering the L3-L4 joint open, all the hard work is done. All the manipulator has to do is gently push the spinous process of the destabilized L3 to the left.

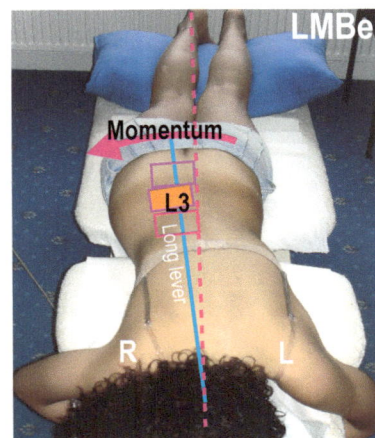

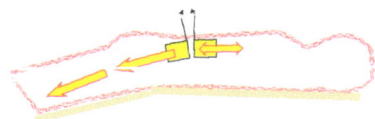

Figure LMBf

Bayliss Advanced Lumbar
PPT: L5-Left-Right

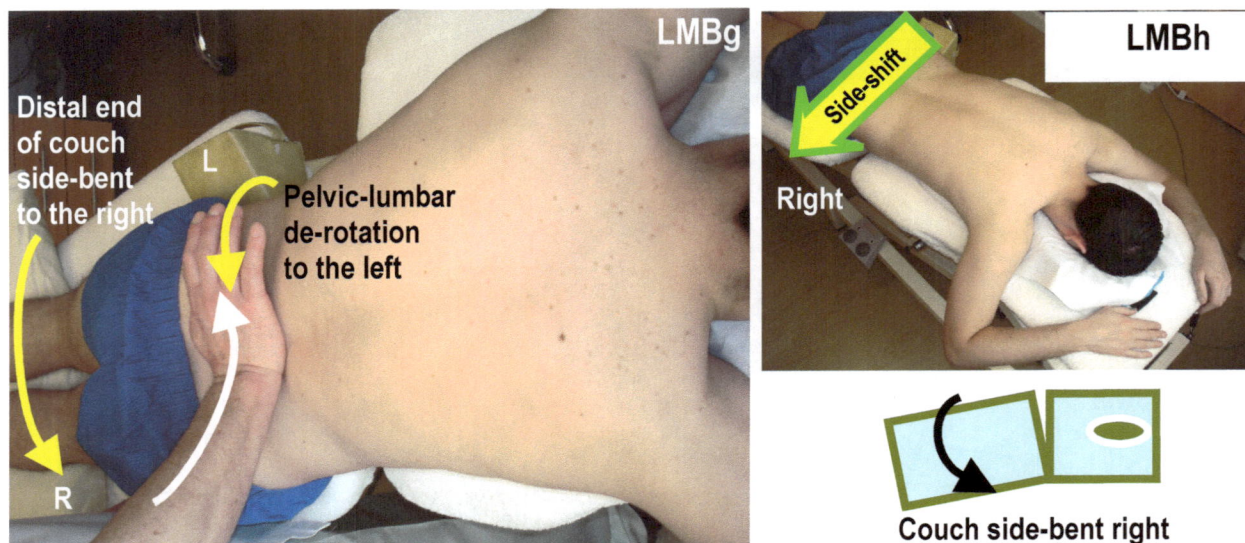

This is a similar long lever technique to the one shown on the previous page, the only difference being that pelvic rotation and side-bending are countered. This makes this is a superior technique but requires that the manipulator has a couch that is capable of side-bending.

Technique:
The patient adopts a relaxed prone position on the couch with their pelvis side-shifted to the right. The distal end of the couch is lowered and a block is placed under the left A.S.I.S. See **figure LMBh.** Though not shown the right arm could optionally be placed on the couch parallel to the torso. The manipulator stands to the right side of the patient, adjacent to the lumbar vertebra to be manipulated. In this case, see **figure LMBg**, L5 is subluxated with rotation to the right in flexion, awaiting manipulation.

The subluxated joint is located by running the pad of the thumb against the side of the spinous process as shown in **figure LMBb** on the previous page. The distal half of the couch is side-bent to the right. The manipulator then uses the pad of their thenar eminence, as shown in **figure LMBg**, to make a gentle sideways push to the left against the side of the spinous process of L5. The manipulator's hand experiences a slight feeling of 'give', which is all that is needed for the joint to slip back into place. Usually there is no click or thud. This technique can be is used to correct the lumbar vertebrae between L2-L5.

How does the technique work?
The lowered legs, as shown in **figure LMBf** on the previous page, pull on the lumbar vertebrae in an inferior direction and open the facets between L5 and the sacrum. The side-shift to the right creates the driving force for L5 to de-rotate to the left. The rotation of the pelvis to the left also encourages L5 to de-rotate. Finally the side-bending of the distal end of the couch approximates the right facets of L5 with those of the superior right sacrum With all these forces lined up, all the manipulator has to do is gently push the spinous process of the destabilized L5 to the left.

Bayliss Basic Lumbar PPT:
L3-Right-Right

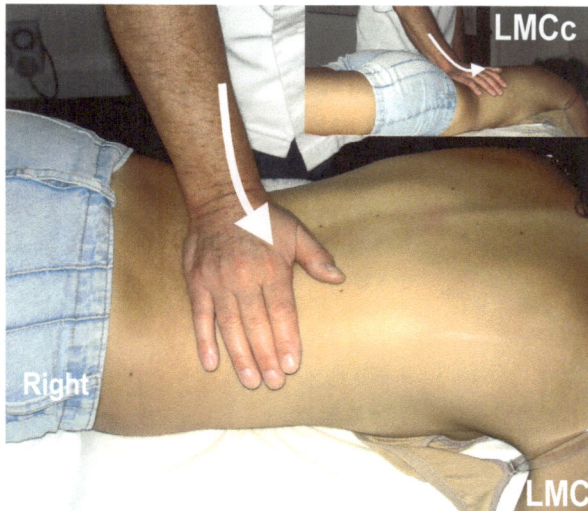

LMCc

Right

LMC

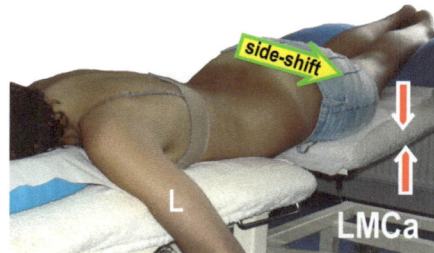

side-shift

L

LMCa

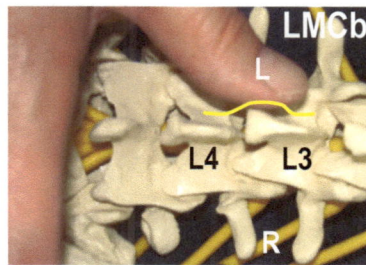

LMCb

L

L4   L3

R

The side of the subluxated spinous process is palpated using the pad of the thumb. The thrust could be made with the thumb. Ensure that L3 is in extension and not flexion.

This is a long lever technique and is very similar to the technique used for correcting the thoracic vertebrae.

Technique:
The patient adopts a relaxed prone position on a flat couch with their pelvis side-shifted to the left See **figure LMCa.** Though not shown the left arm could optionally be placed on the couch parallel to the torso. The manipulator stands to the left side of the patient, adjacent to the lumbar vertebra to be manipulated. In this case L3 is subluxated with side-bending and rotation to the right in extension, awaiting manipulation.

The subluxated joint is located by running the pad of the thumb against the side of the spinous process, see **figure LMCb.** The manipulator then uses the pad of their thenar eminence, as shown in **figures LMC** and **LMCc** to make a gentle sideways push to the right against the side of the spinous process. The manipulator's hand experiences a feeling of 'give', which is all that is needed for the joint to slip back into place. Usually there is no click or thud. This technique can be used to correct lumbar vertebrae between L1-L5.

How does the technique work?
The legs, as shown in **figure LMCf** place an upward force that flexes (backward bends) the lumbar vertebrae and therefore approximates the facets. With the sacroiliac and all the vertebrae below side-shifted to the left and the extended legs levering the L3-L4 joint closed, all the hard work is done. All the manipulator has to do is gently push the spinous process of the destabilized L3 to the right.

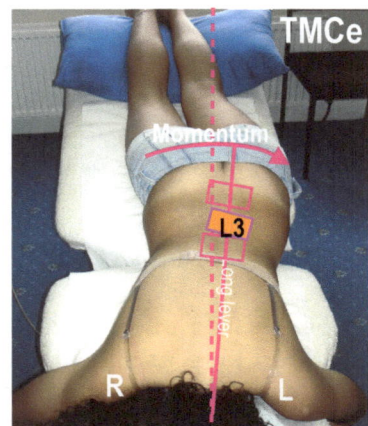

TMCe

Momentum

L3

R   L

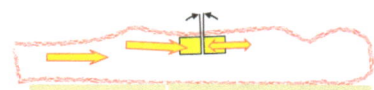

Figure TMCf

185

Bayliss Advanced Lumbar
PPT: L3-Right-Right

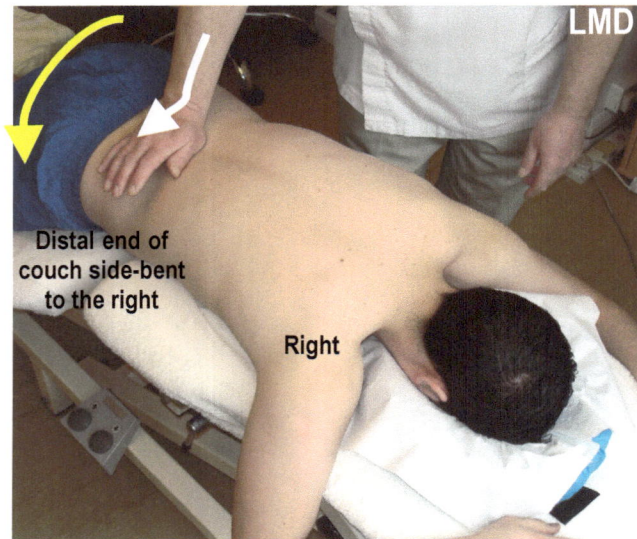

Distal end of couch side-bent to the right

Right

LMD

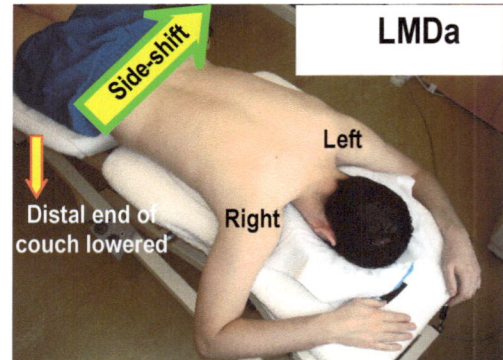

Side-shift

Left

Distal end of couch lowered

Right

LMDa

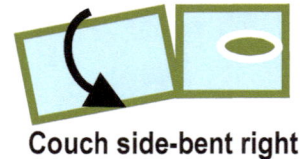

Couch side-bent right

This is an exaggeration long lever technique and is a superior technique to the one on the previous page. Again the couch must be capable of side-bending.

Technique:
The patient adopts a relaxed prone position on the couch with their pelvis side-shifted to the left and the distal end of the couch is lowered. See **figure LMDa** above. The manipulator stands to the left side of the patient, adjacent to the lumbar vertebra to be manipulated. In this case, see **figure LMD**, L3 is subluxated with rotation and side-bending to the right, awaiting manipulation.

The subluxated joint is located by running the pad of the thumb against the side of the spinous process as shown in **figure LMCb** on the previous page. The distal end of the couch is side-bent to the right and the forces focused at the L3/L4 joint. The manipulator then uses the pad of their thenar eminence, as shown in **figure LMD**, to make a gentle sideways push to the right against the side of the spinous process of L3. The manipulator's hand experiences a slight feeling of 'give', which is all that is needed for the joint to slip back into place. At this point the couch is brought back into the mid-line. This technique can be is used to correct lumbar vertebrae between L2-L5 locked in side-bending.

How does the technique work?
The lowered legs, as shown in **figure LMDa**, extend (forward bend) the lumbar vertebrae and place a parting force on their facets. The side-shift to the right creates the driving force for L3 to side-shift to the left. This lessens the fixation and torsion within the subluxated right facets and allows for a small amount of play. The side-bending of the distal end of the couch levers the right L3 facets further superiorly, thus exaggerating the side-bending at L3. With all the forces lined up all the manipulator has to do is gently push the spinous process of the destabilized L3 to the right, and on feeling the 'give' of the fixation breaking the distal end of the couch should immediately be brought back into the mid-line to re-align L3 in extended neutral.

Bayliss Advanced Lumbar PPT:
L1-left-left

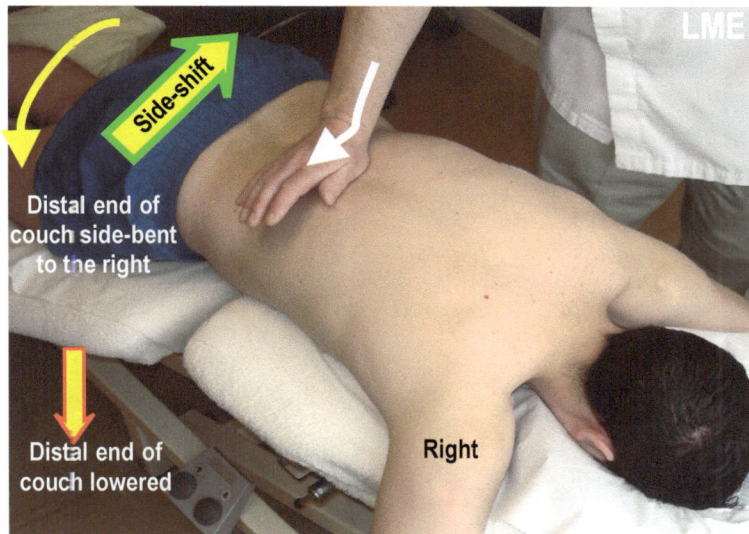

Side-shift

Distal end of couch side-bent to the right

Distal end of couch lowered

Right

LME

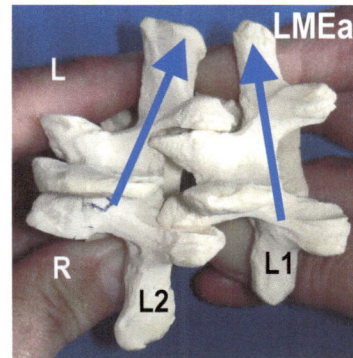

L

R

L2

L1

LMEa

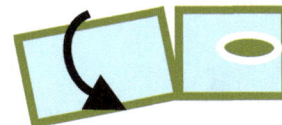

Couch side-bent right

This is an long lever 'breaking' technique and is a superior technique to the one on page 185 because more forces are countered. Again a couch capable of side-bending is needed. L1-left-left is found in the L3-right-right subluxation pattern, see page 126. L1-right-right is a reversal of this.

Technique:
The patient adopts a relaxed prone position on the couch with their pelvis side-shifted to the left and the distal end of the couch is lowered. See **figure LME** above. The manipulator stands to the left side of the patient, adjacent to L1/L2. L1 is subluxated with rotation and side-bending to the left, awaiting manipulation.

The subluxated joint is located by running the pad of the thumb against the side of the spinous process, the same way to that shown in **figure LMCb** on page 185. The distal end of the couch is side-bent to the right to focus parting forces at the L1/L2 joint. The manipulator then uses the pad of their thenar eminence, as shown in **figure LME**, to make a gentle sideways push to the right against the side of the spinous process of L2. The manipulator's hand experiences a slight feeling of 'give', which is all that is needed for the joint to slip back into place. At this point the couch is brought back into the mid-line. This technique is specific to L1/L2 and can be used in reverse to correct L1 subluxated, right-right.

How does the technique work?
The lowered legs, as shown in **figure LME**, extend (forward bend) the lumbar vertebrae and place a parting force at the L1/L2 joint. The side-shift to the right creates the driving force for L2 to side-shift to the left. This lessens the fixation and torsion within the subluxated right facets and allows for a small amount of play. The side-bending of the distal end of the couch levers the right L1 facet apart, thus exaggerating the side-bending at L1. With all the forces lined up all the manipulator has to do is gently push the spinous process of the destabilized L2 to the right. On feeling the 'give' of the fixation 'breaking' the distal end of the couch should immediately be brought back into the mid-line to re-align L1 in extended neutral.

The Neck and Bayliss
CST Manipulation

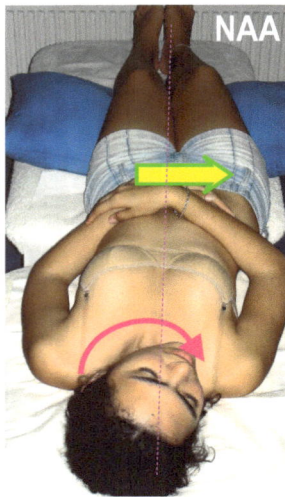

NAA — Knees flexed / Pelvic side-shift right / Arms relaxed / Neck rotation right to the same side as pelvic side-shift

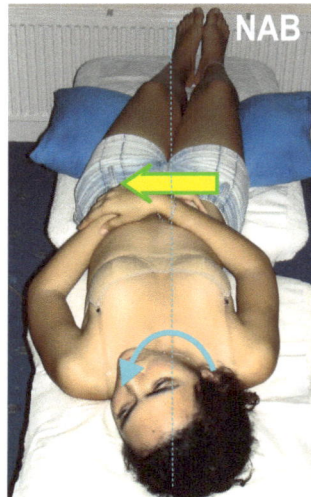

NAB — Knees flexed / Pelvic side-shift left / Arms relaxed / Neck rotation left to the same side as pelvic side-shift

CST is short for 'Co-operative Supine Technique'. It is the name for the protocol when the patient side-shifts their pelvis and co-operates with the manipulator and/or participates in some way.

You can use the neck techniques written up in many manipulation instruction books if you prefer to use a conventional approach. It is surprising how little force is needed to correct neck subluxations when the sacroiliac and spinal joints below are mobile and in true alignment and the pelvis side-shifted. Be aware that there will be an element of force and there will be an audible click.

A word of caution, even though your hear a click you can inadvertently compound a C1/Oct joint subluxation, if you apply your thrust on the wrong side. It is not always easy to identify a patients subluxation pattern. If you are in doubt when it comes to the C1-Ocl joint, it is not the time to take a 50/50 bet on which way the subluxation is locked in. Perform this simple test:

With your patient supine and their neck in A-P/lateral neutral, hold the occipital bone and concentrate the forces against C1. Gently backward bend the occiput and rotate the head in one direction the then the other. The joint will tighten in one direction and not the other. It should be obvious. Your correction should be to the side that offers the least resistance.

Whilst the neck joints are not dependent on side-shift for their movement, the neck and back muscles are. By applying pelvic side-shift in the supine position the muscles on the opposite side to the side-shift become relaxed and offer minimal resistance. This makes the manipulative thrust much easier. The positions are shown in **figures NAA** and **NAB.**

Place the pillow under the patient's knees as this provides knee flexion, which is a prerequisite to any spinal manipulation. Patients do not like hands round their necks and being held in uncomfortable pre-manipulative positions whilst the manipulator postures around preparing themselves. So make your delivery speedy as well as safe. And remember, no excessive force.

Be gentle. Your patients judge you on your neck manipulations more than any other joint.

Bayliss Neck PPT:
in L3-Right-Right Pattern

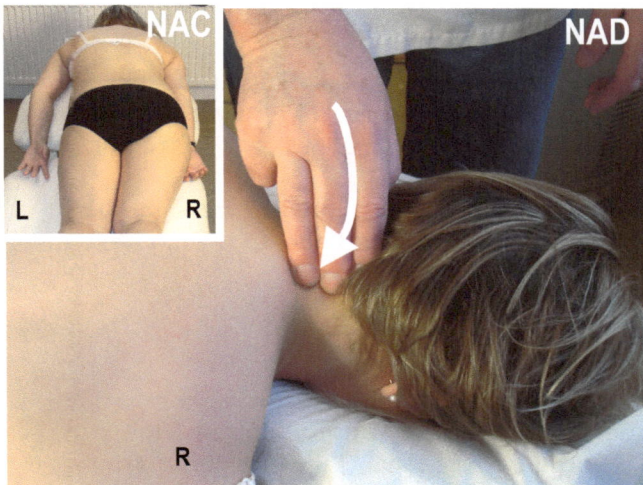

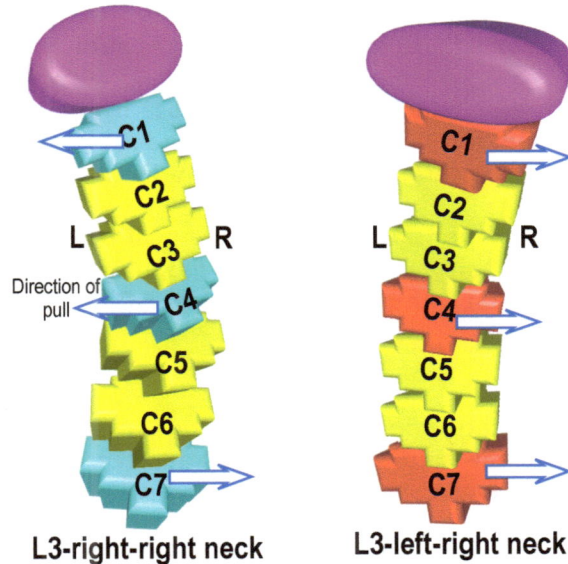

L3-right-right neck   L3-left-right neck

This gentle cervical technique takes very little effort on the part of the manipulator and patients find it a comfortable procedure to have performed on them. In fact patients who have previously experienced traditional neck techniques are often unaware that they have even been manipulated. The procedure uses the slackening of the muscles associated with pelvic side-shift to advantage, and removes the need for any manhandling of the neck. Because the neck is kept in the midline at all times, undue and unnecessary stress to the neck is automatically removed. Logically this has to improve the safety, especially when only a very gentle pull is enough to correct even the most stubborn subluxation.

The technique shown is for the correction of a subluxated C4 joint in the L3-right-right pattern. The technique can be used to correct C4 in the L3-left-right pattern, if the procedure is reversed.

Technique:
The patient adopts a relaxed prone position on a flat, or lowered distal end, couch with their pelvis side-shifted to the right. The proximal end of the couch is then lowered so as to mildly flex the neck in neutral. Both of the patients arms should be parallel to their torso, see **figure NAC**. The manipulator stands to the left of the patients neck. In this case C4 is locked in cervical extension and awaiting manipulation. Having located the subluxated joint with the pad of their thumb against the side of the spinous process, in a similar way to **figure LMCb** on page 185, the manipulator then flexes their fingers and places the pads over the spinous process of C4, as shown in **figure NAD** and makes a very gentle side-ways pull to the left. The manipulator's fingers experience a slight feeling of 'give', which is the joint slipping back into place. There is no click and only an absolute minimal amount of force in needed. This technique is suitable for the manipulation of all of the cervical vertebrae.

As a general rule always start your PPT manipulation in the middle of the neck on the side of the convexity and then go on to correct the C7-C1 joints. The directions of corrections are shown above.

Markers for Assessing
Type of Subluxation Pattern

Differentiation between the two types of subluxation pattern especially when the patient may have encountered additional direct trauma subluxations can be difficult. Here are some pointers.

Place your hands either side of L1. If the left transverse process is posterior on the left and side-bent left the pattern is likely to be part of the L3-right-right pattern. If the right transverse process is posterior on the right and side-bent right it is likely to be part of L3-left-right pattern.

Ask the patient to stand with their aligned feet slightly apart and bend forward from the waist leaving their arms loose and hanging. It is suggested that you read the following text in conjunction with observing **figures RC and RD** below.

L3-Right-Right

If the rib cage veers to the right and the shoulders rotate to the left then the person is likely to have an L3-right-right subluxation pattern. This can be further verified by palpation of the right sacrospinous/sacrotuberous ligaments, which will be tight because this is the site of the primary sacroiliac lesion. In the supine position the patients neck will rotate left with relative ease compared to the right. You can generally side-bend the lumbar to the left.

L3-Left-Right

If the rib cage veers to the left and the shoulders rotate to the right the person is likely to have an L3-left-right subluxation pattern. This can be verified by palpation of the sacrospinous/sacrotuberous ligaments on the left, which will be tight because this is the site of the primary sacroiliac lesion. In the supine position the patients neck will rotate right with relative ease compared to the left. You can generally side-bend the lumbar to the right.

If the patient does not conform to one of these types you should suspect direct trauma, an anatomical or pathological defect or what the 'old Osteopaths' called a "complicated" lesion afflicted to one or more of the vertebrae.

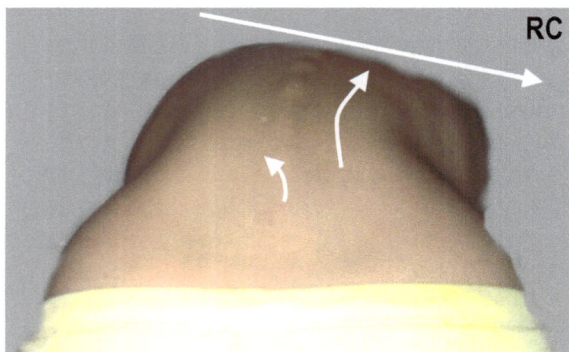

L3-Right-Right

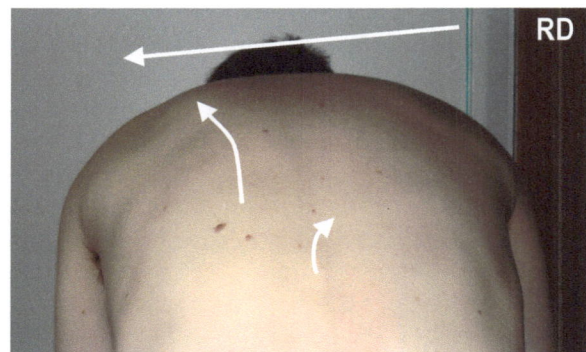

L3-Left-Right

Chapter Sixteen
Physiology of the Rib Cage

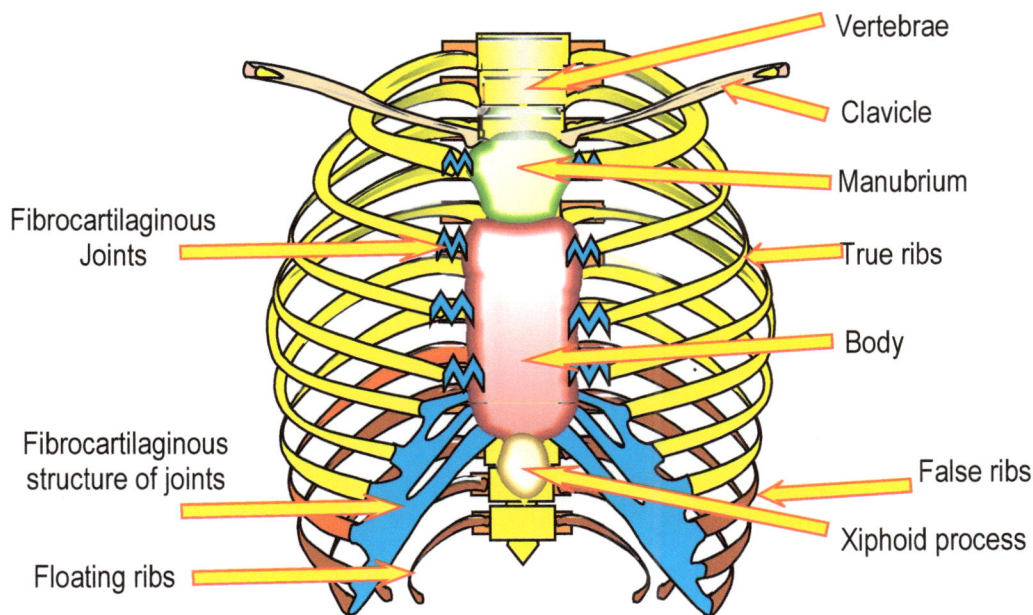

Vertebrae

Clavicle

Manubrium

True ribs

Body

False ribs

Xiphoid process

Fibrocartilaginous Joints

Fibrocartilaginous structure of joints

Floating ribs

Figure 2A
The Rib Cage

There are twenty four ribs; twelve on each side of the spine. Of these twelve, seven are called 'true' ribs and five 'false'. At their anterior the seven 'true' ribs, shown in **figure 2A** coloured yellow attach via cartilage to the manubrium and body and provide an element of stability to the upper vertebrae. Of the 'false' ribs, coloured red, three attach to the lowest part of the anterior rib cage via the hanging cartilage. The last two ribs (11/12) have no anterior attachment and because of this they are named, 'floating ribs'.

Names have been added to the illustration of the ribs cage in **figure 2A** for reference. In most anatomy books the height of the manubrium is shown level with the third vertebra however, it has been lowered slightly in my illustrations to show a little more of T3.

The Xiphoid process, the Body and the Manubrium are known collectively as the Sternum.

The Rib Cage: Breathing

Breathing is a vital function of the body and the rib cage in conjunction with the diaphragm plays an important part in this function. Below is a brief recap on the action taken by the rib cage.

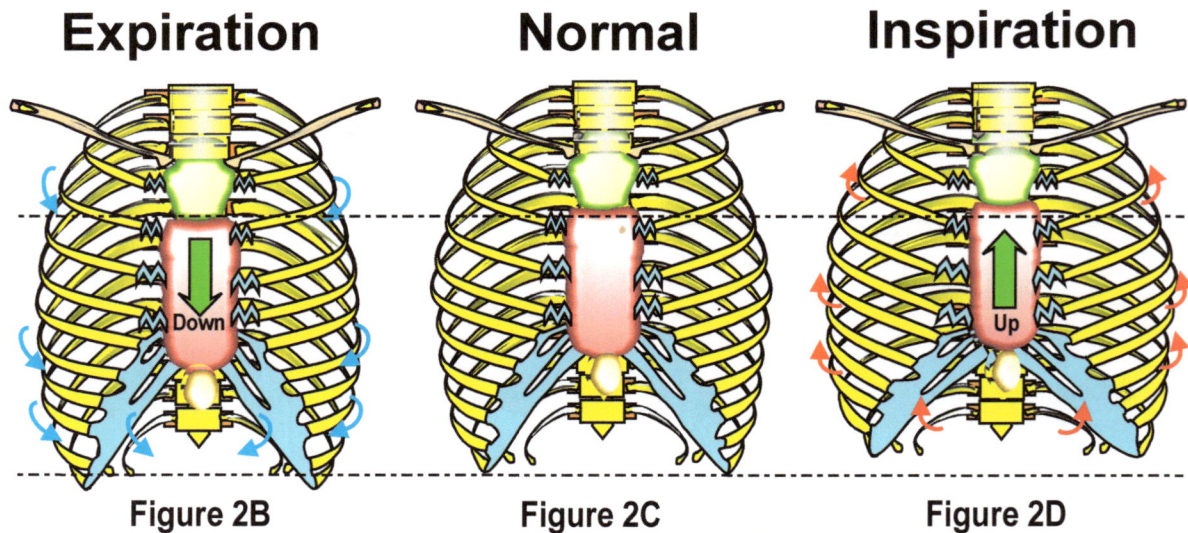

Expiration

Figure 2B

Normal

Figure 2C

Inspiration

Figure 2D

The process of breathing involves a method that has been likened to the trajectory of a bucket handle. This is shown in **figure 2E**. There are two distinct actions taking place 1) the anterior part of the rib is travelling up and down in an arc and 2) the rib itself is rotating horizontally as it completes this.

Inspiration

Figure 2D. The rib cage expands superiorly and laterally, when a person breaths in. This action is aided if the arms are raised above the head.

Expiration

Figure 2B. The rib cage contracts inferiorly and medially when a person breaths out. This action is aided if the arms are loose at the sides.

Figure 2Ee shows how the conical shape of the rib affects the rising and falling of the sternum.

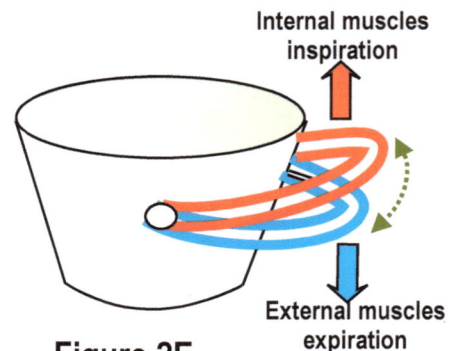

Internal muscles inspiration

External muscles expiration

Figure 2E
Rib bucket handle mechanism

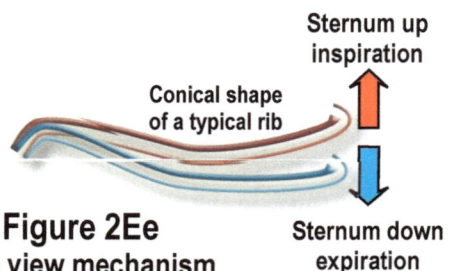

Sternum up inspiration

Conical shape of a typical rib

Sternum down expiration

Figure 2Ee
Side view mechanism

192

Articular Surface of a Typical T7 Rib

Working Rib Theory
Ribs must remain level to function efficiently.

For a rib theory to work, it must fulfil certain criteria. It has to make allowance for keeping the ribs level during the breathing mechanism in neutral, thoracic flexion, side-bending and rotation.

The detailed physiology shown in the following chapters, explains the 'Bayliss rib theory' and how the above criteria can be satisfied.

-

The anterior end of a typical rib at its articulation with the costo-cartridge looks like it has been sawn through, as shown in **figures 2F** and **2G**. In contrast, the posterior end contains facets that give the surface a knobbly appearance.

There are three facets at the posterior end, shown in **figures 2G** and **2H.** Two of these facets are convex in shape and are located at the head of the rib. Their purpose is to articulate with the 'semi-dens' facets located on the bodies of the T7 and T8 vertebrae. The superior facet is angled vertically to articulate with T7 and the inferior facet is angled horizontally to articulate with T8 .

The third tubercle facet is located on the lateral posterior border of the rib. It is off-set inferio-anteriorly and convex horizontally and vertically. The facet articulates with the 'costo-transverse' facet located on the transverse process of the T7 vertebra.

The combination of these three rib joints provides the rib with the stability and the mobility it needs to perform the bucket handle breathing motion whilst in neutral, thoracic flexion, side-bending and rotation.

At the anterior end of the rib the bone fuses with fibrocartilage which in turn fuses with the body of the sternum. This provides the 'true ribs' with large degrees of flexibility that allow superior, inferior, anterior and posterior planes of movement.

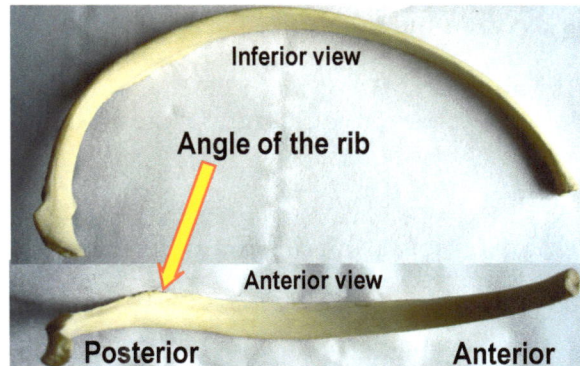

Figure 2F
Overview of a T7 rib

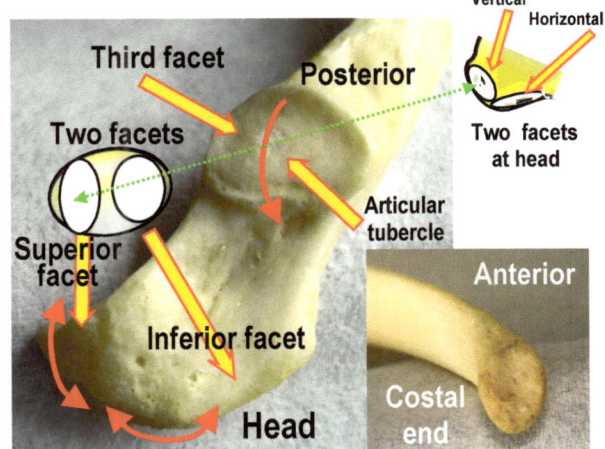

Figure 2G
Head and costal end of T7 rib

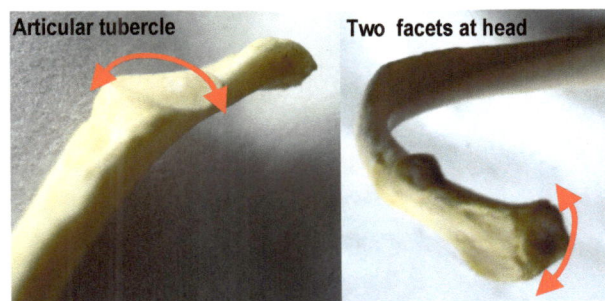

Figure 2H
Posterior facets

Articular Surface of a T1 Rib

The 1st ribs are small, wide and flat, as shown in **figures 2J and 2K**.

At the posterior end of the rib there are three facets. Two at the "head" and the third set back along the neck and off-set laterally. The latter is called the tubercle facet and is shown in **figure 2L**.

The facets at the head of the 1st rib articulate with the superior and inferior facets of the T1 and T2 vertebrae, as shown in **figure 2MA**. The 1st rib forms a canopy over the rib cage and acts as an anchor for some of the neck muscles. It would appear to play only a small role in the breathing mechanism.

Figure 2M shows the 1st rib in relation to its bony surroundings.

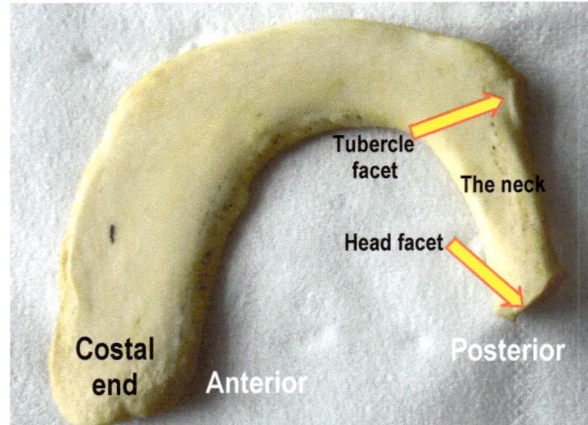

Figure 2J
Aerial view of a T1 rib

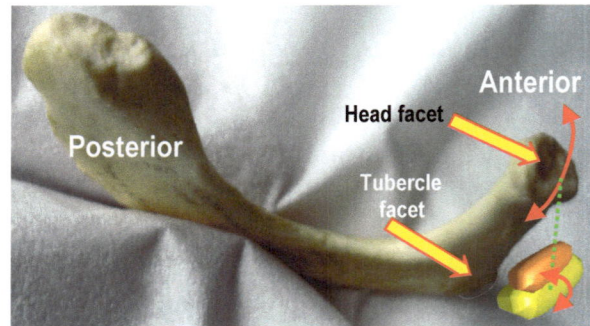

Figure 2K
Medial view of a T1 rib

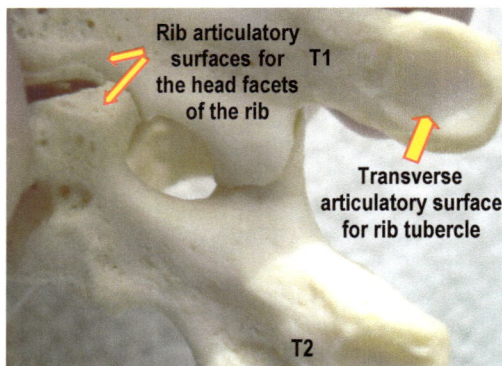

Figure 2MA
Side view of T1-T2 rib facets

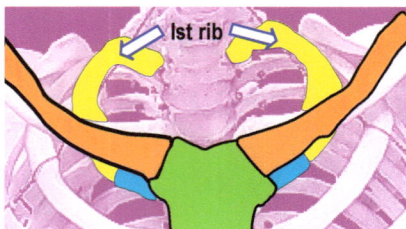

Figure 2M
Anterior view of a T1 rib

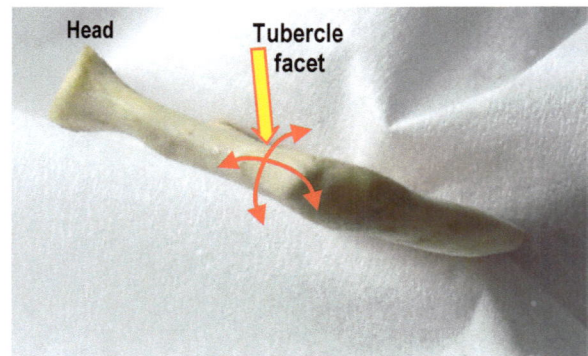

Figure 2L
Posterior view of a T1 rib

194

Rib Attachments to Body
and Transverse Process

Figure 2N is a side-view of the demi-facets of the seventh and eighth vertebrae. Both facets are concave. The upper demi-facets of T7 are more vertical than the lower demi-facets of T8. The eighth demi-facets are predominantly horizontal. Note the proximity of the nerve.

To make it easier to visualize, the angles of the demi-facets are shown in illustration form, in **figure 2P**.

Figure 2Q is a photograph of the transverse facet. It is concave and off-set latro-medially.

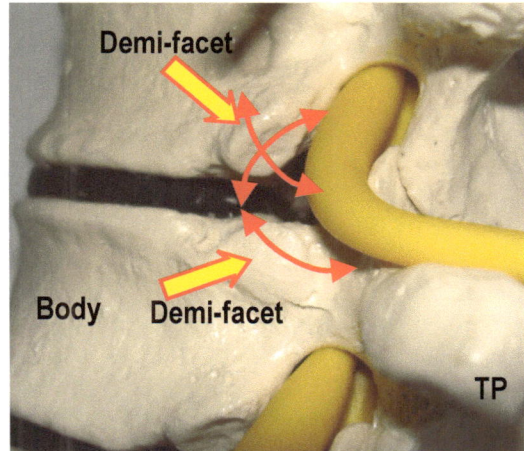

Figure 2N
Side-view of demi-facts

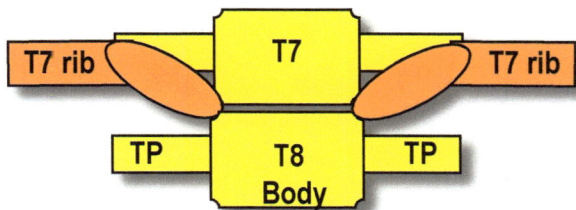

Figure 2P
Illustration of demi-facts

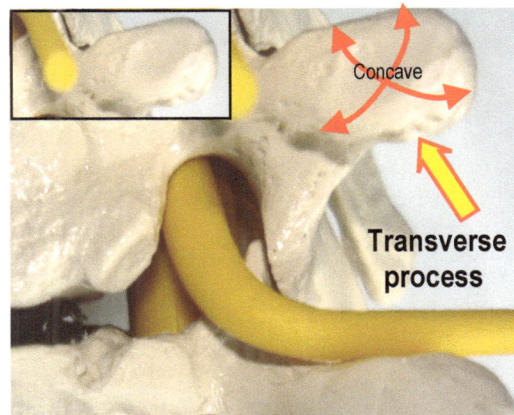

Figure 2R
Facet attachment
posterior View

The combined shape of these three facets allow the seventh rib to synchronously articulate with the seventh vertebra.

The facets are designed to accommodate the breathing action of the ribs in neutral, thoracic flexion together with rotation and side-bending (side-shift)

Figure 2R is a posterior view and illustration of how the seventh ribs attach to the seventh and eighth vertebrae.

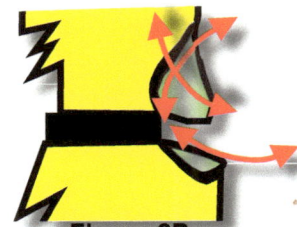

Figure 2Q
Anterior view of the T7
Transverse facet

195

The Rib Articulation During Breathing

Figure 2NA illustrates the articulatory movement of the facets at the head and neck of a typical rib.

During expiration the inferior facet at the head of the rib moves inferiorly against the demi-facet of the vertebra below, whilst swivelling supero-posteriorly over the host concave tubercle facet.

During inspiration the superior facet at the head of the rib moves superiorly against the inferior demi-facet of the host vertebra, whilst swivelling inferio-anteriorly over the tubercle facet.

Figure 2NB is a side-view illustrating the levering effect that the change in facet position combined with muscle contraction has over the position of the ribs. Note that the reason the rib in inspiration goes up at the end is due to the conical shape of the rib, see **figure 2F** on page 193.

Figure 2ND is an aerial view of the rib cage illustrating the expansion and contraction that takes place during the breathing mechanism. This expansion and contraction is due to the conical shape of the ribs.

Figure 2NC is a horizontal cross section through three typical ribs and illustrates how the contraction of the internal and external muscles cause the ribs to behave in a similar manner to the blades of a venetian blind.

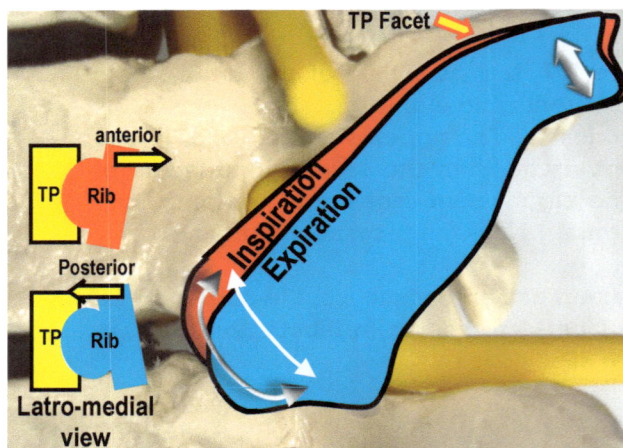

Figure 2NA
Anterior-view and cross section of the movement of a typical rib during the breathing articulation

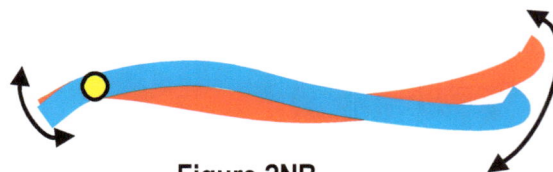

Figure 2NB
Side-view of rib trajectory during breathing

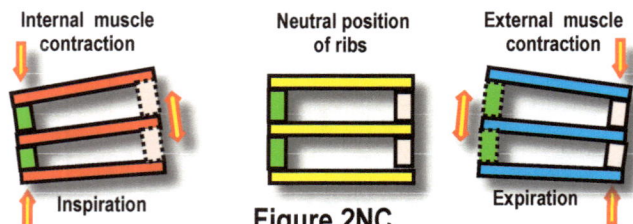

Figure 2NC
Transverse section through ribs during breathing

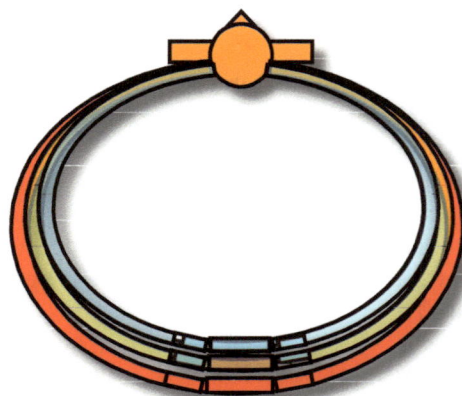

Figure 2ND
View from above of rib expansion and contraction during breathing

Rib Facet Surface Adaptation to Rotation

Figure 2S is a photograph of T7 rotating right in thoracic flexion. In order to complete this action and keep the ribs level and free for inspiration and expiration to take place, the seventh vertebra side-shifts to the right where the facets rotate right around the facets of T8. Note, breathing during thoracic rotation is not as deep as when the thoracic spine is in neutral or forward bending.

Figure 2T illustrates how the design of the demi-facets of T7 and T8 accommodate this side ways movement. In thoracic neutral or forward bending, observe that the head of the seventh rib on the right, swivels superiorly as it gets dragged along with the side-shift. Conversely the left rib swivels inferiorly against the demi-facet of T8 and counters the side-side shift. To make it easier to understand, **figure 2U** illustrates by exaggeration the shape of the demi-facets.

In reality this movement is a degree or so at most thereby allowing the inferior and superior facets to be kept in contact with the vertebral demi-facets, only one rib facet will play a more guiding role.

Figures 2V and **2W** illustrate the plane of movement the demi-facets offer to facilitate the rotational, vertical and side-ways movements of the ribs whilst they remain symmetrical and level.

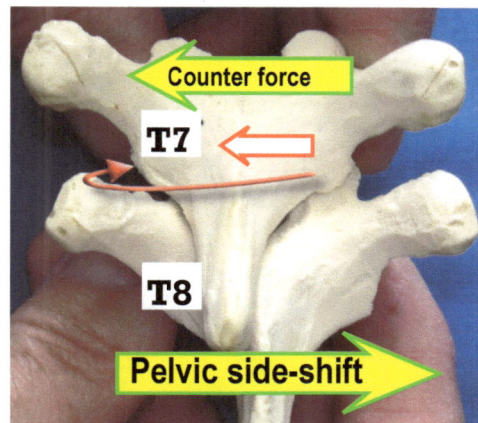

Figure 2S
Posterior view of
T7 vertebral rotation

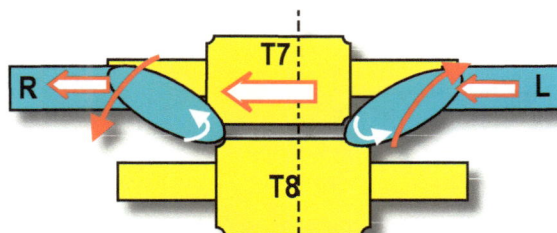

Figure 2T
Anterior view of rotation in
Neutral showing T7 rib accommodation

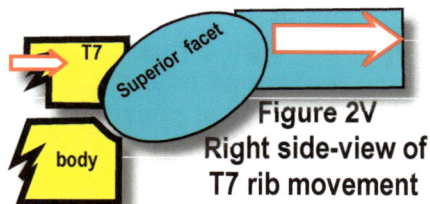

Figure 2V
Right side-view of
T7 rib movement

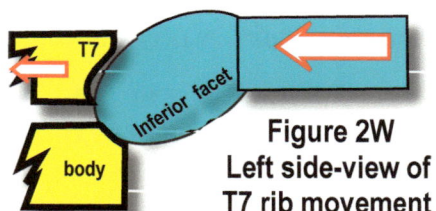

Figure 2W
Left side-view of
T7 rib movement

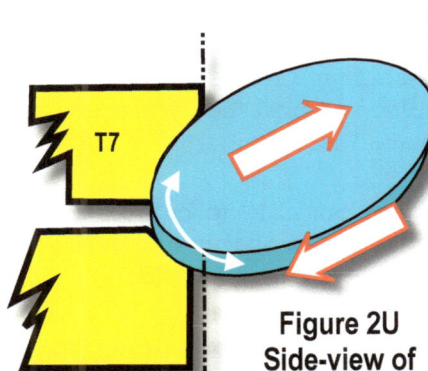

Figure 2U
Side-view of
T7-T8 rib facets

Rib Adaptations in
Flexion Rotation

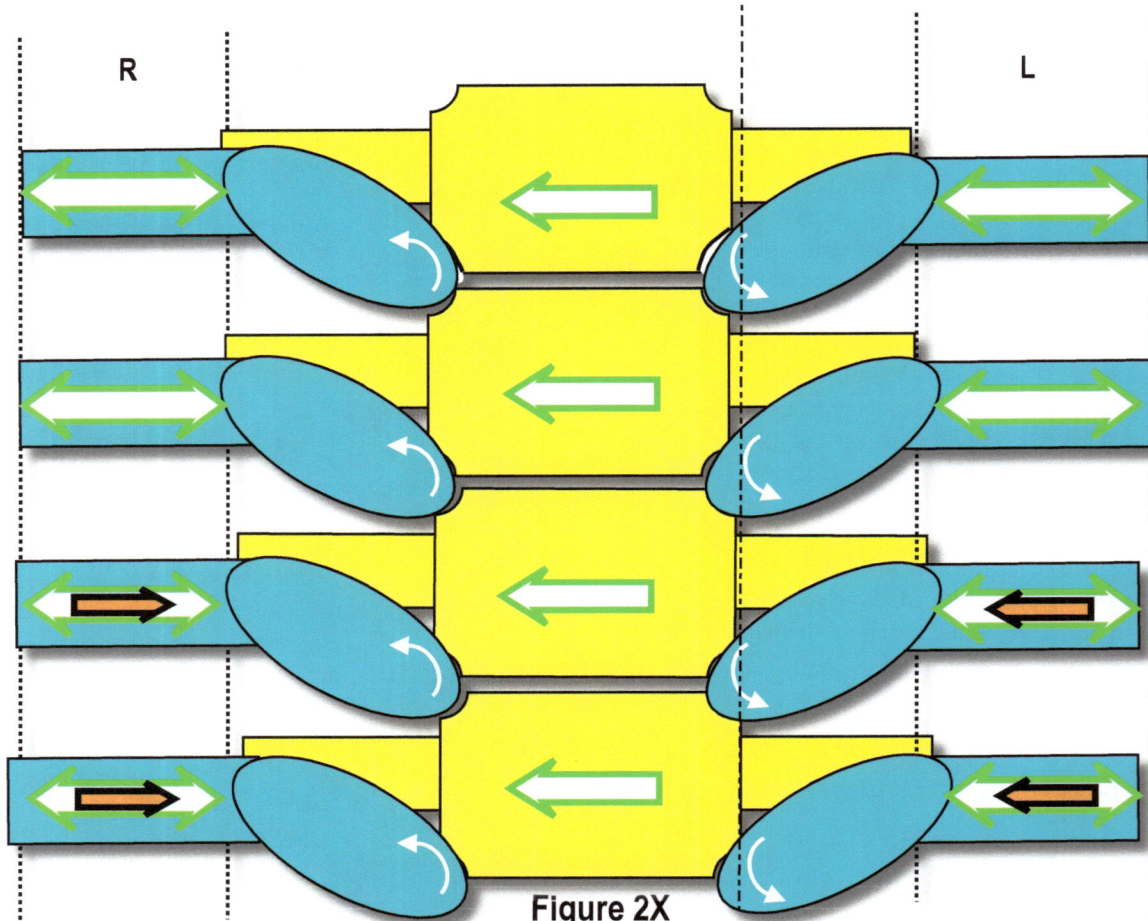

Figure 2X
Anterior view
Group flexion rotation
and rib accommodation

Figure 2X illustrates the overall positioning of the ribs and vertebrae during rotation right in thoracic flexion. Note that the ribs attempt to remain parallel and in position as the vertebrae side-bend (side-shift) and rotate. The arrows have been drawn in to represent the general counter forces the ribs place against the vertebrae. The arrows on the previous page showed the forces the vertebrae placed on the ribs.

However, it is not possible to completely compensate for the lateral side-shift at the lower vertebrae. This is most probably one of the main reasons why false and floating ribs allow more flexibility than true ribs. See page 78.

Where there is more flexibility there is more chance of problems arising and as the diaphragm attaches to the lower ribs and utilizes their increased flexibility, so the correct seating and articulation of the ribs becomes very important.

Chapter Seventeen
Physiology of the Manubrium and Clavicle

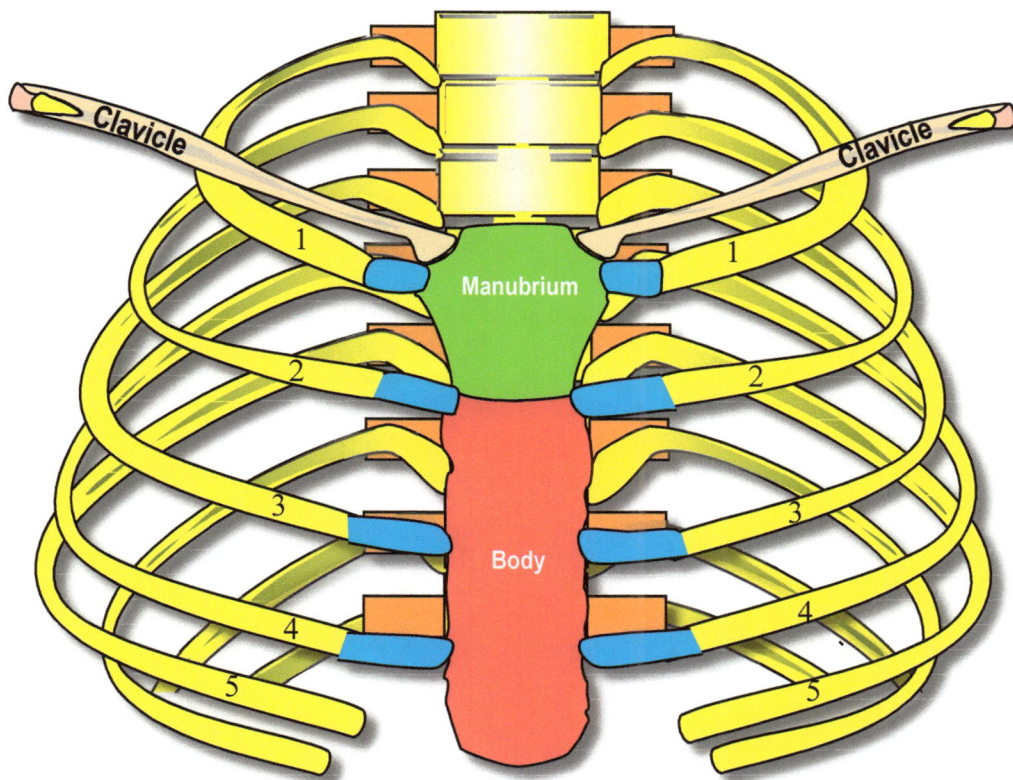

Figure 3A
Anterior view from slightly above
of the manubrium and clavicle bones

The sternum comprises of three bones: The "Manubrium", the "Body" and the "Xiphoid process". This chapter is about the top bone, the manubrium and its articulation with the clavicle bones, as illustrated in **figure 3A**.

The Manubrium

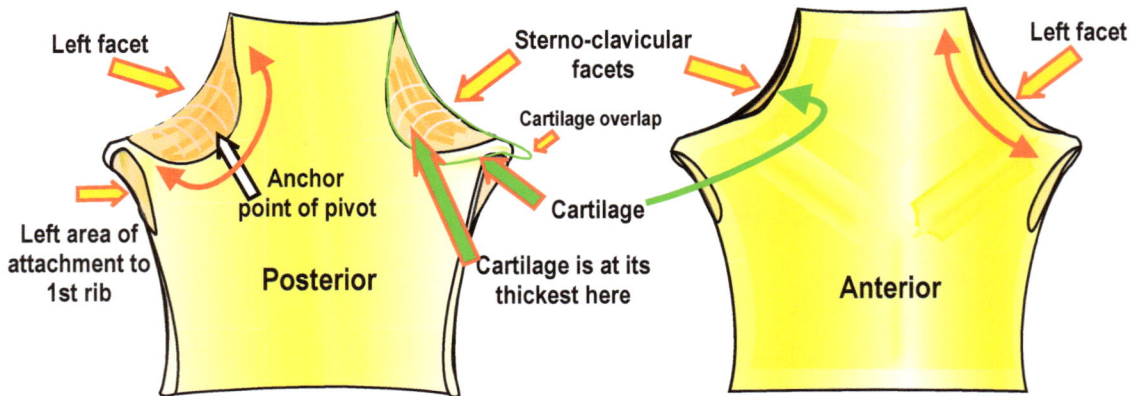

Figure 3B
Posterior and anterior views of the manubrium

Cut into the superior surface of the manubrium there is a facet at either side, as illustrated in **figure 3B**. These facets are covered by cartilage and articulate with the sternal ends of the clavicle bones. The cartilage, shown in green, extends down the facets where it forms a slippery barrier between the clavicle and 1st rib.

The cartilage is thicker at the posterior part of the facet. Therefore, from an engineering point of view this is the most likely area for the point of pivot. See **figure 3D**.

Figure 3C shows photographs of the left side of the manubrium and further illustrates the differences in the angles of the posterior and anterior facets. As can be seen, the posterior part of the sterno-clavicular facet slopes inferiorly and medially. Notice how close it is to the costal-cartilage of the 1st rib.

Figure 3D shows illustrations and a photograph of the sloping angle of the sterno-clavicular articular facets. The cross section is taken through the point of pivot, as shown in **figure 3B** and illustrates the convex shape of the facet.

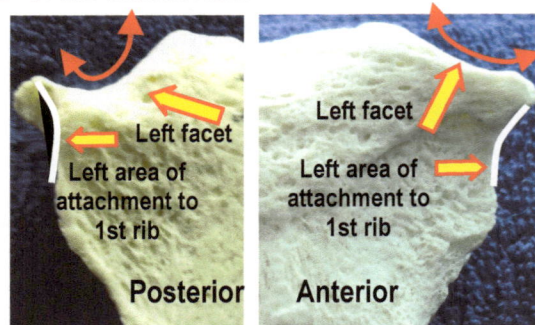

Figure 3C
Posterior and anterior views of the left side of the manubrium

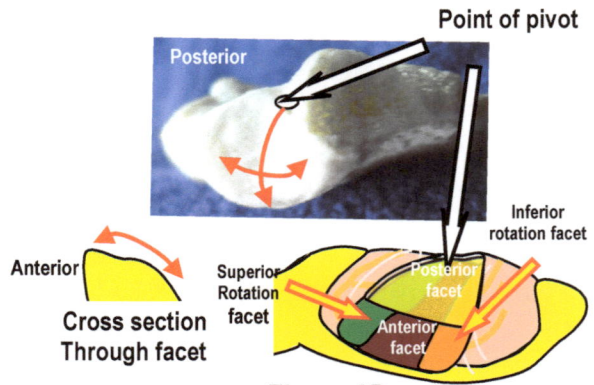

Figure 3D
Sterno-clavicular facets

200

The Clavicle

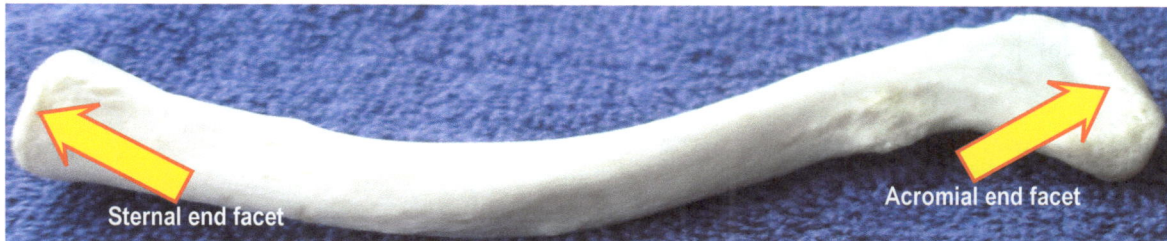

Figure 3E
Aerial view of a left clavicle

Figure 3E is an aerial view of a left clavicle bone. The clavicle has facets at either end.

The medial end articulates with the manubrium and the lateral end with the acromial angle of the acromial process of the scapula.

Figure 3F illustrates the angles of the facet at the acromial end. Generally, the facet is inclined inferiorly and shaped like a rounded over-hanging precipice, though this shape can vary. Across its antero-posterior border it is generally convex. In some people there is a meniscus between this facet and the acromion facet.

Figures 3G shows by illustration and photograph the complex surface contours of the clavicle facet at its sternal end.

The clavicle uses the thickened cartilage at the posterior part of the facet to anchor and pivot. This allows three basic planes of trajectory.

1) The facet contours shown in illustration "B" create a shape that can create a sideways rocking action along the antero-lateral and postero-medial surface.

2 and 3) The facet contours shown in photograph "A" show the swivel like trajectory the facets follow when rotation takes place.

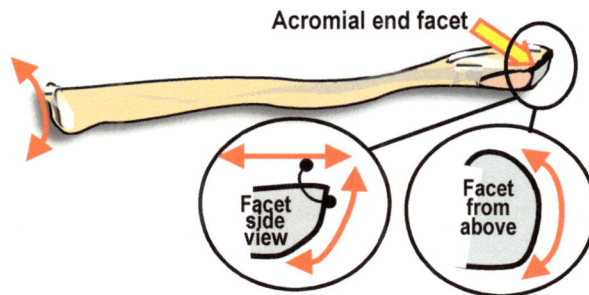

Figure 3F
Anterior view of a left clavicle

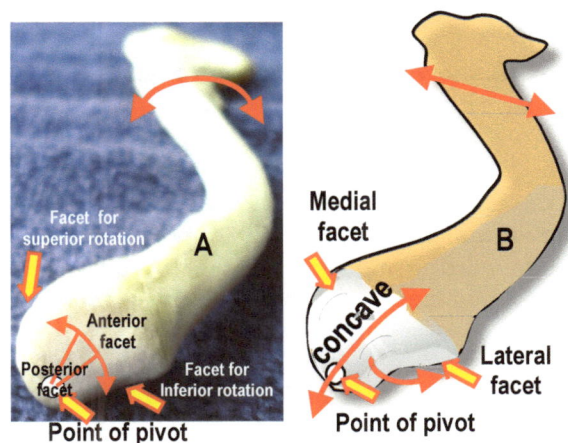

Figure 3G
View of sternal end of left clavicle

201

The Sterno-Clavicular Joint:
Side-Bending and Rotation

Figure 3H shows three photographs of the sterno-clavicular joint during clavicular side-bending.

Figure 3HA shows the joint in neutral for comparison purposes.

Figure 3HB shows the plane of movement when the clavicle side-bends postero-inferiorly. During this movement the facets of the clavicle engage at the posterior part (the pivot point) of the manubrial facet and rock in the line of the trajectory illustrated in **figure 3D** on page 200.

Figure 3HC shows the plane of movement when the clavicle side-bends antero-superiorly. During this movement the facets of the clavicle engage at the anterior part of the manubrial facet and rock in the line of trajectory illustrated in **figure 3D** on page 200.

Figure 3J shows three photographs of the sterno-clavicular joint during clavicular rotation. Again the same anchor point of pivot is used and works in a similar way to the axis of a singular central windscreen wiper.

Figure 3JA shows the joint in neutral and is for comparison only.

Figure 3JB shows the plane of movement when the clavicle rotates superiorly. During this movement the facets of the clavicle rotate and slide medially over the anterior part of the manubrial facet, as shown in **figure 3D** on page 200.

Figure 3JC shows the plane of movement when the clavicle rotates inferiorly. During this movement the facets of the clavicle rotate and slide laterally over the anterior part of the manubrial facet, as shown in **figure 3D** on page 200.

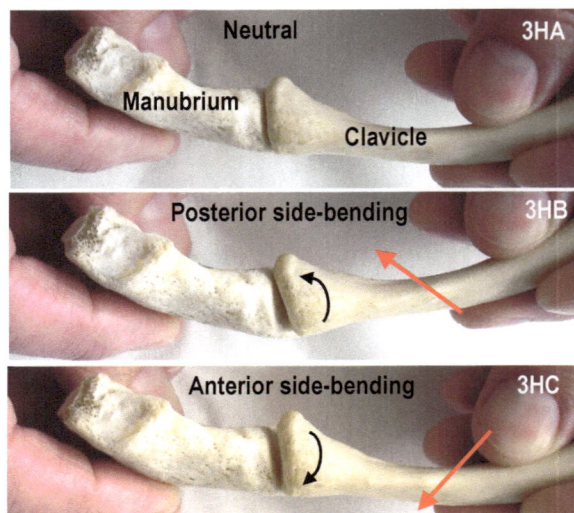

Figure 3H
View from above of the sterno-clavicular joint side-bending

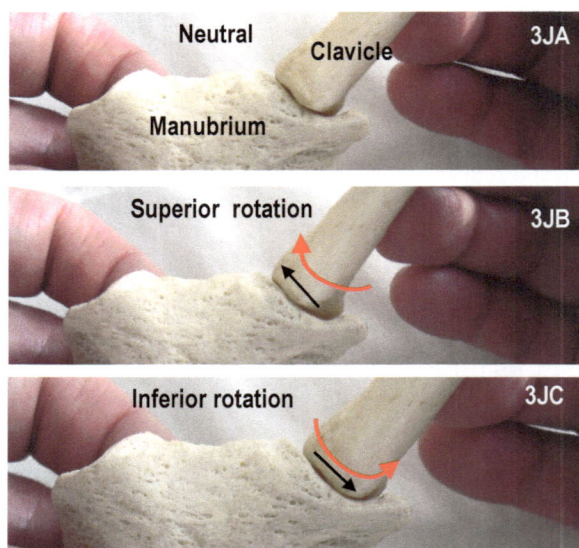

Figure 3J
Anterior view of the sterno-clavicular joint rotating

The Clavicle:
Side-Bending and Rotation

This page should be read and compared with the previous page.

Figure 3K shows three photographs of the acromion end of the clavicle during clavicular side-bending anteriorly and posteriorly.

Figure 3KA shows the joint in neutral for comparison purposes.

Figure 3KB shows the plane of movement when the posterior part of the manubrial facet is engaged. The distal end of the clavicle side-bends along an inferior-posterior plane.

Figure 3KC shows the plane of movement when the anterior part of the manubrial facet is engaged. The distal end of the clavicle side-bends along an supero-anterior plane.

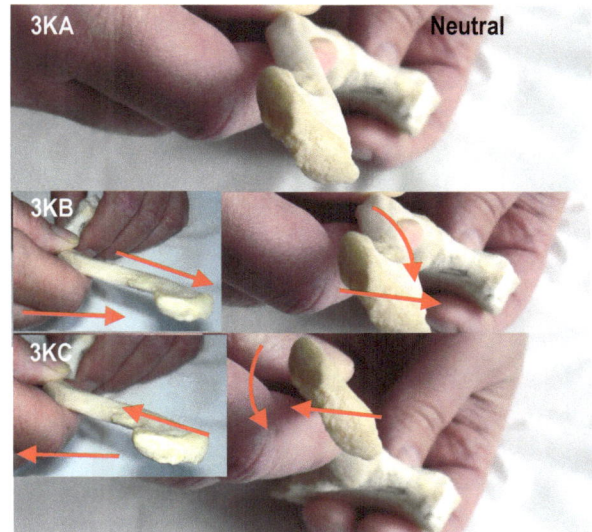

Figure 3K
Lateral view from above of the
sterno-clavicular joint side-bending

Figure 3L shows three photographs of the acromion end of the clavicle during clavicular inferior and superior rotation.

Figure 3LA shows the joint in neutral and is for comparison only.

Figure 3LB shows the plane of movement at the distal end of the clavicle during superior rotation. During this movement the facets of the clavicle arc medially along the anterior manubrial facet. See **figure 3GA** on page 201.

Figure 3LC shows the plane of movement at the distal end of the clavicle during inferior rotation. During the movement the facets of the clavicle arc laterally along the anterior manubrial facet. See **figure 3GA** on page 201.

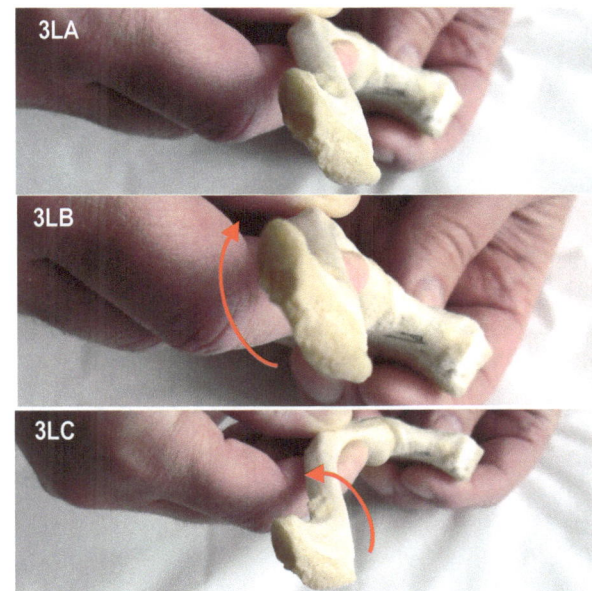

Figure 3L
Lateral view from above of the
sterno-clavicular joint rotating

In Summary

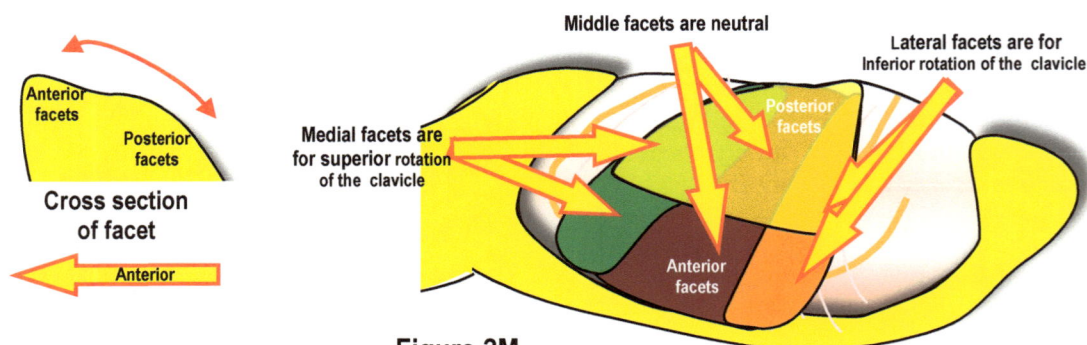

Figure 3M
The manubrium facet surface areas

To summarize, the manubrial facets can be divided into six continuous segments:

When the clavicle engages with the middle posterior and anterior facets, the arm hangs in neutral. This means that the palmer surface of the hand will face the upper thigh.

When both the medial posterior and anterior facets are engaged the arm hangs in neutral and the palmer surface of the hand faces anteriorly.

When both the lateral posterior and anterior facets are engaged the arm hangs in neutral and the palmer surface of the hand faces posteriorly.

When the posterior middle facet is singularly engaged the arm moves in extension with the palmer surface of the hand in neutral.

When the posterior medial facet is singularly engaged the arm moves in extension with the palmer surface of the hand facing anteriorly.

When the posterior lateral facet is singularly engaged the arm moves in extension with the palmer surface of the hand facing posteriorly.

When the anterior medial facet is singularly engaged the arm moves in flexion with the palmer surface of the hand facing anteriorly.

When the anterior lateral facet is singularly engaged the arm moves in flexion with the palmer surface of the hand facing posteriorly.

Chapter Eighteen
Physiology of the
Acromio-Clavicular Joint and
Scapula

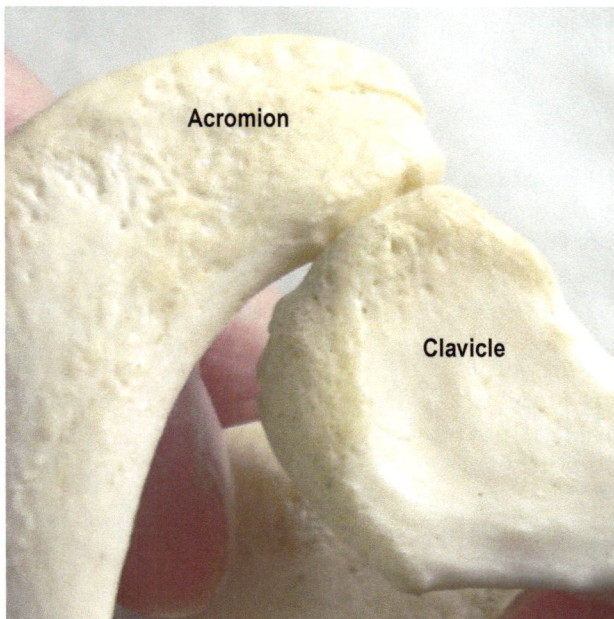

Figure 4A
Aerial view of
the sterno-clavicular joint

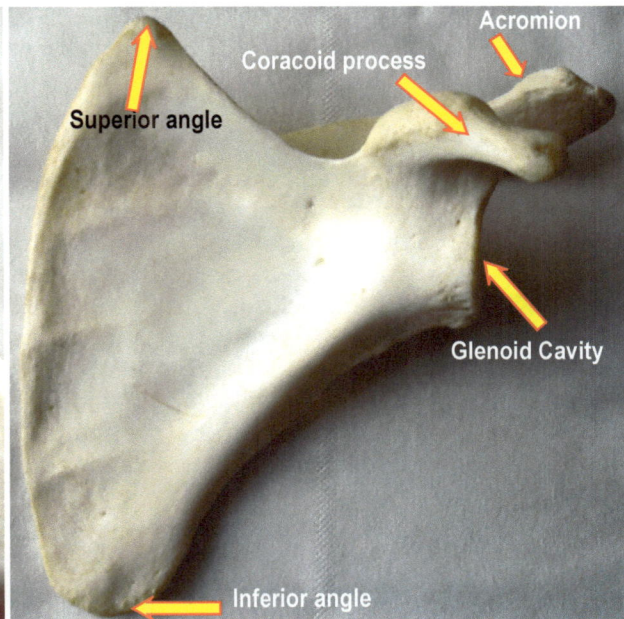

Figure 4B
Anterior view of
scapula

The acromio-clavicular joint as shown in **figure 4A** is simple and multi-purpose. The articulation of the joint provides an antero-posterior arc together with supero-inferior rotation of the scapula.

For reference purposes **Figure 4B** is an anterior photograph of a left scapula. The scapula is 'strapped' to the body by muscles which provide it with considerable mobility. It makes physical joint contact with the lateral end of the clavicle at the sterno-clavicular joint and with the head of the humorous at the gleno-humeral joint.

Overview of the
Acromio-Clavicular Ligament

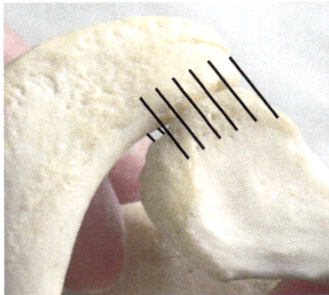

Figure 4C
Aerial view of
The sterno-clavicular
ligaments

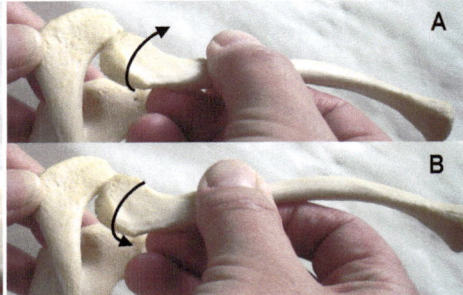

Figure 4D
Aerial view of
The sterno-clavicular joint
incorrect rotation

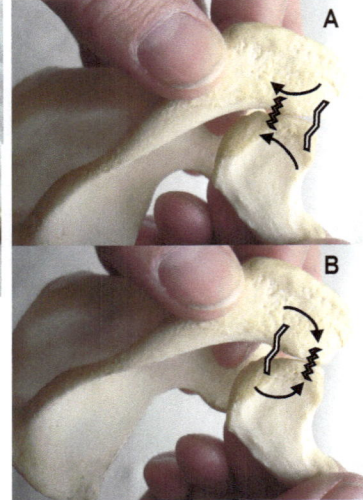

Figure 4E
Aerial view of
The sterno-clavicular joint
horizontal side-bending

Although the acromio-clavicular articular facets and ligaments look simple they are very cleverly designed and provide a dual function. The fibres of the coraco-clavicular ligaments run in a medial to lateral direction, above and below the joint, as shown in **figure 4C**. With such a ligament configuration, obvious rotation as that shown in **figures 4D A** and **B** would have the ligaments at a disadvantage and lead to a buckling of the joint. Nature would be unlikely to have allowed this type of vulnerability to have evolved. Therefore, it can be deduced that this is not the way the acromio-clavicular accommodates arm rotation.

Figure 4E, **A** and **B** illustrate how the ligaments make allowance for a horizontal side-bending swivel type action. This action is required when the arm moves along an antero-superior (flexion) or inferio-posterior (extension) plane of direction. As can be seen, this movement fits in perfectly with the line of the ligaments.

Figure 4F, **A** and **B** illustrate how the line of the ligament fibres make allowance for vertical side-bending. It will be explained later in this chapter why vertical side-bending is integral to arm rotation.

In summary, the position of the ligament and the line of its fibres accommodate both side-bending horizontally and vertically, either independently, or at the same time.

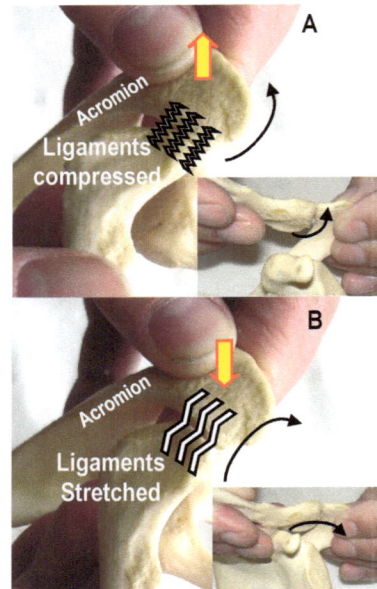

Figure 4F
Aerial view of
The sterno-clavicular joint
vertical side-bending

Acromio-clavicular Joint Movements

Figures 4GA, B and **C** illustrate the action that takes place at the acromio-clavicular joint during arm movements.

Figure 4GA shows the joint in neutral. When the arm is in neutral the arm and hand hang at the side of the body with the palmer surface of the hand facing the thigh.

Figure 4GB shows the joint in extension. The arm and hand with the palmer surface facing medially moves posteriorly and medially. The scapula moves inferiorly and posteriorly drawing the lateral end of clavicle along with it in the same plane. At the apex of this movement the anterior section of the acromio-clavicular joint side-bends open.

Figure 4GC shows the joint in flexion. The arm and hand with the palmer surface facing medially moves anteriorly, laterally and superiorly. The scapula moves superiorly and anteriorly drawing the lateral end of the clavicle along with it in the same plane. At the apex of this movement the posterior section of the acromio-clavicular joint side-bends open.

Figure 4HA illustrates the acromio-clavicular joint in neutral.

Figure 4HB illustrates the acromion side-bending in a vertical plane inferiorly when the arm is extended.

Figure 4HC illustrates the acromion side-bending in a vertical plane superiorly when the arm is flexed.

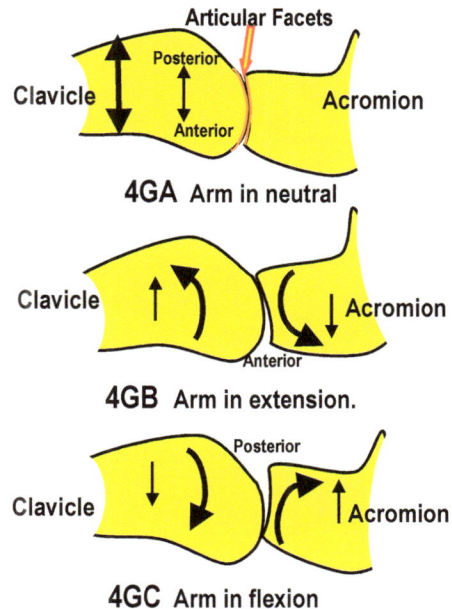

4GA Arm in neutral

4GB Arm in extension.

4GC Arm in flexion

Figure 4G
Aerial view of the right sterno-clavicular joint showing horizontal side-bending

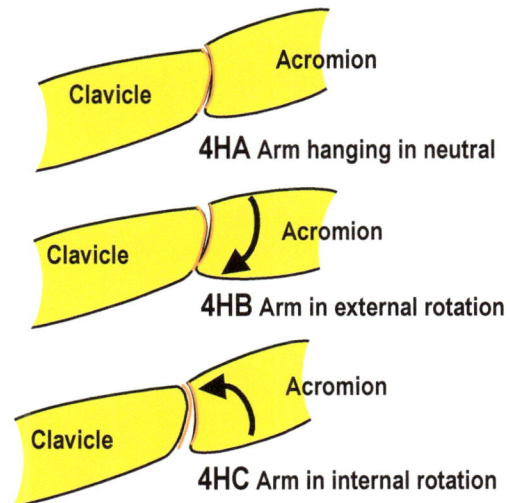

4HA Arm hanging in neutral

4HB Arm in external rotation

4HC Arm in internal rotation

Figure 4H
Anterior view of the right sterno-clavicular joint showing vertical side-bending

Arm Rotation and the Scapula

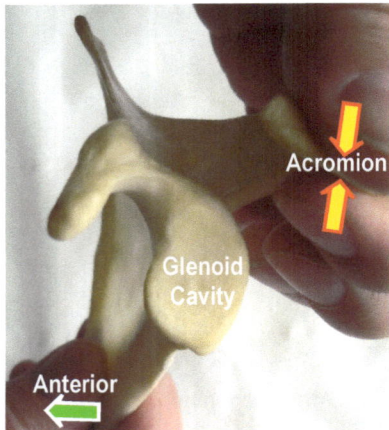

Figure 4J
Side-view of
the scapula in neutral

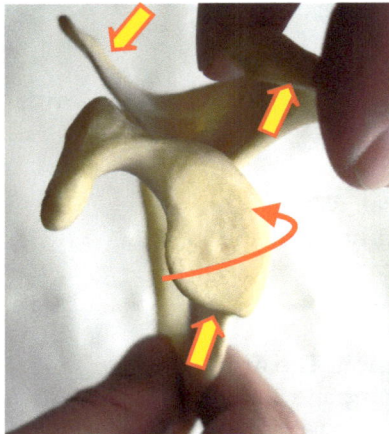

Figure 4K
Side-view of
the scapula in external rotation

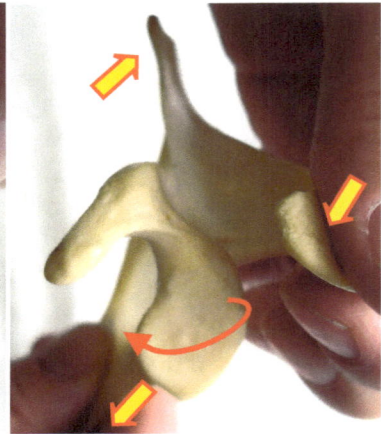

Figure 4L
Side-view of
the scapula in internal rotation

Try this experiment: With your arm hanging loose in neutral at your side. Be aware of the height of your shoulder and make finger tip contact with your thigh. If you internally rotate your hand your finger tips and shoulder will move inferiorly. If you externally rotate your arm your shoulder and fingers will move superiorly. Most arm rotation comes from the gleno-humeral joint. However, the scapula also has an important role to play in these movements.

Figure 4 M is a side-view of the glenoid cavity and the acromion. Note that the angle of the acromion is off-set. Therefore, supero-lateral and inferio-medial rotational movements at the acromio-clavicular joint will produce superior and inferior rotational movements at the glenoid cavity.

These rotational movements are illustrated in **figures 4J**, **4K** and **4L.** When gleno-humeral and acromio-clavicular rotation has taken place, further rotation takes place at the sterno-clavicular joint.

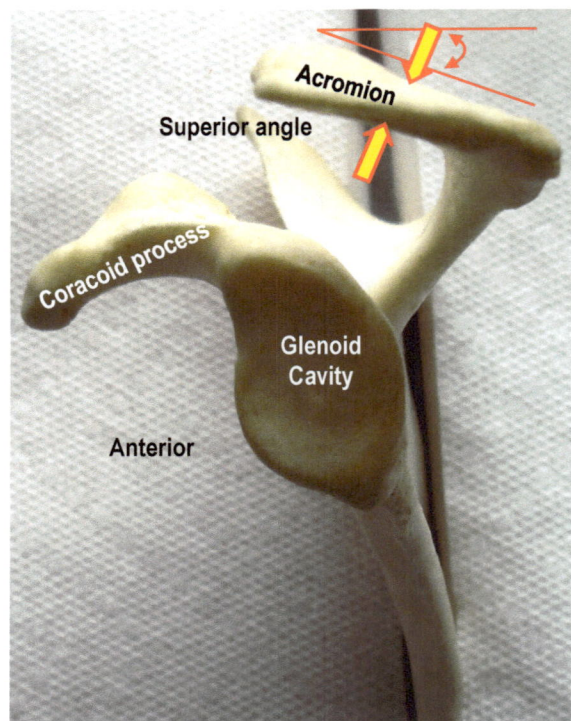

Figure 4M
Side-view of
the scapula

208

Chapter Nineteen
Rib Cage and Clavicle
Subluxations

Ribs can become subluxated in either inspiration or expiration, as illustrated in **figures TSHa,b** and **c,** and **TSEa,b** and **c,** and was explained in chapter 12.

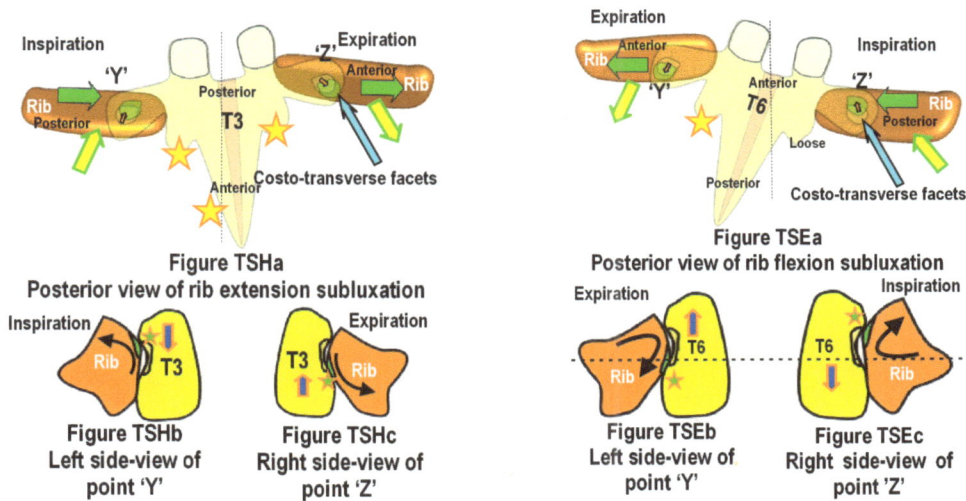

Figure TSHa
Posterior view of rib extension subluxation

Figure TSHb
Left side-view of point 'Y'

Figure TSHc
Right side-view of point 'Z'

Figure TSEa
Posterior view of rib flexion subluxation

Figure TSEb
Left side-view of point 'Y'

Figure TSEc
Right side-view of point 'Z'

Because ribs move in a similar way to blades of a venetian blind it only takes one blade to lock and go out of alignment, as shown in **figure 5A**, to cause the surrounding blades to become entangled and displaced. If more than one blade lock and go out of alignment, the disarray as will be shown later in this chapter, will cause the rib cage and sternum to distort. This could theoretically effect the efficiency of the breathing mechanism and would definitely distort the symmetry and therefore, the efficiency of the shoulder girdle.

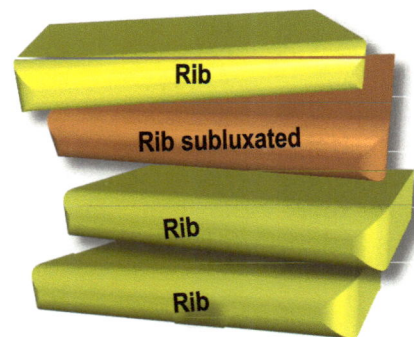

Figure 5A
Illustration of rib misalignment

Rib Displacements in Flexion and Extension

Figures 5AA and **5AAA** illustrate the facet positioning within a flexion subluxation. The right 7th rib, shown in red, is pulled superiorly and away from the demi-facets with a consequent loss of stability. The reason it is pulled laterally is due to the pull of the ligaments at the transverse facet of T7. If it were not for these ligaments the rib would dislocate. The left rib, shown in blue is pushed inferiorly and becomes lodged against the superior demi-facet of T8. This entrapment locks the rib and causes a band of rib rigidity around that side of the torso.

Figures 5AB and **ABA** illustrate the positions of the 7th ribs subluxated in extension. Extension subluxations are more serious than flexion subluxations because two violations of the thoracic laws of movement take place.

1) The vertebra rotates in the opposite direction to that intended while at the same time compressing the subluxated vertebra against its neighbour below. See chapter twelve.

2) The compression placed on the ribs leaves no room to manoeuvre. Therefore, when side-shift takes place the ribs on either side of T7 are pushed into the side of the demi-facets where they lock. This locking results in a band of rigidity around the trunk far more rigid than that found in ribs subluxated in thoracic flexion.

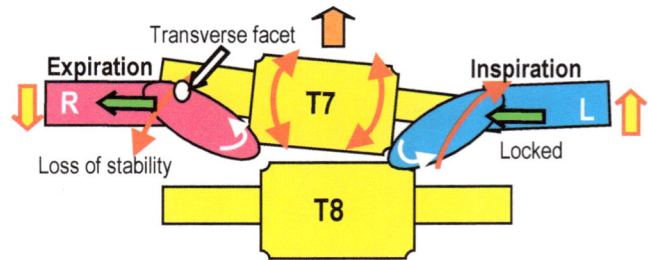

Figure 5AA
Anterior view of rotation left within flexion subluxation showing T7 rib displacement

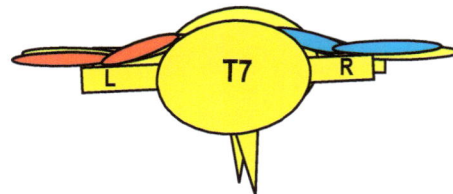

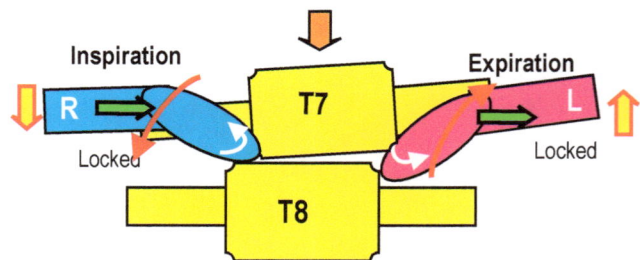

Figure 5AAA
Aerial view of rotation left in flexion subluxation showing T7 rib displacement

Figure 5AB
Anterior view of rotation right within extension subluxation showing T7 rib displacement

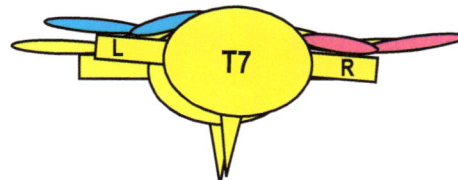

Figure 5ABA
Aerial view of rotation right with in extension subluxation showing T7 rib displacement

210

Rib Displacements in Flexion and Extension

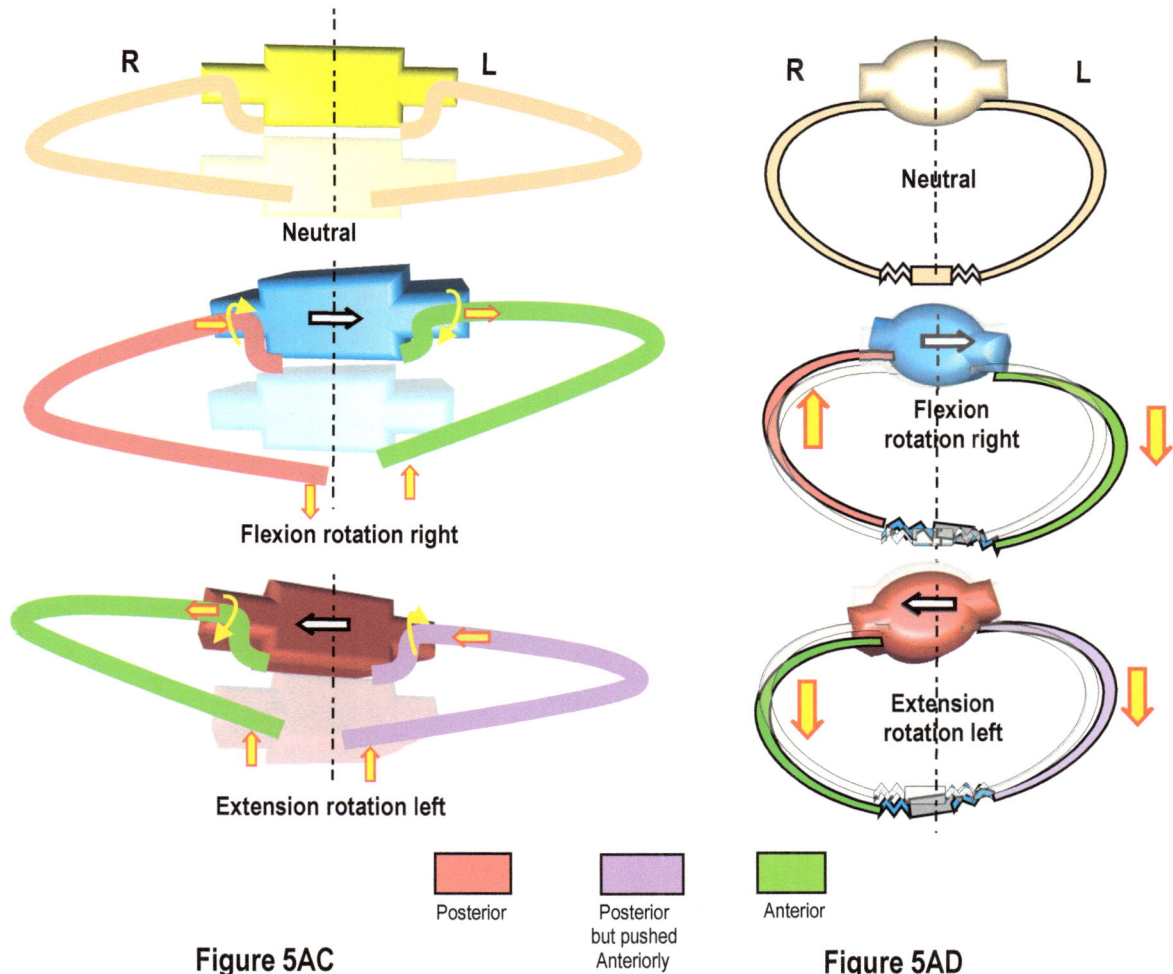

R ... **L**

Neutral

Flexion rotation right

Extension rotation left

Neutral

Flexion rotation right

Extension rotation left

Posterior

Posterior but pushed Anteriorly

Anterior

Figure 5AC
Anterior view of rib distortions in flexion and extension

Figure 5AD
Aerial view of rib distortions in flexion and extension

Figures 5AC and **5 AD**, which are self explanatory, show the extent to which the ribs become distorted when certain vertebrae become subluxated. The distortions have been exaggerated for clarity, nevertheless they are not as far from reality as it may at first seem.

Above; these distortions will affect the alignment of the sternum and therefore the general symmetry of the rib cage and have implications for the correct seating and alignment of the clavicle.

Below; these distortions have serious consequences regarding the efficiency of the diaphragm.

Rib Cage Distortions in the
L3-Right-Right Subluxation Pattern

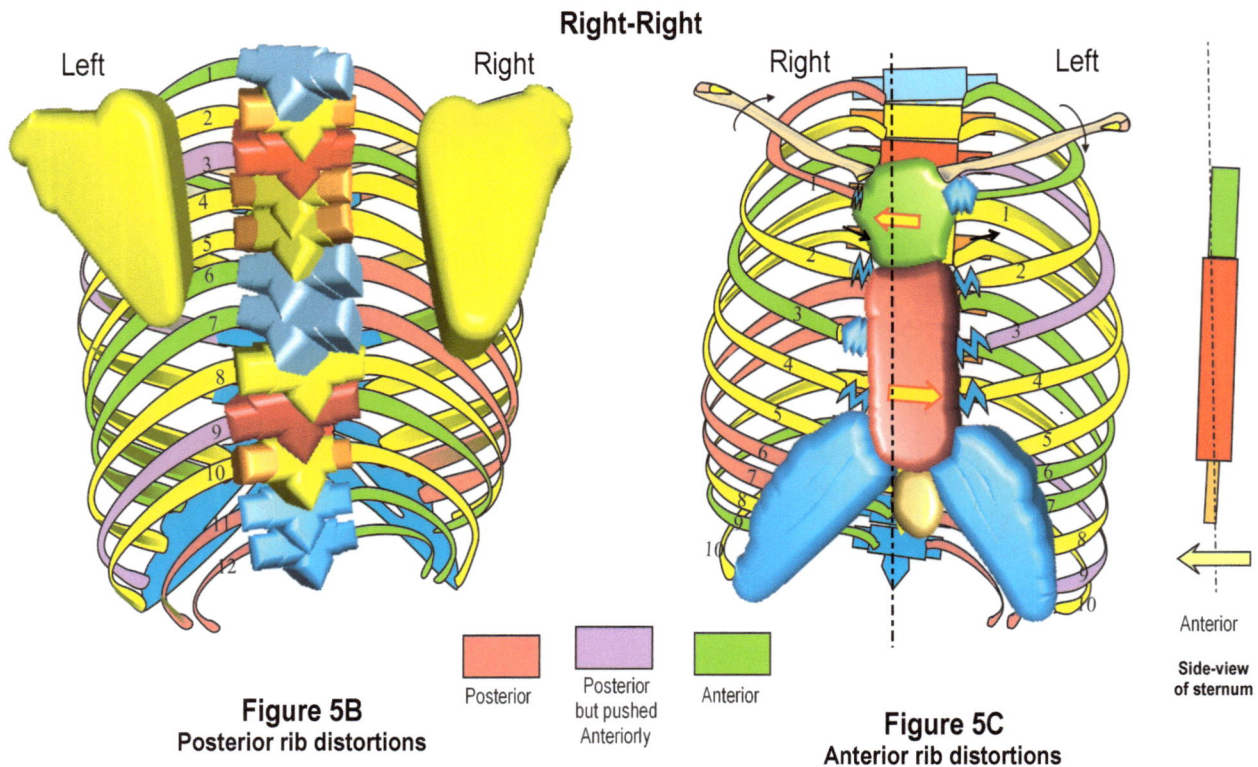

Right-Right

Left

Right

Right

Left

Figure 5B
Posterior rib distortions

Posterior

Posterior
but pushed
Anteriorly

Anterior

Figure 5C
Anterior rib distortions

Anterior

**Side-view
of sternum**

The illustrations above are based upon the conclusion subluxation pattern illustrated on page 152. The red ribs are those that subluxated and became levered posteriorly. The purple ribs are those that should be posterior but due to the angle of the corresponding vertebral transverse process become levered anteriorly. The green ribs are those that became levered anteriorly.

Figure 5B shows the subluxation pattern and the effect this pattern inflicts on the rib cage. It looks grossly distorted with obvious general rotation to the left and oblique side-bending that splits the rib cage at T8. When I first drew this I thought that it must be a mistake but when I compared it to the L3-right-right model it fitted exactly.

Figure 5C shows the subluxation pattern and the effect the ribs subluxations have on the sternum. Note that the sternum has become side-sifted to the right around the inferior ribs and to the left at the manubrium. It has also incurred an element of rotation to the right.

This displacement has a direct effect on the seating of the clavicle bones and therefore has implications for the alignment and efficiency of the shoulder joints.

Rib Cage Distortions in the
L3-Right-Right Subluxation Pattern

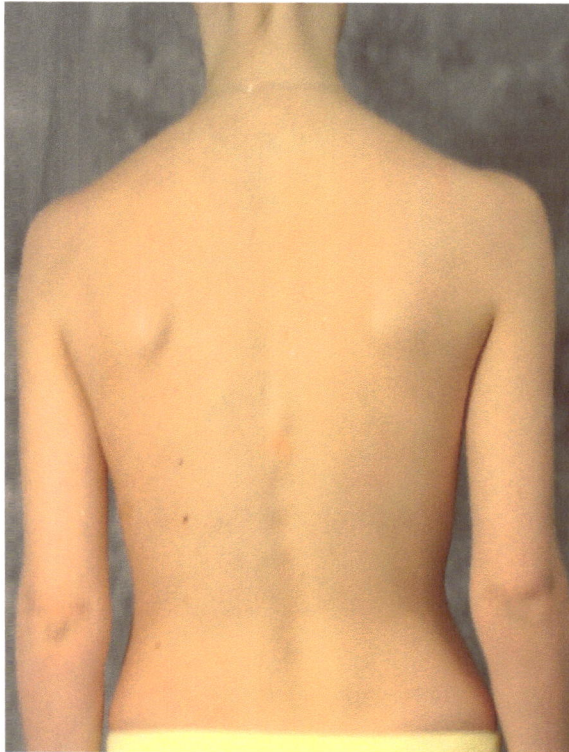

Figure 5D
Posterior rib distortions

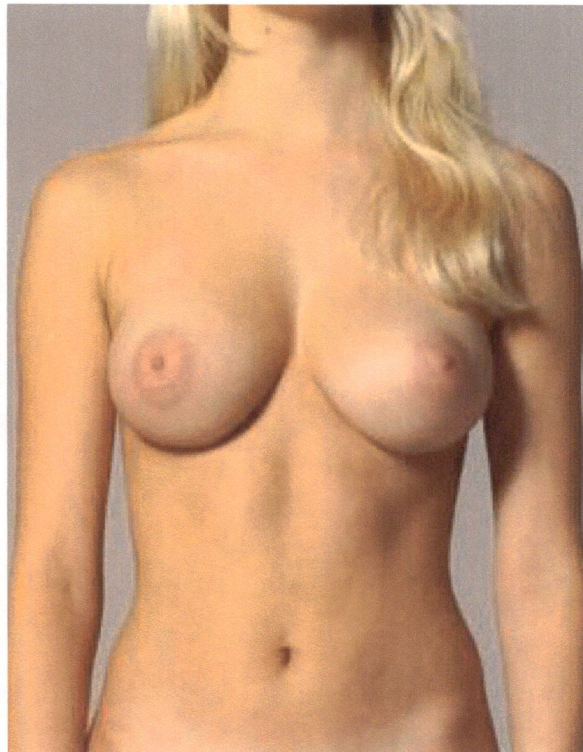

Figure 5E
Anterior rib distortions

Compare the above photographs with the illustrations on the previous page and a marked similarity can be seen.

Look particularly at the waist lines of both young women. Remember, the diaphragm attaches to this area and so it is of particular importance.

Observe the protruding clavicle on the right in **figure 5E** and how it squares and tightens the shoulder posteriorly. This posterior pull causes the right arm to be drawn backwards and the elbow to flex.

Rib Cage Distortions in the
L3-Left-Right Subluxation Pattern

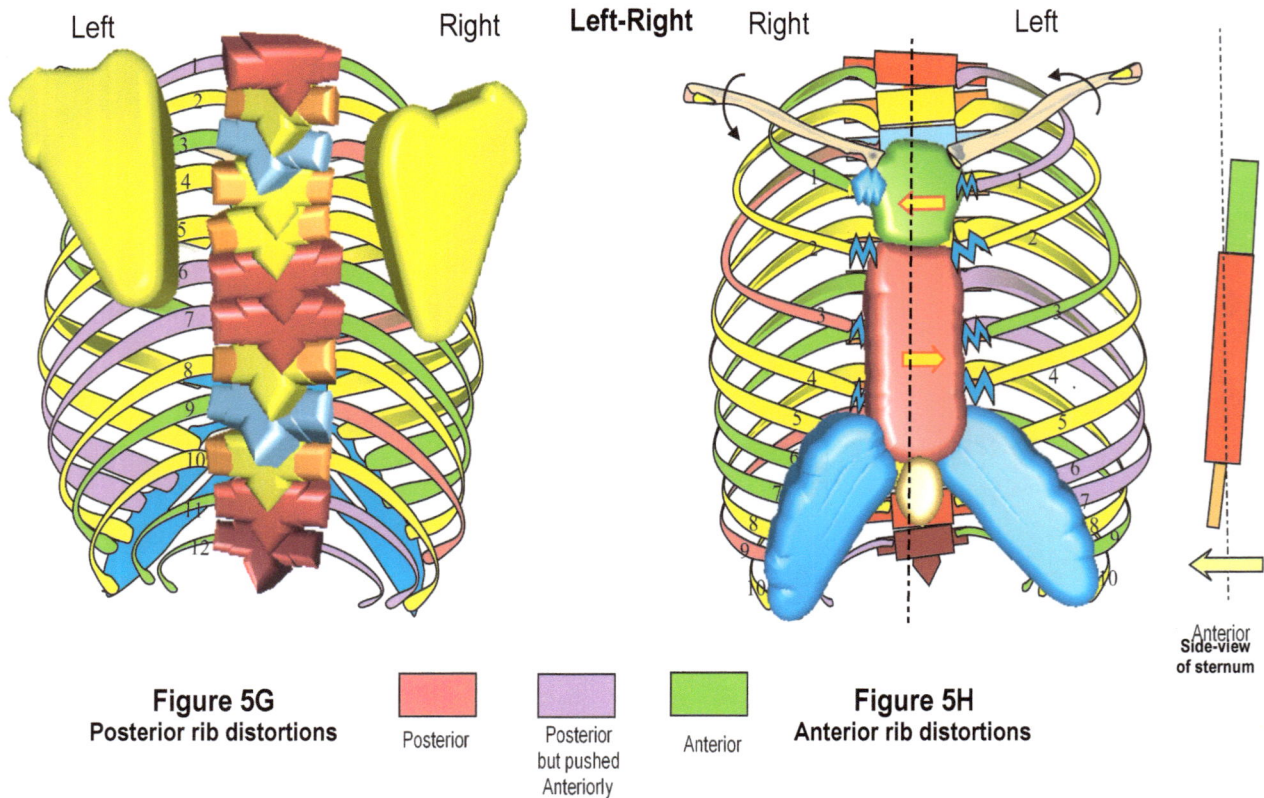

Figure 5G
Posterior rib distortions

Posterior | Posterior but pushed Anteriorly | Anterior

Figure 5H
Anterior rib distortions

Anterior
Side-view of sternum

The illustrations above are based upon the conclusion subluxation pattern illustrated on page 153. The red ribs are those that subluxated and became levered posteriorly, the purple ribs should be posterior but due to the angle of the corresponding vertebral transverse process became levered anteriorly. The green ribs are those that became levered anteriorly.

Figure 5G shows the subluxation pattern and the effect this pattern inflicts on the rib cage. It looks distorted with obvious general rotation to the left and oblique side-bending that splits the rib cage at T8. This illustration fits exactly with the L3-left-right model.

Figure 5B shows the subluxation pattern and the effect the rib subluxations have on the sternum. Note that the sternum has side sifted and side-bent to the left. It has also incurred an element of rotation to the left.

This displacement has a direct effect on the seating of the clavicle bones and therefore has implications for the alignment and efficiency of the shoulder joints.

Rib Cage Distortions in the L3-Left-Right Subluxation Pattern

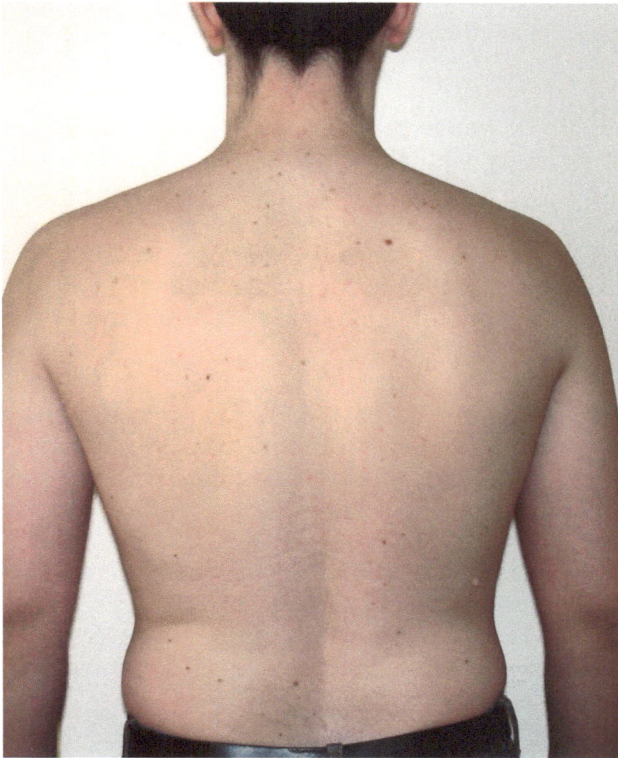

Figure 5J
Posterior rib distortions

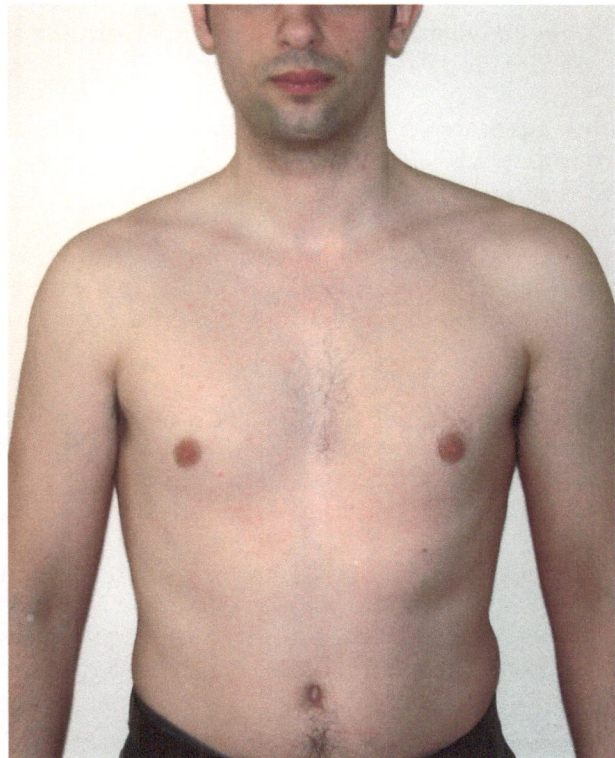

Figure 5K
Anterior rib distortions

Compare the photographs above with the illustrations on the previous page and a marked similarly can be seen.

Look particularly at Dan's waist line. The diaphragm attaches to this area and so this distortion is of particular importance.

Compare **figure 5k** with **figure 5E** on page 213 and notice how the mid-line of the rib cage side-bends and rotates to the left in the L3-left-right pattern and how it side-bends and rotates to the right in the L3-right-right pattern.

In the photographs of all the models they are standing on both legs with their feet in alignment.

Direct Trauma to Ribs

Ribs can become subluxated by other causes than spinal misalignment and for completeness this has been included.

From the chapters on how the thoracic vertebrae articulate, it was explained why thoracic backward bending and rotation are prohibited in normal physiology and why if attempted the joint/s and rib/s subluxate.

Some every day tasks can put extreme levering forces on the ribs and cause them to severely subluxate. This type of trauma can result in extreme sharp pain and breathing difficulties for the person. Direct trauma rib subluxations can occur in both inhalation, which is the more common, and exhalation.

To recap on the mechanics, in thoracic backward bending if the intension of the person is to rotate right, the thoracic vertebrae depending on its integrity at the time will either block this movement or rotate the vertebrae to the opposite side, left.   This means that any forced rotation to the right will lever and force the ribs in a non-physiological manner that risks their severe subluxation.

As the arms are usually the guiding rotational force, rib trauma subluxations tend to be found higher up the rib cage, between T7 and T1. They do occur below this at around T9-T10 but are much less common. Below are some photographs of Lindsey completing some of the every day tasks that people regularly do that can lead to direct trauma rib subluxations.   They all involve backward leaning and rotation.

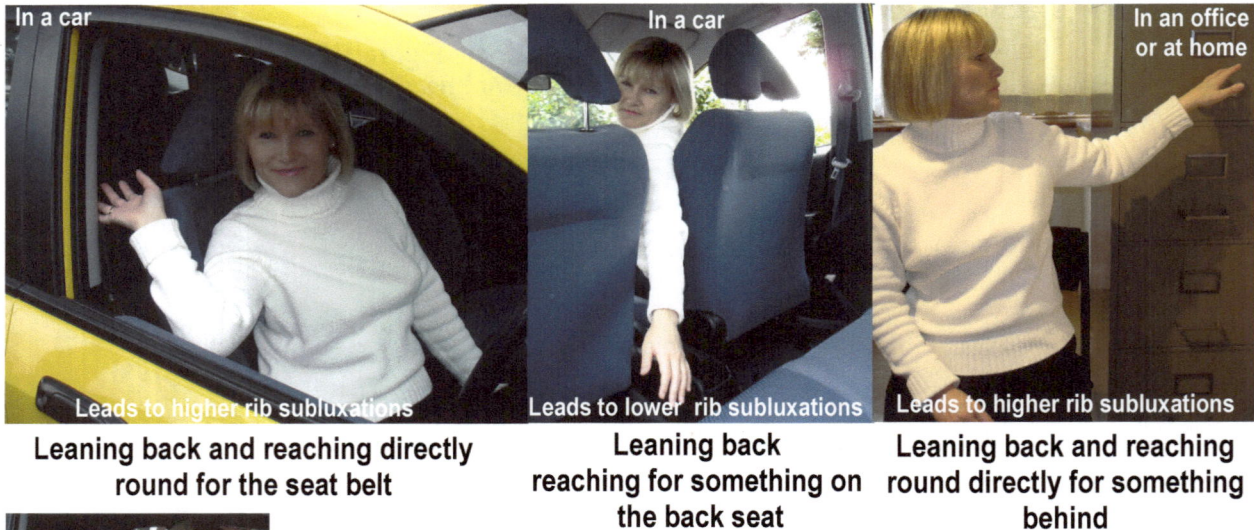

In a car
Leads to higher rib subluxations

Leaning back and reaching directly round for the seat belt

In a car
Leads to lower rib subluxations

Leaning back reaching for something on the back seat

In an office or at home
Leads to higher rib subluxations

Leaning back and reaching round directly for something behind

Showing how to put a seat belt on. Lean forward and bring the furthest arm round.

Clavicle Misalignments

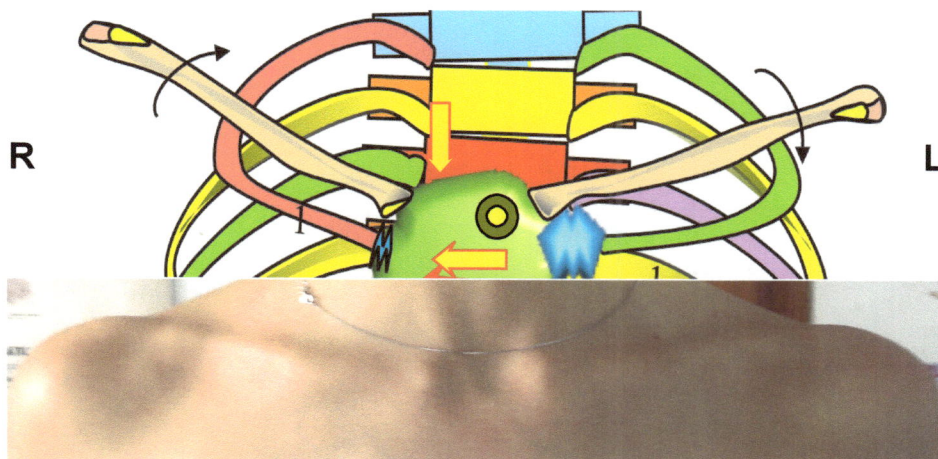

Figure 5L
Clavicle misalignments in the L3-right-right
Subluxation pattern distortions

Key:
◎=Anterior

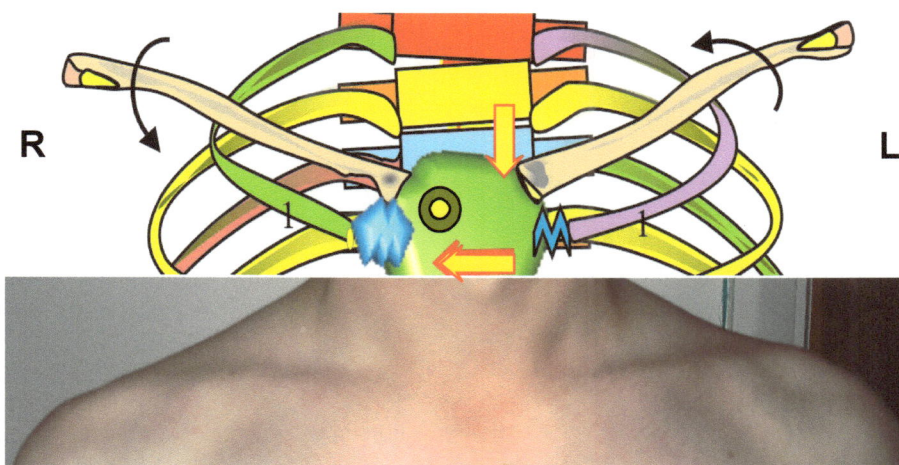

Key:
◎=Anterior

Figure 5M
Clavicle misalignments in the L3-left-right
Subluxation pattern distortions

In **figure 5L**, **L3-R-R**, observe the distorted position of the manubrium. It has side-shifted, side-bent and rotated to the right and altered the seating of the clavicle bones.   The right clavicle is angled higher than the left. Note that the right shoulder is anterior.

In **figure 5M**, **L3-L-R**, observe the distorted position of the manubrium. It has side-shifted right, side-bent and rotated to the left and altered the seating of the clavicle bones. The left clavicle is angled higher than the right. Note that the right shoulder is anterior.

Clavicle Rotated Superiorly and Laterally

Figure 5N is anterior view of the left side of the sterno-clavicular joint for reference purposes.

The illustrations apply to the sterno-clavicular subluxations that can present on the left side in the L3-left-right subluxation pattern and on the right in the L3-right-right pattern.

Figure 5P shows the manubrium rotated posteriorly on the affected side caused by the leverage exerted on the body of the sternum by the myriad of rib subluxations below.

This rotation causes the posterior part of the manubrial facet to part away from the posterior part of the clavicle facet. This parting destabilizes the joint.

Figure 5Q shows the secondary force of side-bending placed on the sterno-clavicular joint by the distortion of the sternal body.

The manubrium on the affected side is forced to side-bend inferiorly. This causes the already destabilized anterior facets of the clavicle to swivel medially along the anterior margin of the manubrial facet towards point A. At the same time the posterior part of clavicle facet is forced to swivel towards point B. At this point the joint locks in subluxation.

This subluxation places the medial facet of the clavicle medially and therefore upwards against the manubrial facet..

This is a sterno-clavicular subluxation, in other words the manubrium becomes displaced against the clavicle, not the other way round.

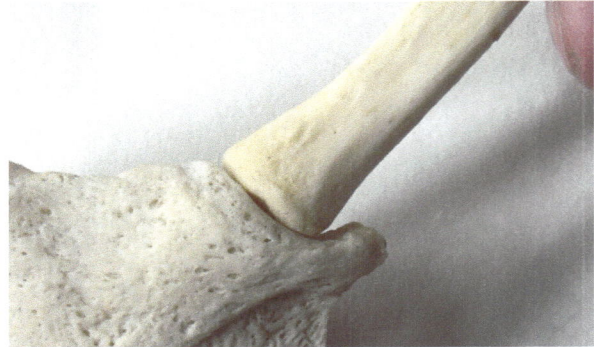

Figure 5N
Clavicle in Neutral

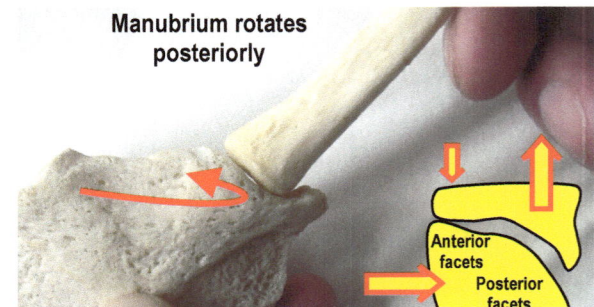

Manubrium rotates posteriorly

Anterior facets

Posterior facets

Figure 5P
Anterior view of manubrium when forced to rotate posteriorly

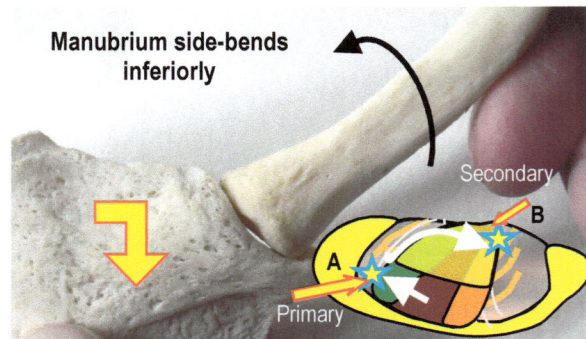

Manubrium side-bends inferiorly

Secondary

B

A

Primary

Figure 5Q
Anterior view of manubrium when forced to side-bend

218

Clavicle Rotated Inferiorly and Medially

Figure 5R is an anterior view of the left side of the sterno-clavicular joint for reference purposes.

The illustrations apply to the sterno-clavicular subluxations that can present on the right side in the L3-left-right subluxation pattern and on the left in the L3-right-right pattern.

Figure 5S shows the manubrium rotated anteriorly on the affected side. This rotation was caused by the leverage exerted on the body of the sternum by the myriad of rib subluxations. As the manubrium moves anteriorly on the effected side, the anterior areas of the facets of both the manubrium and the clavicle become parted. This parting destabilizes the joint.

Figure 5T shows the secondary superior force of side-bending that is also inflicted on the sterno-clavicular joint by the unruly forces placed on the body of the sternum by the myriad rib subluxations.

This causes the already destabilized posterior facet of the clavicle to side-shift medially up the posterior manubrial facet towards point A. At the same time the anterior part of the clavicle facet swivels laterally along the anterior margin towards point B where the joint locks in subluxation.

This subluxation also causes the medial facet of the clavicle to rotate inferiorly and therefore downwards against the manubrial facet.

This is a sterno-clavicular subluxation; in other words the manubrium becomes displaced against the clavicle, not the other way round.

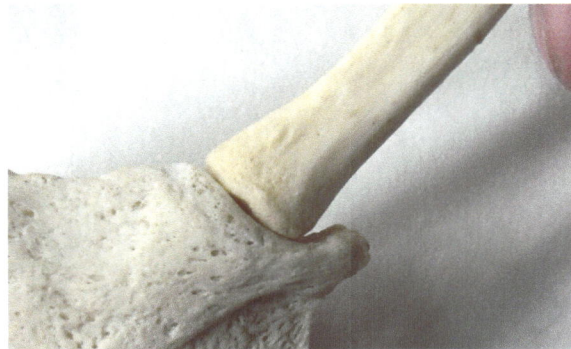

Figure 5R
Clavicle in Neutral

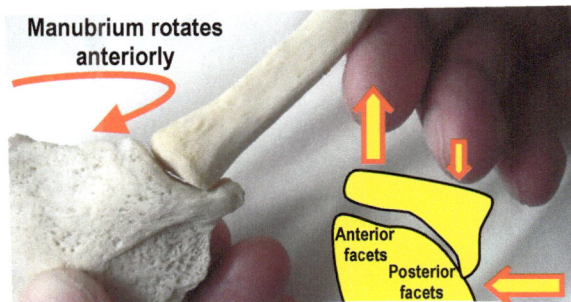

Manubrium rotates anteriorly

Anterior facets
Posterior facets

Figure 5S
Anterior view of manubrium when forced to rotate posteriorly

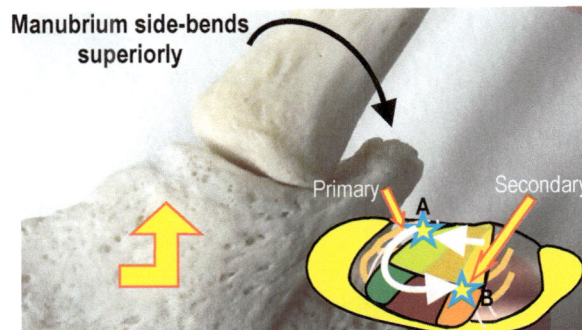

Manubrium side-bends superiorly

Primary   Secondary
A
B

Figure 5T
Anterior view of manubrium when forced to side-bend

219

Displacement of the Acromion in L3-Right-Right Pattern

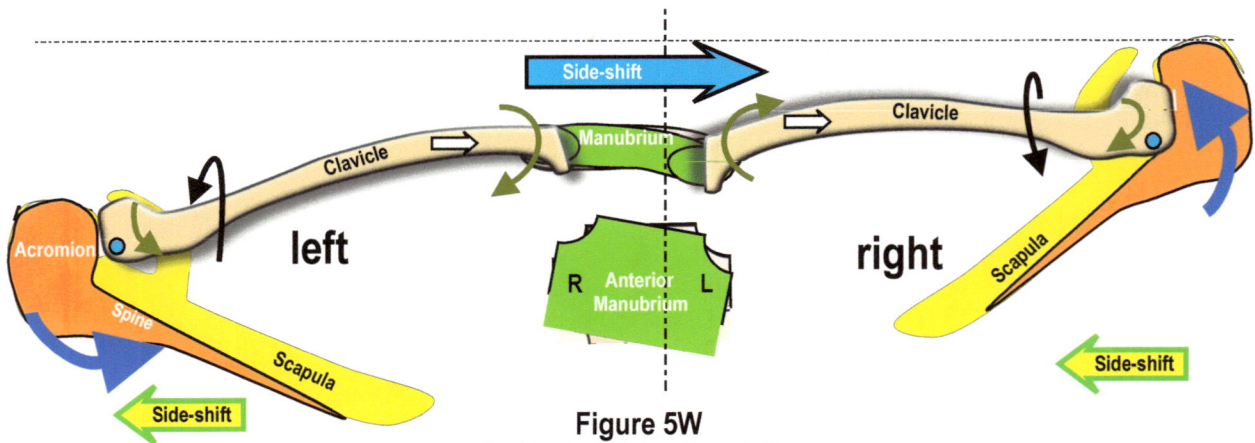

Figure 5W
Aerial view of shoulder girdle in the L3-right-right pattern

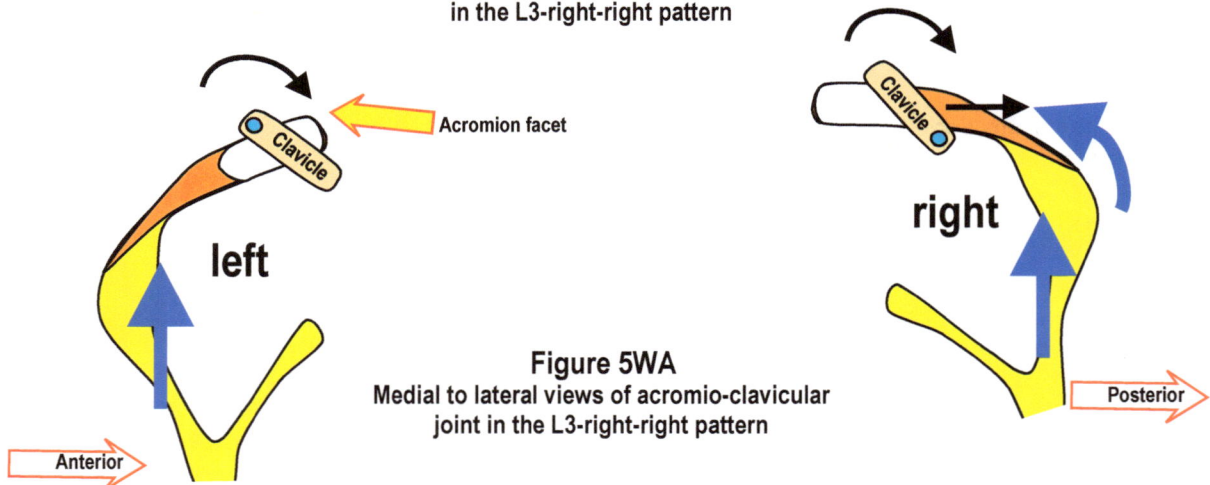

Figure 5WA
Medial to lateral views of acromio-clavicular joint in the L3-right-right pattern

In Chapter 12 it was demonstrated how the scapula becomes misaligned. This has serious implications on the alignment of the acromio-clavicular joint.

L3-right-right

The above illustrations have been drawn to show the positions of the facets at the acromio-clavicular joint.

Both the left and right scapulae are raised with a general side-shift to the left. This side-shift exerts side-shift forces to the right at the manubrium. See **figure 5L** on page 216 and page 152.

Both scapula bones are rotated to the left. See **figure 5W.** Because the side-shift forces exerted on the scapula are to the left, see **figure 17A** page 132, the right scapula and therefore the right acromio-clavicular joint becomes the focus of most of the force.

Displacement of the Acromion in L3-Left-Right Pattern

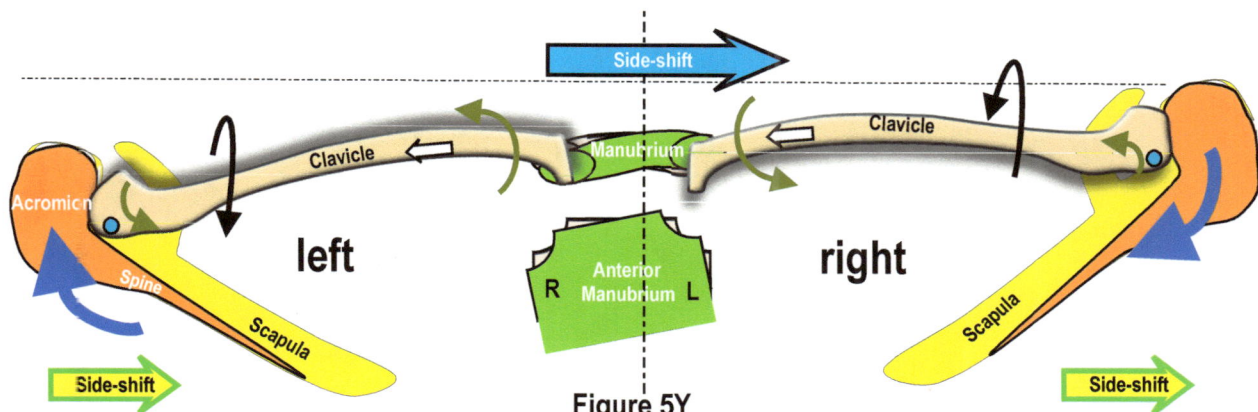

Figure 5Y
Aerial view of shoulder girdle
in L3-left-right pattern

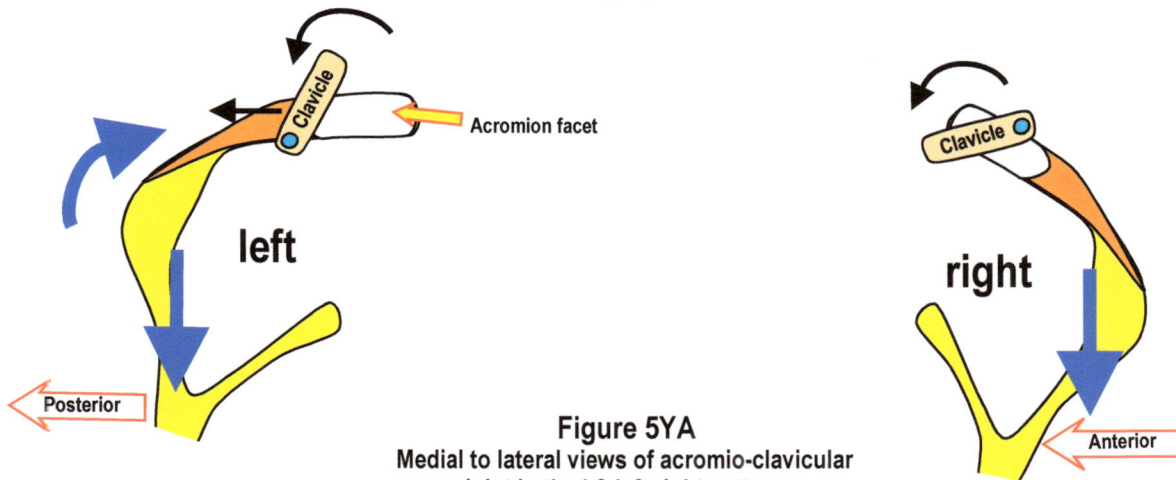

Figure 5YA
Medial to lateral views of acromio-clavicular
joint in the L3-left-right pattern

L3-left-right

The above illustrations have been drawn to show the positions of the facets at the acromio-clavicular joint.

Both the left and right scapulae are lowered with a general side-shift to the right. This side-shift moves round the torso and exerts side-shift forces to the left at the manubrium. See **figure 5M** on page 216 and page 153.

Both scapula bones are rotated right, see **figure 5Y**. Because the side-shift forces exerted on the scapula are to the right, see **figure 17C** page 139, the left scapula and therefore the left acromio-clavicular joint becomes the focus of most of the force.

Aids to Diagnosis

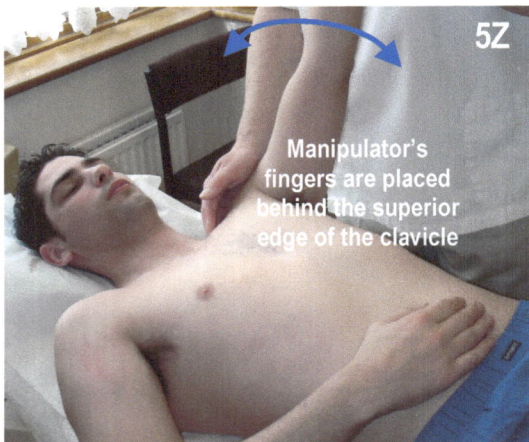

5Z Manipulator's fingers are placed behind the superior edge of the clavicle

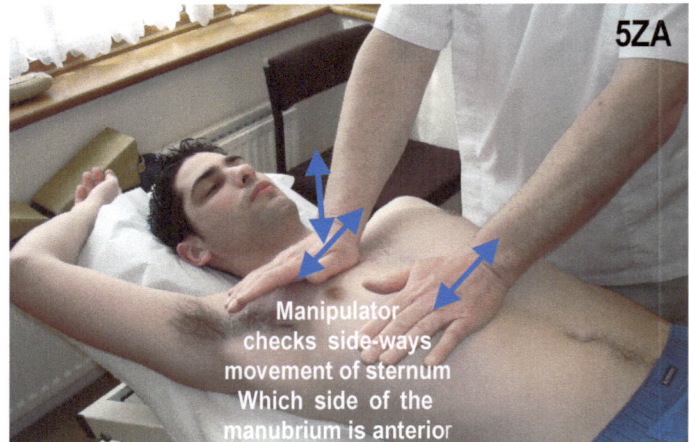

5ZA Manipulator checks side-ways movement of sternum Which side of the manubrium is anterior

Due to complications of trauma etc, rib cage and shoulder diagnosis may need verification. **Figure 5Z** shows how the angle of the clavicle can be checked. Both sides are compared. With an inferior clavicle resistance is felt when the arm is raised. To check the distortion of the sternum, **figure 5ZA** shows how the direction can be diagnosed. Check for side-ways movement. The side that feels easiest to move is the side the rib cage is veering. By putting the results of these two tests together, the angles of the manipulation can be confirmed.

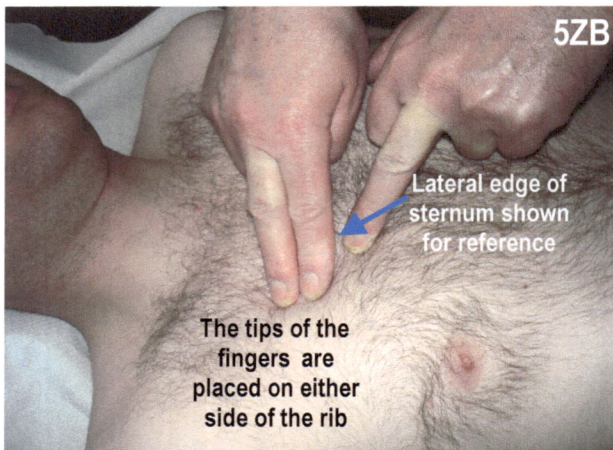

5ZB Lateral edge of sternum shown for reference

The tips of the fingers are placed on either side of the rib

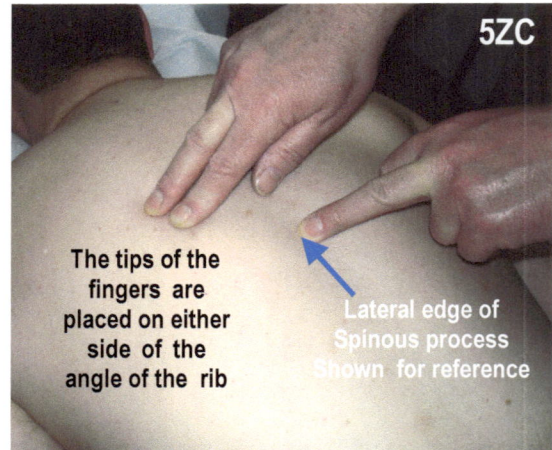

5ZC The tips of the fingers are placed on either side of the angle of the rib

Lateral edge of Spinous process Shown for reference

Again due to complications of trauma etc. the diagnosis of whether a rib is locked in inhalation or exhalation may need verification. **Figure 5ZB** and **5ZA** show the position the manipulators fingers should be placed. The patient is then asked to breath in or out. If the patient breaths in and the rib does not move the rib is locked in exhalation. If the patient breaths out and the rib does not move the rib is locked in inspiration.

The displaced angle of the subluxated rib feels like the head of a pea. It can be difficult to locate with up to a ¼ of an inch of soft tissue above. Palpation requires considerable skill, but it can be done.

222

Chapter Twenty
CST and CPT
Rib Cage Manipulation

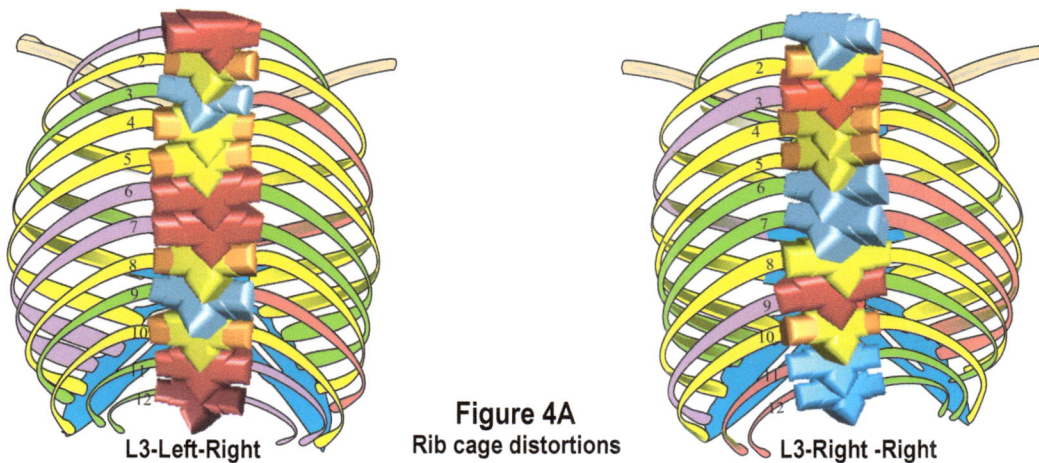

Figure 4A
Rib cage distortions

L3-Left-Right

L3-Right -Right

CST stands for <u>C</u>o-operative <u>S</u>upine <u>T</u>echnique and CPT stands for <u>C</u>o-operative <u>P</u>rone <u>T</u>echnique.

Secondary rib cage and shoulder joint distortions follow on when the sacroiliac joints become subluxated and these distortions have the potential to affect the efficient function of the breathing mechanism.

Unfortunately, rib cage and shoulder joint distortions by their very nature, double back and compound the locking of the already subluxated spine. Each area locks-in the previous area. With this catch 22 situation taking place it makes it very difficult to know where to start. But a start has to be made. This is where the science behind this type of manipulation becomes exciting.

A lot of manipulation takes place during a single treatment session if 'true alignment' is your goal and not every patient wants this. When PPT's CPT's and CST's are correctly applied, only a minimal trauma footprint is left behind so that in a single treatment session every joint in the spine and torso can be manipulated several times, when necessary, with minimal after affect.

The chest is a very sensitive and painful area to palpate and often patients can feel uncomfortable during palpation and in particular during stretching articulation techniques. However, because CST's are so quick and gentle, discomfort is minimal.

Bayliss Manipulation
Rib Expiration Technique

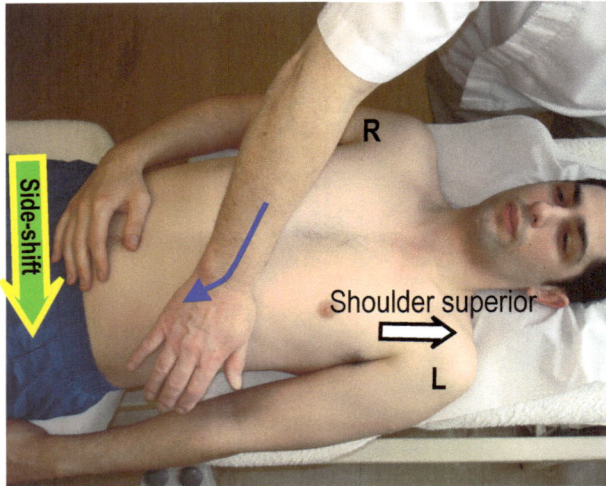

Figure 6A
Anterior view of patient
receiving CST rib manipulation

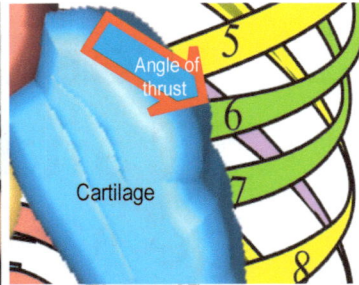

Figure 6B
Anterior views T6 and T7

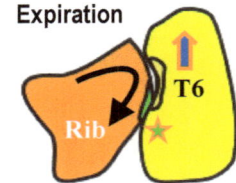

Figure TSEb
Left side-view of
point 'Y'

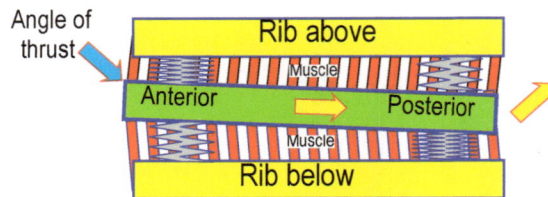

Figure 6C
Side-view of subluxated rib

This rib expiration correction technique uses the subluxated rib as a long lever. For this reason very little force is needed. The technique can be used for correcting ribs locked in both flexion and extension. The patient whilst co-operating has no control over when the manipulation will be made therefore, they are less likely to tense prior to the gentle push.

Technique
The patient is placed in a supine position on a flat couch with their left shoulder raised. Their knees are supported and flexed by a pillow and their pelvis side-shifted to the left, as shown in **figure 6A**. The manipulator asks the patient to breath in, 'inspiration'. A gentle push in then made in a posterior inferio-lateral direction, using the hypothenar eminence, against the superior surface of the rib. This is shown in **figures 6A, B** and **C**.

How does it work
The ribs are made malleable by the pelvic side-shift left which causes all of the individual vertebrae up the spine to attempt to shift towards the right. This is away from the subluxated rib and therefore this lessens the tension within the vertebral/rib subluxation.

The raised left shoulder opens and lifts the rib cage on the left. When the patient breaths in the anterior part of the ribs move superiorly. A push is then made in a posterior inferior lateral direction, as shown in **figure 6C,** (the mechanics of this are explained in **figure 6D)** and this pushes the posterior end of the rib medially and superiorly to mate correctly with the corresponding vertebrae.

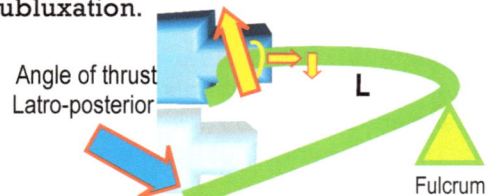

Figure 6D
Anterior views of T6
Showing angle of thrust

Bayliss Rib Manipulation
Inspiration Technique

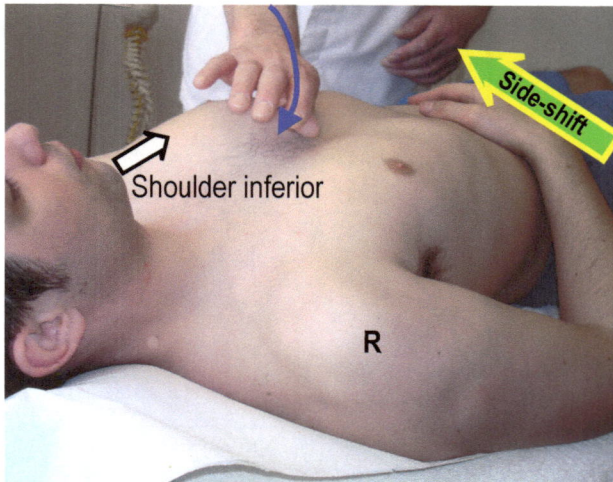

Figure 6F
Anterior view of patient
receiving CST rib manipulation

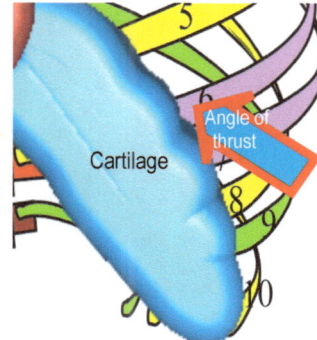

Figure 6G
Anterior views T6 and T7

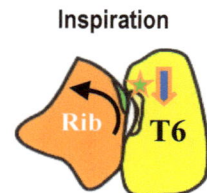

Figure TSHb
Left side-view of
point 'Y'

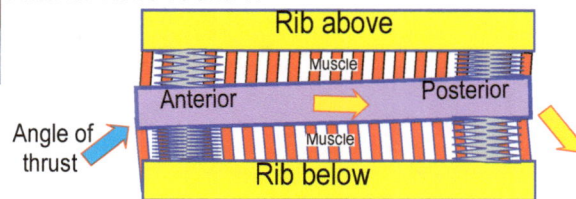

Figure 6H
Side-view of subluxated rib

This rib inspiration correction technique is only suitable for ribs subluxated in extension. The rib is used as a long lever and for this reason very little force is needed.

Technique
The patient is placed in a supine position on a flat couch with their left shoulder lowered. Their knees are supported and flexed by a pillow and their pelvis side-shifted to the left with their left arm at their side. The manipulator stands to the left side of the table parallel to the patients abdomen. The patient is then asked to breath out, 'expiration'. A supero-medial push is then made against the anterior surface of the rib. Only a light push is needed and is shown in **figures 6F, G** and **H.** Note that the palmer surface of the hand is steeply angled to avoid any accidental contact with breast tissue.

How does it work
The rib is made malleable by the pelvic side-shift to the left which causes all the individual vertebrae up the spine to attempt to shift towards the right. This is away from the rib, and therefore removes the tension from the joint.

The lowered left shoulder closes the rib cage on the left. When the patient breaths out the anterior part of the ribs move inferiorly. A gentle push is then made in a supero-medial direction, as shown in **figure 6H,** (the mechanics of this are explained in **figure 6J),** and this pushes the posterior end of the rib laterally and inferiorly to mate correctly with the corresponding vertebrae.

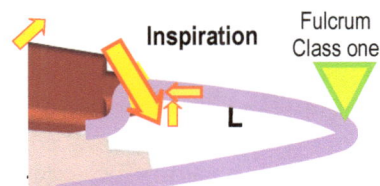

Figure 6J
Anterior view of T6
Showing angle of thrust

Rib Trauma Manipulation
Technique in Inspiration

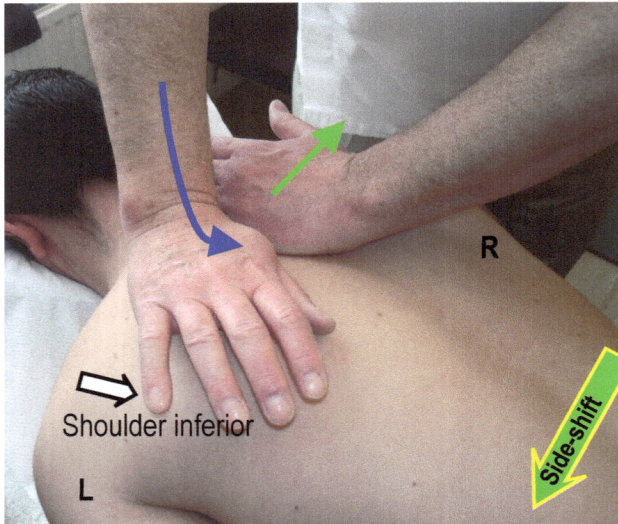

Figure 6K
Posterior view of patient
receiving CPT rib manipulation

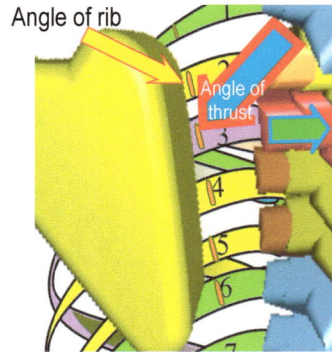

Figure 6L
Posterior view of T3

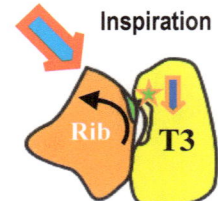

Figure TSHb
Left side-view of
point 'Y'

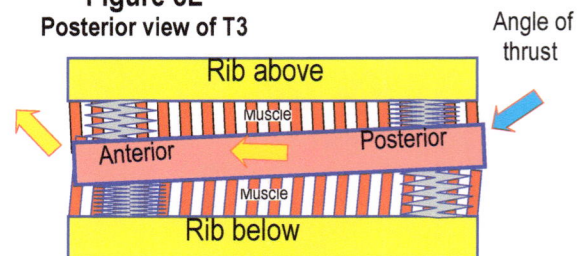

Figure 6M
Side-view of subluxated rib

This correction technique is suitable for ribs subluxated in inspiration caused by inappropriate lever or trauma. The rib is used as a short lever and for this reason a little force is needed.   The patient while co-operating has no control over when the manipulation will be made, therefore they are less likely to tense before the thrust. This is a fairly standard technique the only difference is that the pelvis is side-shifted to the left, which reduces the trauma of the manipulation.

Technique

The patient is placed in a prone position on a flat couch with their shins supported by a pillow to flex their knees. Their pelvis is side-shifted to the left, as shown in **figure 6K** and the left shoulder is lowered. The manipulator stands to the right side the table parallel with patients shoulder. The patient is then asked to breath out, 'expiration'.   The heel of the manipulators left hand stabilizes the spinous process of the vertebra at the same time as the thenar eminence of the right hand makes the thrust against the superior angle of the rib in an anterior latro-inferior direction, as shown in **figures 6K, L** and **M.**

How does it work

The Pelvic side-shift to the left causes the T3 vertebra to side-shift to the right and therefore away from the subluxated rib. The combination of the lowered arm and the patient breathing out causes the ribs to move generally inferiorly. This therefore highlights the angle of the rib locked in inspiration. The thrust, made in a latro-inferior direction, wrenches the rib away from the vertebra in a direction that allows the rib to reseat against the vertebrae. There can be an audible click.

Rib Trauma Manipulation
Technique in Expiration

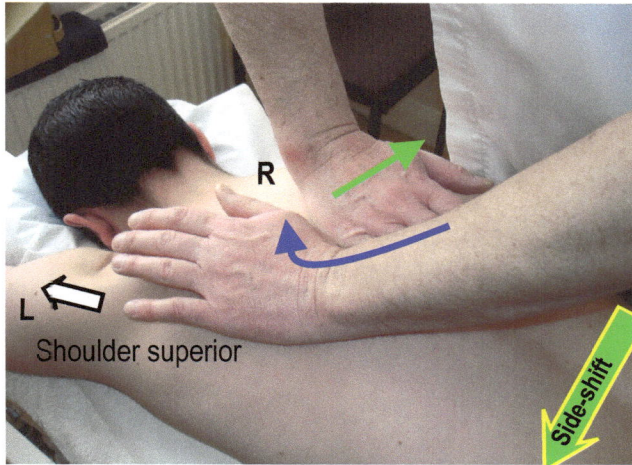

Figure 6KA
Posterior view of patient
receiving CPT rib manipulation

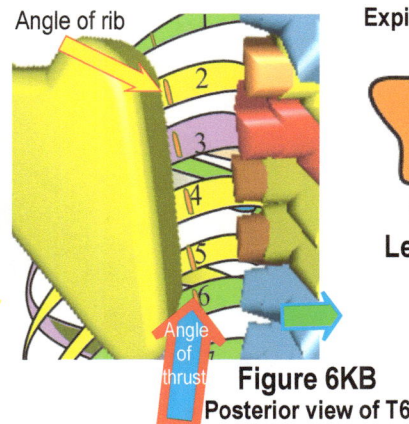

Figure 6KB
Posterior view of T6

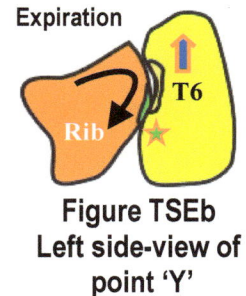

Figure TSEb
Left side-view of point 'Y'

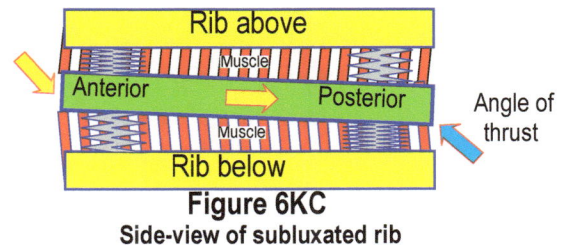

Figure 6KC
Side-view of subluxated rib

This correction technique is suitable for ribs subluxated in expiration caused by inappropriate lever or trauma. The rib is used as a short lever and for this reason a little force is needed. The patient while co-operating has no control over when the manipulation will be made, therefore they are less likely to tense before the thrust. This is a fairly standard technique, with added knee flexion and pelvic side-shift to make the manipulation less traumatic.

Technique
The patient is placed in a prone position on a flat couch with their shins supported by a pillow to flex their knees. Their pelvis is side-shifted to the left, as shown in **figure 6KA** and the left shoulder and arm are raised. The manipulator stands to the right side the table parallel with patients torso. The patient is then asked to breath in, 'Inspiration'. The heel of the manipulators left hand stabilizes the spinous process of the vertebra, while at the same time the thenar eminence of their right hand makes the thrust against the inferior angle of the rib in a medio-superior direction, as shown in **figures 6KA** and **6KB.**

How does it work
The Pelvic side-shift to the left causes the T6 vertebra to side-shift to the right and therefore away from the subluxated rib. The combination of the raised arm and the patient breathing in causes the ribs generally to move superiorly. This therefore highlights the angle of the rib locked in expiration. The thrust, made in a medio-superior direction, wrenches the rib away from the vertebra in the direction that allows the rib to reseat against the vertebrae. There can be an audible click. In this type of subluxation the angle of the rib is hidden, therefore it can be difficult to locate a rib subluxated in expiration.

Bayliss Rib Manipulation
Elevated First Rib

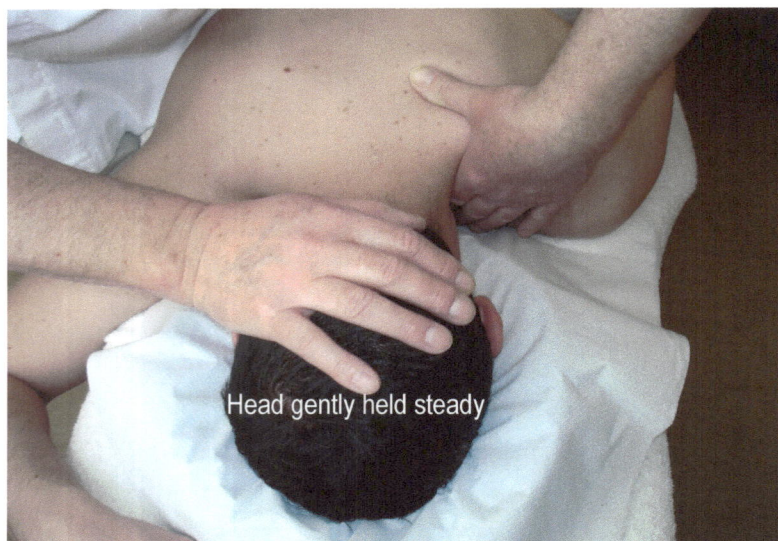

Figure 6MA
Posterior view of patient
receiving CPT rib manipulation

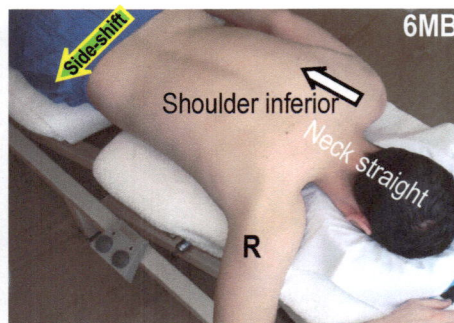

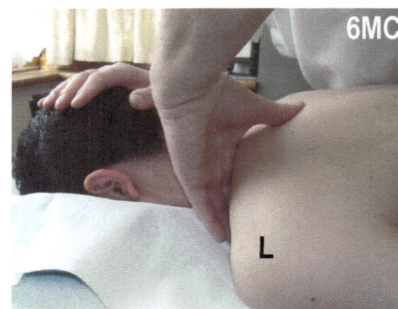

This rib technique is suitable for correcting a subluxated 1st rib locked in elevation. Unlike most 1st rib correction techniques the neck and head are kept in the mid-line and only a gentle push is needed. This keeps the neck safe.

Note. T1 must be aligned before attempting this manipulation.

Technique
The patient is placed in a prone position on a flat couch with their shins supported by a pillow to flex their knees. Their pelvis is side-shifted to the right, as shown in **figure 6MB** and the left shoulder is lowered. The patients right arm should be at a minimum of 90 degrees.

The manipulator stands to the left side the table parallel with patients lower torso. The patient is then asked to breath out, 'expiration'. The manipulators right hand stabilizes the head and neck ensuring that they are kept in the mid-line while the thenar eminence of the left hand makes contact with the supero-medial part of the 1st rib. The thrust is made in an inferior medial direction. See **figures 6MA** and **6MB.**

How does it work
The Pelvic side-shift to the right destabilizes the subluxated 1st rib. The combination of the lowered arm and the patient breathing out causes the ribs on the left to generally move inferiorly. This highlights any ribs locked in inspiration. The gentle push is made in an inferior medial direction, as shown in **figure 6MD** and allows the 1st rib to effortlessly reseat.

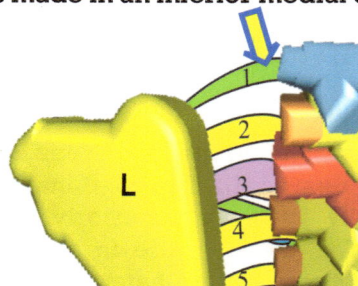

Figure 6MD
Posterior view showing angle of thrust

Bayliss CST Inferiorly Rotated Clavicle Acromio-Clavicular Manipulation

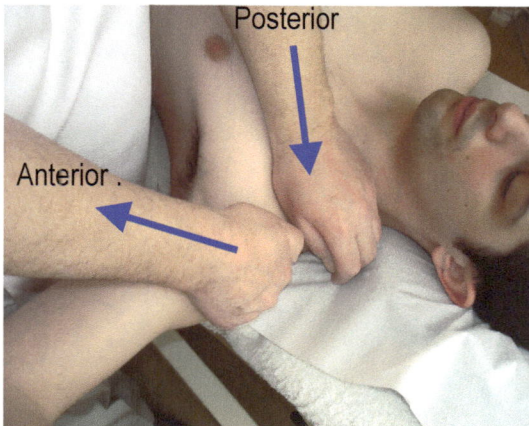

Figure 6N
Acromio-clavicular manipulation

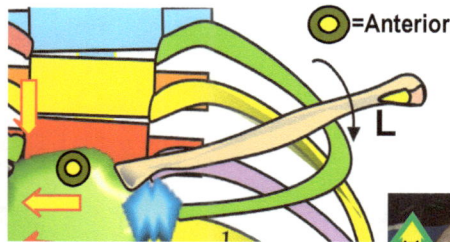

=Anterior

Figure 6P
Anterior view showing the
inferior rotation of the left clavicle

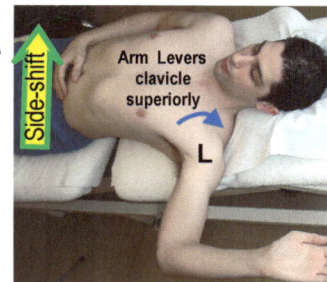

Side-shift

Arm Levers clavicle superiorly

L

Figure 6Q
Position prior to manipulation

This technique is used to correct a left acromio-clavicular joint subluxated in the L3-right-right subluxation pattern.

This is a simple CST manipulation to correct an inferiorly rotated clavicle on the left. In the L3-left-right subluxation pattern the exact same procedure is carried out on the right shoulder.

Technique
The patient adopts a supine position on a flat couch. A pillow is placed under their knees to induce mild knee flexion and the pelvis side-shifted to the right. The left elbow is bent and the forearm raised parallel with the head with the palmer surface of the hand upward, as shown in **figure 6Q**. The manipulator stands to the side of the left shoulder and places the heel of their left hand over the anterior surface of the left clavicle while the right hand is placed under the humeral head. The joint is then gently aligned by pushing down (posteriorly) on the clavicle while the right hand pulls the humeral head in the opposite direction (anteriorly).

How does it work
The pelvic side-shift to the right destabilizes the left acromio-clavicular joint, making the joint malleable. The raised left arm rotates the clavicle superiorly and correctly aligns it with acromion process.

As can be seen from **figure 6R** the lateral end of the clavicle is anterior in relation to the acromion. By gently pushing down on the clavicle and upwards on the humeral head the joint is sliced and eased back into place.

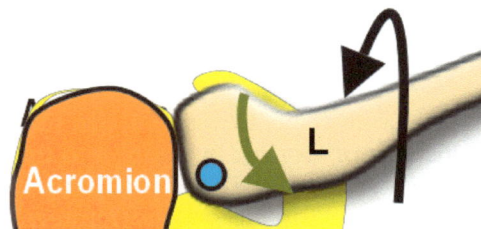

Acromion

L

Figure 6R
View from above of the left
acromio-clavicular joint

229

Bayliss CST Superiorly Rotated Clavicle Acromio-Clavicular Manipulation

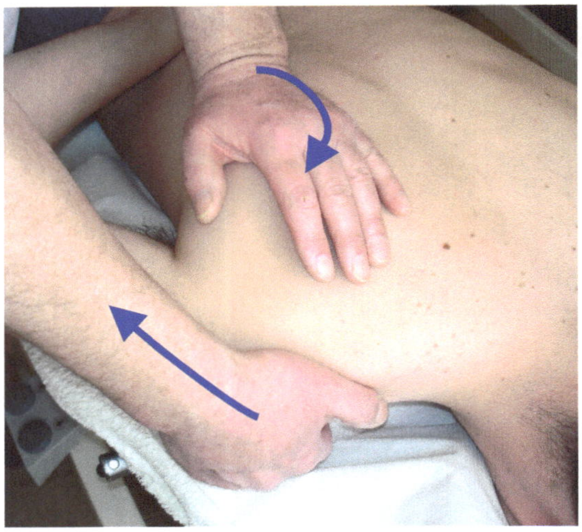

Figure 6S
Acromio-clavicular manipulation

=Anterior

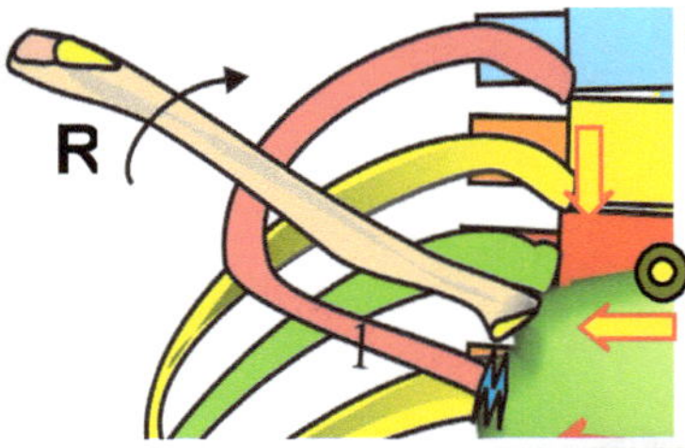

Figure 6T
Anterior view showing the superior rotation of the right clavicle

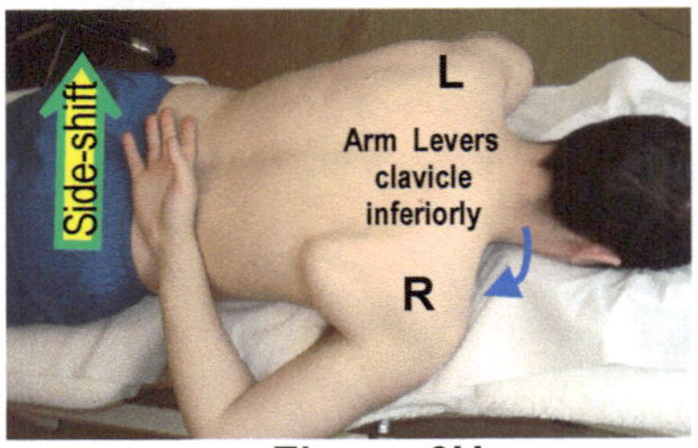

Side-shift

L

Arm Levers clavicle inferiorly

R

Figure 6U
Position prior to manipulation

This technique is used to correct a right acromio-clavicular joint subluxated in the L3-right-right subluxation pattern. This is a simple CPT manipulation to correct a superiorly rotated clavicle on the right.

In the L3-left-right subluxation pattern the exact same procedure is carried out on the left shoulder. The left scapula can be guided inferiorly to refine the technique. See **figure 17C** on page 139 for the reason.

Technique
The patient adopts a prone position on a flat couch. A pillow is placed under their shins to induce mild knee flexion and the pelvis side-shifted to the left. The right arm is either placed along side the torso or behind the back, as shown in **figure 6U**. The manipulator stands to the side of the right shoulder and places their right hand under the humeral head and their left hand over at medial border of the right scapula. The joint is then gently aligned by pulling the humeral head up (posteriorly) while the right hand pushes the scapula laterally and anteriorly in such a way as to toggle the scapula posteriorly at its lateral border.

How does it work
The pelvic side-shift to the left destabilizes the right acromio-clavicular joint, making the joint malleable. The neutral position of the arm rotates the clavicle inferiorly and correctly aligns it with acromion process.

As can be seen from **figure 6V** the lateral end of the clavicle is posterior in relation to the acromion. By toggling and laterally side-shifting the scapula whilst gently pulling up on the humeral head the joint is sliced and eased back into place.

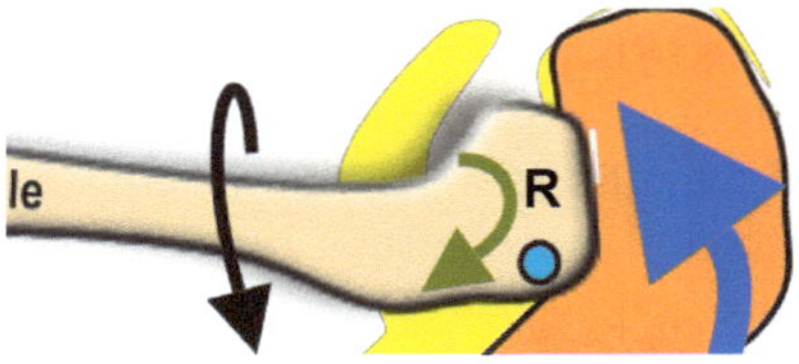

le

R

Figure 6V
View from above of the right acromio-clavicular joint

Bayliss CST
Sterno-Clavicular-Rib Cage Manipulation

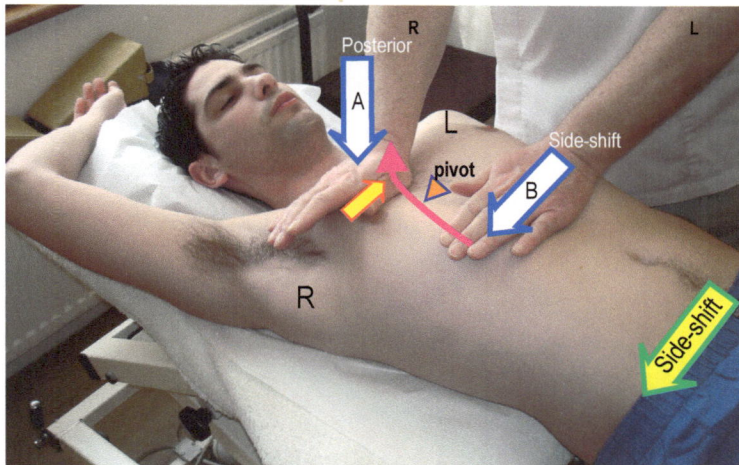

Figure 6W
Sterno-clavicular manipulation

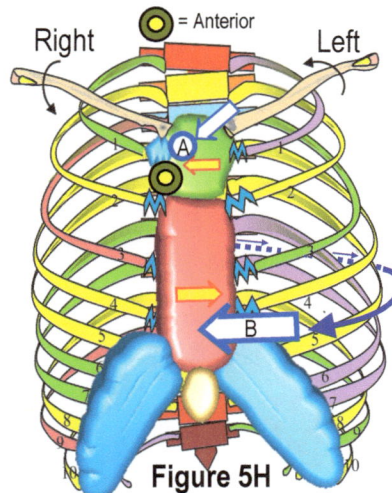

Figure 5H
Anterior rib distortions in
the L3-left-right pattern

This is a sterno-clavicular technique and as the name suggests the emphasise of the correction should be placed on correcting the position of the sternum relative to the clavicle, not the other way round. The L3-left-right rib cage subluxation pattern in being used as an example. In the L3-right-right subluxation pattern the left arm would be raised.

Technique
The patient adopts a supine position on a flat couch and raises their right arm parallel to their head, as shown in **figure 6W**. The left arm is positioned in neutral to the side of the torso. A pillow is placed under the patient knees to induce mild knee flexion and the pelvis side-shifted to the right. The manipulator stands to left of the patients torso and places the heel of their left hand against the left side of the body of the sternum, just above the xiphoid process, shown as 'B' in **figure 5H**. At the same time they place the heel of their right hand over the right anterior part of the manubrium, at point 'A' shown in **figure 5H**. In one movement the body of the sternum is gently pushed to the right and the manubrium posteriorly. A slight feeling of give is experienced as the sternum and sterno-clavicular joints re-align.

How does it work
The upper left side of the sternum is made malleable by the side-shift of the pelvis to the right. The raised right arm attempts to de-rotate the right clavicle subluxated inferiorly and the left arm held in neutral at the side de-rotates the left subluxated clavicle superiorly. The pelvic side-shift to the right, causes the lower thoracic vertebrae and ribs to side-shift to the left. This force is carried round the rib cage so that at the front the ribs tend to side-shift towards the right. Note, if the pelvic side-shift were to the left the upper ribs would move towards the left.

The side-ways push to the right on the sternum is aided by the lower rib side-shift to the right. This combined force causes the sternum to act as a long lever and swivel the manubrium, which is being eased posteriorly by the manipulators right hand, to the left. In doing this all the forces are aligned and therefore the sternum, rib cage and the sterno-clavicular joints unlock and reseat in their correct and mobile position.

Skeleton
L3-Right-Right Subluxation Pattern

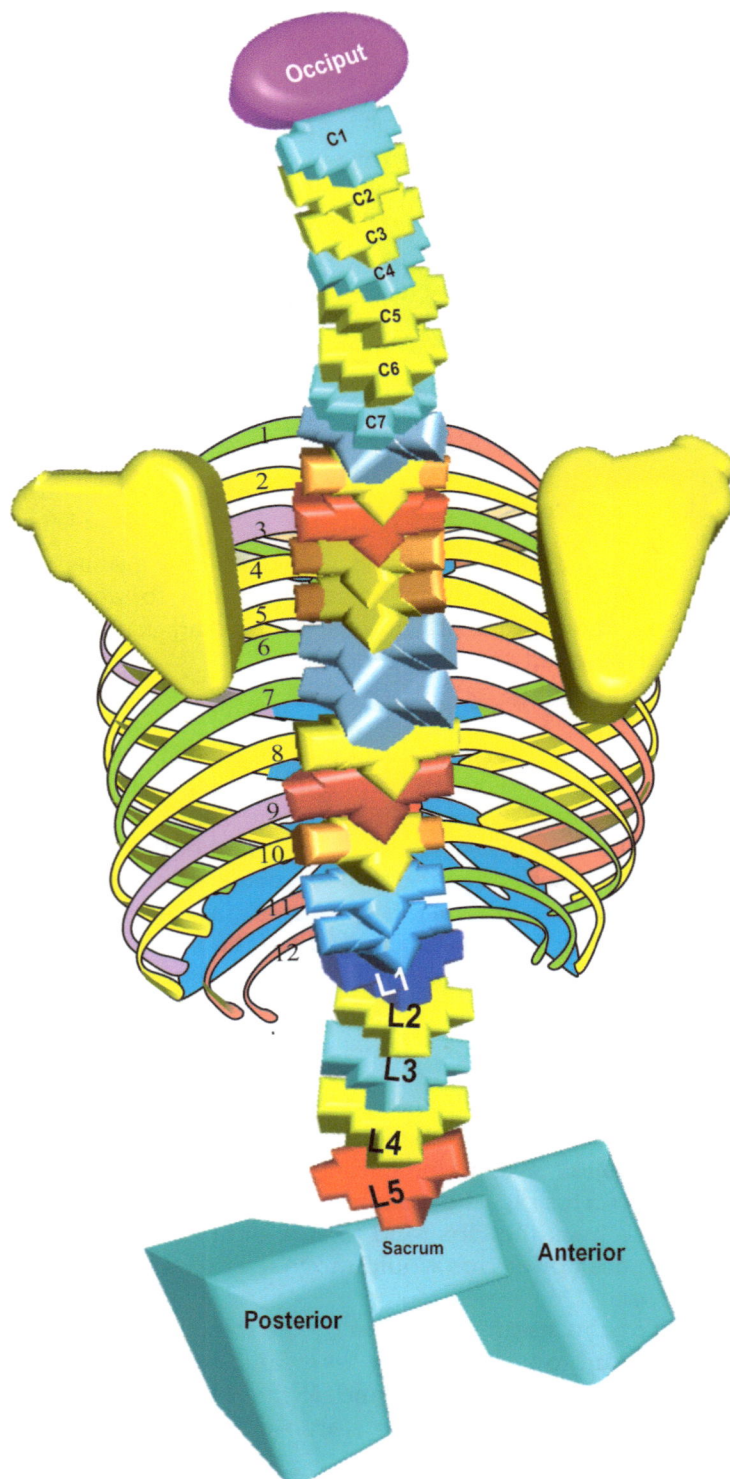

Skeleton
L3-Left-Right Subluxation Pattern

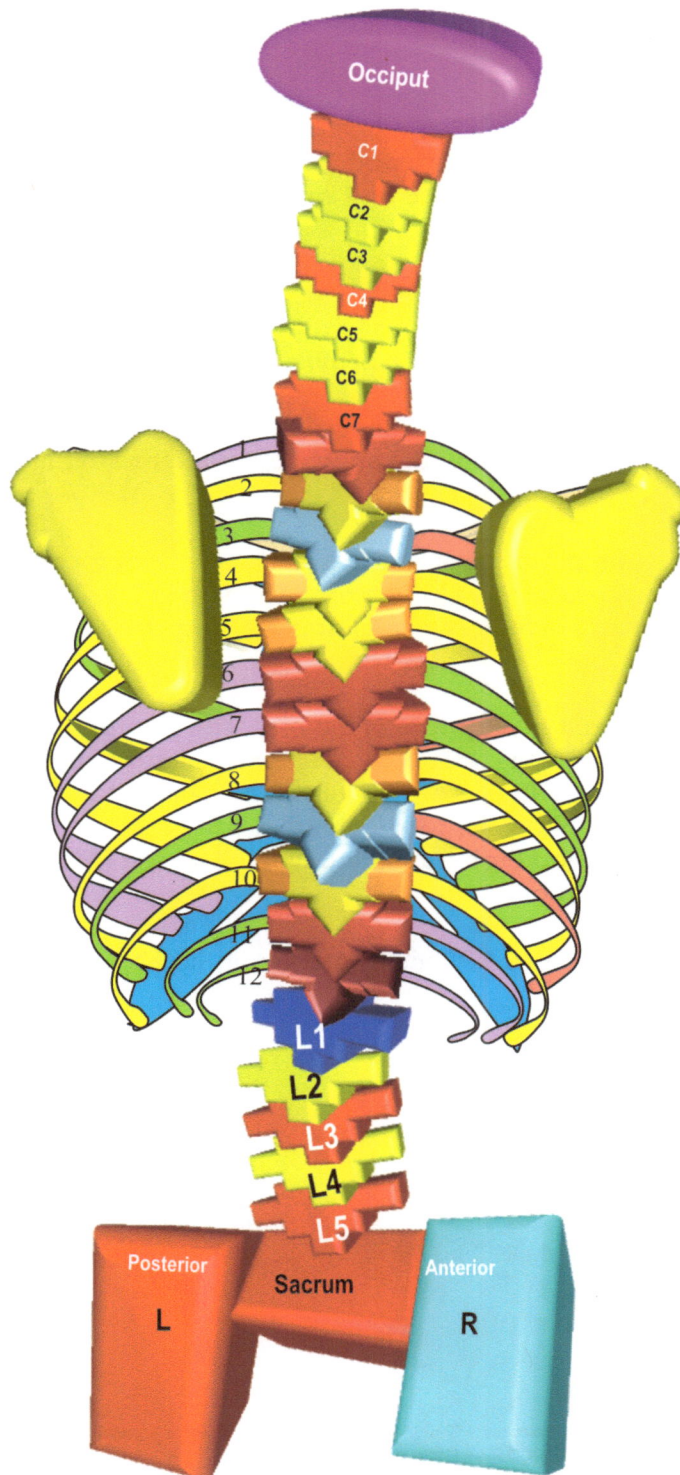

Where do we go from here?

A new door has opened in the history of
spinal mechanics and manipulation

With this new understanding of the how spine, sacroiliac, ribs and shoulder joints articulate and how these same joints subluxate, a new era in the science of spinal mechanics has begun.

The monopoly of muscle based treatments so favoured by the medical professions is ebbing to give way to a more structured and scientific approach to the treatment of joint and nerve pain.

Some critics claim manipulation is dangerous and should never be practiced. In future they will not be able to accuse professional manipulators who use PPT's CPT's and CST's of this. Why? because these techniques leave only a small trauma footprint behind; usually less than that of a standard massage.

In an Osteopathic patient research survey 50% of the research group did not know that they had been manipulated, and those that did felt the manipulation was less traumatic than conventional techniques. 100% felt PPT's were effective and caused them no anxiety and pain. 89% said that would be more likely to recommend a friend to a therapist using these techniques. 94% felt PPT's relieved their pain effectively. 72% felt PPT's relieved their pain faster than conventional manipulation.

So where do the professions who use PPT manipulation at the heart of their treatments go from here? *Forwards, with pride.*

Research survey by J.R.Bayliss completed by patients in summer 2006. A small group of 27 patients were chosen at random by the order they attended the clinic were asked to take part in the PPT survey. Of these eighteen filled in the questionnaire and returned it anonymously that is 67%. The research survey was only meant as a toe test in the water.

Another title by the author of this book to help you to expand your knowledge of spinal mechanics is:

DVD: Spinal Mechanics and Bony Locking *For Heath Professionals*

If a picture is worth a thousand words, a moving picture is worth many many more. To see the close up movement of joints, from many angles, helps the viewer to more clearly understand and appreciate how the sacroiliac and spinal joints articulate and subluxate.

The DVD is 1 hour and 38 minutes long and presented from the point of view of posture dysfunction. The two models are again sited for reference.

The DVD is available through: www.spinalmechanics.com

References:

Gray's Anatomy Edition 36 by Williams & Warwick published by Churchill Livingstone

The Anatomy Coloring Book by Wynn Kapit/Lawrence M. Elson published by Churchill Livingstone

The Physiology of the Joints Volume 3 The Trunk and the Vertebral Column By I. A. Kapandji published by Churchill Livingstone

Journal of Osteopathic Medicine volume 7 Number 1 Clinical Considerations of Sacroiliac Anatomy by M.C.McGrath April 2004 published by Research media Pty Ltd/ Journal of Osteopathic medicine

Joint Motion: Method of Measuring and Recording published by American Academy of Orthopaedic Surgeons

Principles of Osteopathic Technic By H Fryette.

Osteopathy: Notes on the Technique and Practice by John Wernham published by The Maidstone Osteopathic Clinic

An Illustrated Manual of Osteopathic Technique by John Wernham and Mervyn Waldman: published by The Maidstone Osteopathic Clinic

Interactive Spine: Chiropractic Edition. CD ROM published by Primal

Spinal Mechanics and Bony Locking *for Health Professionals.* DVD by John Bayliss DO published by John Bayliss

PPT Manipulation Patient Research Survey Preliminary Findings by J.R.Bayliss publication by spinalmechanics.com